BIOCERAMICS: PROPERTIES, PREPARATION AND APPLICATIONS

BIOCERAMICS: PROPERTIES, PREPARATION AND APPLICATIONS

WOLFFE KOSSLER
AND
JACOB FUCHS
EDITORS

Nova Biomedical Books
New York

Library of Congress Cataloging-in-Publication Data

Bioceramics : properties, preparation, and applications / Wolffe Kossler and Jacob Fuchs.
p. ; cm.
Includes bibliographical references and index.
ISBN 978-1-60741-056-0 (hardcover : alk. paper)
1. Ceramics in medicine. I. Kossler, Wolffe. II. Fuchs, Jacob, 1959-
[DNLM: 1. Biocompatible Materials. 2. Ceramics--therapeutic use. 3. Ceramics--chemistry. QT 37.5.C4 B6165 2009]
R857.C4.B573 2009
610.28'4--dc22

2009010498

Published by Nova Science Publishers, Inc. ✝ New York

Contents

Preface

Ceramic materials that are specially developed for use as medical and dental implants are termed bioceramics. Bioceramics can have structural functions as joint or tissue replacements, can be used as coatings to improve the biocompatibility of metal implants, and can function as resorbable lattices which provide temporary structures and a framework that is dissolved, replaced as the body rebuilds tissue. Some ceramics even feature drug-delivery capability. This book presents current research and cutting edge thinking in this field. It begins with an overview of the significance of calcium orthophosphates for humankind, specifically for dental and bone grafting applications. The development of granulate systems of calcium phosphate-based drugs with controlled drug release kinetics is examined as well. This is an increasingly important area of research because of the prevalent rates of infection in bone and dental surgery. In order for bioactive glasses or ceramics to bond to living bone, the formation of a bone-like apatite layer on their surfaces must occur. This book also presents two different methods for the synthesis of these bioceramic materials.

Chapter I - In early 1980-s, researchers discovered self-setting calcium orthophosphate cements, which are a bioactive and biodegradable grafting material in the form of a powder and a liquid. Both phases after mixing form a viscous paste that after being implanted sets and hardens within the body as either a non-stoichiometric calcium deficient hydroxyapatite (CDHA) or brushite, sometimes blended with unreacted particles and other phases. As both CDHA and brushite are remarkably biocompartible and bioresorbable (therefore, *in vivo* they can be replaced with a newly forming bone), calcium orthophosphate cements represent a good correction technique of non-weight-bearing bone fractures or defects and appear to be very promising materials for bone grafting applications. Besides, these cements possess an excellent osteoconductivity, molding capabilities and easy manipulation. Nearly perfect adaptation to the tissue surfaces in bone defects and a gradual bioresorption followed by new bone formation are additional distinctive advantages of calcium orthophosphate cements. Besides, reinforced formulations are available; those in a certain sense might be described as calcium orthophosphate concretes. The discovery of self-setting cements and concretes has opened up a new era in the medical application of calcium orthophosphates; several commercial formulations have already been introduced as a result. Many more compositions are in experimental stages. In this review, an insight into calcium orthophosphate cements, as excellent biomaterials suitable for both dental and bone grafting application, has been provided.

Chapter II - The present overview is intended to point the readers' attention to the important subject of calcium orthophosphates. This type of materials is of the special significance for the human beings because they represent the inorganic part of major normal (bones, teeth and antlers) and pathological (*i.e.* those appearing due to various diseases) calcified tissues of mammals. For example, atherosclerosis results in blood vessel blockage caused by a solid composite of cholesterol with calcium orthophosphates. Dental caries and osteoporosis mean a partial decalcification of teeth and bones respectively that results in replacement of a less soluble and harder biological apatite by more soluble and softer calcium hydrogenorthophosphates. Therefore, the processes of both normal and pathological calcifications are just an *in vivo* crystallization of calcium orthophosphates. Similarly, dental caries and osteoporosis might be considered as *in vivo* dissolution of calcium orthophosphates. Conversely, due to a great chemical similarity with the biological calcified tissues, many calcium orthophosphates possess remarkable biocompatibility and bioactivity. Materials scientists extensively use this property to construct artificial bone grafts that are either entirely made of or only surface-coated by the biologically relevant calcium orthophosphates. For example, self-setting hydraulic cements made of calcium orthophosphates are helpful in bone repair, while titanium substitutes covered by a surface layer of calcium orthophosphates are used for hip joint endoprostheses and tooth substitutes. Porous scaffolds made of calcium orthophosphates are very promising tools for tissue engineering applications. In addition, calcium orthophosphates of a technical grade are very popular mineral fertilizers. There is a great significance of calcium orthophosphates for the humankind and, in this paper, an overview on the current knowledge on this subject is provided. To assist and guide the readers, a great number of references to the related publications detalizing various specific aspects of the matter has been collected.

Chapter III - Biomedical scientific community is currently demanding new nanotechnological advances for the development of third generation bioceramics that promote bone tissue regeneration. Much effort is being devoted to the design of scaffolds with three-dimensional (3D) interconnected hierarchical porosity that allows new bone in-growth.

Recently, silica-based ordered mesoporous materials have been proposed as starting materials for the manufacture of 3D scaffolds for bone tissue engineering. The outstanding textural properties of mesoporous materials, such as high surface areas and pore volumes and narrow pore size distributions, make these matrices excellent candidates for local controlled delivery systems of biologically active molecules. These molecules include different drugs to treat bone infection, inflammation or diseases and diverse osteogenic agents such as amino acids, peptides, proteins or growth factors, which can promote new bone formation. The structural and textural properties of host mesoporous matrices can be tailored depending on the targeted guest-molecule. Moreover, their silanol-rich surfaces can undergo chemical functionalization with different organic groups, allowing a better control over molecule loading and release kinetics.

On the other hand, the *in vitro* bioactive behavior of mesoporous silicas has been demonstrated; since the growth of an apatite-like layer onto their surfaces is observed when they are in contact with simulate body fluids. This apatite is quite similar to the mineral phase of bone, leading to a bioactive bond that would ensure the implant-tissue integration. Recently, in an effort to accelerate bioactive responses, the synthesis of mesoporous glasses, which exhibit the excellent textural properties of mesoporous materials and chemical compositions similar to those of bioactive sol-gel glasses, has been reported. Mesoporous glasses have shown extraordinary *in vitro* behaviors, such as biomimetic bone mineralization and the fastest bioactive response reported so far.

The recent advances in mesoporous materials as bioceramics for bone tissue regeneration are reviewed in this chapter. Moreover, a critical discussion of the current possibilities of these materials for biomedical purposes together with the future perspectives is also carried out.

This chapter describes the general properties and the different synthesis methods of mesoporous materials. Moreover, the recent nanotechnological advances to enhance the bioactive behavior and controlled delivery capability of mesoporous matrices for bone tissue regeneration applications are also tackled. In addition, the recently developed strategies to design 3D scaffolds starting from mesoporous materials for bone tissue engineering are reviewed. Finally, a critical discussion of the current possibilities of these materials for biomedical purposes together with their future perspectives is also carried out.

Chapter IV - Granulate systems for the delivery and application of drugs are claimed to have enhanced bioavailability, predictable therapeutic response, greater efficacy and safety, and controlled and prolonged drug release time. Therefore, the development of granulate systems of calcium phosphate-based drugs (e.g. antibiotics, antimicrobial agents, growth factors, etc.) with controlled drug release kinetics have increasingly become an important area of research, in view of the prevalent rates of infection in bone and dental surgery. Further, porous calcium phosphate ceramics are also expected to play important roles in treating bone problems with the emerging tissue engineering approach, as it involves loading proper cells into porous ceramics (scaffolds) and implanting the cell-loaded scaffolds into a host body for achieving bone tissue regeneration. Porous spherical HAp granules of 50-2000 μm diameter have been produced by the dispersion of well-mixed HAp/polymer slurry in a dispersion medium for example. Several studies have reported the development of HAp granulates by various techniques with irregular or spherical geometry. Various studies have been conducted using different polymers (such as gelatin, collagen, chitosan, etc.) as matrices for the preparation of HAp microbeads and researchers have recently reported that HAp microspheres were prepared by using oil-in-water emulsions and solvent evaporation technique. We herein will report the preparation and characterization of porous calcium phosphate beads from two kinds of new strategy route. One is that porous bead prepared by alginate-interacting Ca ions mechanism on addition of a pore-forming PE powder by sintering process, another one is by water-in-oil emulsions in higher temperature and fast condensation shaping technique.

Chapter V - The $CaO - SiO_2$ or $CaO - SiO_2 - P_2O_5$ ceramic materials can be applied for biomedical applications due to the bioactive character. The essential condition for bioactive glasses or ceramics to bond to living bone is the formation of a bone-like apatite layer on their surfaces. The bioceramic materials can be synthesized by two methods: by classic melt-quenching process starting from inorganic powders ⌈*e.g.* $CaCO_3$, SiO_2, P_2O_5⌋ and by sol-gel technique starting from metal alkoxides ⌈ *e.g.* $Si(OR)_4$⌋ or inorganic salts ⌈$Ca(NO_3)_2$⌋.

One of the most important advantages of the sol-gel technique is the low energy requirement, much lower than that of conventional powder or melting technologies; <1000 °C in contrast to 1500-2000 °C. In addition, the sol–gel processing allows one to produce gel glasses with compositions lying within the liquid–liquid immiscibility dome of several silicate systems.

For example as with many multicomponent glasses, only a certain range of $CaO - SiO_2$ compositions can be melting derived. According to some published results, the bioactivity of the sol-gel derived glass-ceramics is unambiguously better than that of ceramics prepared by quenching of melts. The increase in bioactivity can be explained by the great differences in the textural properties of the materials synthesized by different techniques. The crystallinity and porosity out of the texture parameters influence strongly the bioactivity. The structure of a higher porosity obtained by sol-gel method can more fit the porous bone tissues than the compact one. The amount and position of crystalline particles (*e.g.* carbonates) can be much easier controlled via sol-gel than melting processes.

Chapter VI - Injectable calcium phosphates cements (ICPC) are an alternative to calcium phosphates preforms, such as granules or blocks, and other bone substitute materials that can not be molded to the defect site they have to fill. In addition they are potential candidates for minimal invasive surgery. Several approaches have been used to accomplish this task. Here we review two approaches that have been studied by two different research groups and that are amply used. The first approach uses the formation of one or more calcium phosphate compounds when mixing a liquid solution, containing or not calcium or phosphate ions, with calcium phosphate compounds. Then, the dissolution-precipitation mechanism, and growth of crystals, governs the setting of the material. The second approach is a composite one, which uses calcium phosphate as a filler material in a polymer matrix; in this situation the stiffness of the cement depends on the polymer properties. The actual state of the art, biphasic concept, mechanical and physical properties, control of porosity, drug delivery capacities, in vivo tests, as well as the future trends and differences for these two approaches are discussed.

Chapter VII - An AlTiN ceramic coating was deposited on the surface of biomedical Ti6Al4V alloy by high ionic pulse (H.I.P) technology; The electrochemical corrosion test indicated that the Ti6Al4V-AlTiN coating material basically kept to a passivation state in the range of current density $-0.4 \sim 0.25 A/m^2$, but the current density increased suddenly at 0.5V potential while Ti6Al4V alloy sample tested, and its oxidation film broken; The chemical immerssion test also displayed that the coated material effectively blocked the release of Al and V ions; And the property of biofriction and wear of AlTiN coating in simulated serum lubrication at 37^0C was investigated and compared with that of non-coating Ti6Al4V alloy. It shows that under the same conditions, the wear loss of the sample deposited AlTiN was 1.2% of the substrate, and the friction coefficient was only 0.007. A significant approach to the mechanism of the property is discussed with the aid of SEM, EDS and XRD.

Short Communication - Nearly 40 years of intensive research on bone regeneration, biomaterials, material characteristics and predictable medical results led to a number of different synthetic bone substitution and bone regeneration materials. Due to their risks of immunoresponse, inflammation and disease transfer caused by remaining proteins, xenografts (from other animals, e.g. cows) or allografts (chemically treated bone from human cadavers) should be avoided. Even if autologous bone is still used in most of the clinical cases, an increasing number of bone defects is filled with resorbable synthetic biomaterials from β-tricalcium phosphate (β-TCP). In the past years over 600.000 cases were treated with the β-TCP biomaterial Cerasorb® (curasan AG, Kleinostheim, Germany) in the whole skeletal system. Different sizes, shapes and porosities were manufactured specifically adapted to the clinical case so that today the knowledge about the use of β-TCP is elevated.

In: Bioceramics: Properties, Preparations and Applications ISBN: 978-1-60741-056-0
Editors: W. Kossler, J. Fuchs, pp. 1-65

Chapter I

Calcium Orthophosphate-Based Biocements and Bioconcretes

Sergey V. Dorozhkin*
Kudrinskaja sq. 1-155, 123242 Moscow, Russia

Abstract

In early 1980-s, researchers discovered self-setting calcium orthophosphate cements, which are a bioactive and biodegradable grafting material in the form of a powder and a liquid. Both phases after mixing form a viscous paste that after being implanted sets and hardens within the body as either a non-stoichiometric calcium deficient hydroxyapatite (CDHA) or brushite, sometimes blended with unreacted particles and other phases. As both CDHA and brushite are remarkably biocompartible and bioresorbable (therefore, *in vivo* they can be replaced with a newly forming bone), calcium orthophosphate cements represent a good correction technique of non-weight-bearing bone fractures or defects and appear to be very promising materials for bone grafting applications. Besides, these cements possess an excellent osteoconductivity, molding capabilities and easy manipulation. Nearly perfect adaptation to the tissue surfaces in bone defects and a gradual bioresorption followed by new bone formation are additional distinctive advantages of calcium orthophosphate cements. Besides, reinforced formulations are available; those in a certain sense might be described as calcium orthophosphate concretes. The discovery of self-setting cements and concretes has opened up a new era in the medical application of calcium orthophosphates; several commercial formulations have already been introduced as a result. Many more compositions are in experimental stages. In this review, an insight into calcium orthophosphate cements, as excellent biomaterials suitable for both dental and bone grafting application, has been provided.

* E-mail: sedorozhkin@yandex.ru

Keywords: calcium orthophosphate, cement, concrete, self-setting, hydraulic, injectable, bone grafting, dental, reinforced, calcium deficient hydroxyapatite, brushite, bioceramics, biomaterials, osteoconductivity, bioresorbability, materials science.

1. Introduction

Calcium orthophosphates have been studied as bone repair materials for the last 80 years. The first *in vivo* use of calcium orthophosphates was performed in 1920; that time the researchers implanted tricalcium phosphate (TCP) into animals to test its efficacy as a bone substitute [1]. In the following years, some other calcium orthophosphates were tested on animals to investigate their effect on the healing of nonunions [2]. However, it was 1951, when for the first time hydroxyapatite (HA) was implanted in rats and guinea pigs [3]. Those attempts might be characterized as initial medical trials with the first generation of bone substituting biomaterials. However, it was already the 1970-s, when other calcium orthophosphates were synthesized, characterized, investigated and tried in medicine [4-10]. The list of known calcium orthophosphates, including their standard abbreviations and the major properties, is shown in Table 1 [11].

The possibility to obtain a monolithic calcium orthophosphate ceramics at ambient or body temperature via a cementation reaction was put forward by LeGeros et al [12] and Brown and Chow [13-16] in the early 1980-s[1]. Currently this type of materials is known as *calcium phosphate cements* (commonly referred to as CPC), and, due to their suitability for repair, augmentation and regeneration of bones, they might be named as calcium phosphate *bone* cements (occasionally referred to as CPBC) [19]. However, in order to stress the fact, that these cements consist either entirely or essentially of calcium *ortho*phosphates, this review is limited to consideration of calcium orthophosphate cements only. Due to a good bioresorbability, calcium orthophosphate cements belong to the second generation of bone substituting biomaterials [20]. These cements are blends of amorphous and/or crystalline calcium orthophosphate powder(s) with an aqueous solution, which might be distilled water, phosphate-buffered saline (PBS), an aqueous solution of sodium orthophosphate (~ 0.25M), orthophosphoric acid, 0.5 M aqueous solution of citric acid [21] or even revised simulated body fluid (rSBF) [22]. After the powder(s) and the solution are mixed together, a viscous and mouldable paste is formed that sets to a firm mass within a few minutes. When the paste becomes sufficiently stiff, it can be placed into a defect as a substitute for the damaged part of bone, where it hardens *in situ* within the operating theatre. The proportion of solid to liquid or the powder-to-liquid (P/L) ratio is a very important characteristic because it determines bioresorbability and injectability. As the paste is set and hardened at room or body temperature, direct application in healing of bone defects became a new and innovative treatment modality in the end of the XXth century.

---

[1] There is an opinion [17] that the self-setting calcium orthophosphate cements for orthopedic and dental restorative applications have first been described in the early 1970-s by Driskell *et al.* in US Patent No. 3913229 [18].

Table 1. Existing calcium orthophosphates and their major properties. The solubility is given as the logarithm of the ion product of the given formulae (excluding hydrate water) with concentrations in mol/l [11]

Ca/P ionic ratio	Compound	Chemical formula	Solubility at 25 °C, $-\log(K_s)$	Solubility at 37 °C, $-\log(K_s)$	pH stability range in aqueous solutions at 25°C
0.5	Monocalcium phosphate monohydrate (MCPM)	$Ca(H_2PO_4)_2 \cdot H_2O$	1.14	data not found	0.0–2.0
0.5	Monocalcium phosphate anhydrous (MCPA)	$Ca(H_2PO_4)_2$	1.14	data not found	[c]
1.0	Dicalcium phosphate dihydrate (DCPD), mineral brushite	$CaHPO_4 \cdot 2H_2O$	6.59	6.63	2.0–6.0
1.0	Dicalcium phosphate anhydrous (DCPA), mineral monetite	$CaHPO_4$	6.90	7.02	[c]
1.33	Octacalcium phosphate (OCP)	$Ca_8(HPO_4)_2(PO_4)_4 \cdot 5H_2O$	96.6	95.9	5.5–7.0
1.5	α-Tricalcium phosphate (α-TCP)	α-$Ca_3(PO_4)_2$	25.5	25.5	[a]
1.5	β-Tricalcium phosphate (β-TCP)	β-$Ca_3(PO_4)_2$	28.9	29.5	[a]
1.2–2.2	Amorphous calcium phosphate (ACP)	$Ca_xH_y(PO_4)_z \cdot nH_2O$, n = 3–4.5; 15–20% H_2O	[b]	[b]	~5–12 [d]
1.5–1.67	Calcium-deficient hydroxyapatite (CDHA)[e]	$Ca_{10-x}(HPO_4)_x(PO_4)_{6-x}(OH)_{2-x}$ [f] $(0<x<1)$	~85.1	~85.1	6.5–9.5
1.67	Hydroxyapatite (HA)	$Ca_{10}(PO_4)_6(OH)_2$	116.8	117.2	9.5–12
1.67	Fluorapatite (FA)	$Ca_{10}(PO_4)_6F_2$	120.0	119.2	7–12
2.0	Tetracalcium phosphate (TTCP), mineral hilgenstockite	$Ca_4(PO_4)_2O$	38–44	37–42	[a]

[a] These compounds cannot be precipitated from aqueous solutions.

[b] Cannot be measured precisely. However, the following values were found: 25.7±0.1 (pH=7.40), 29.9±0.1 (pH=6.00), 32.7±0.1 (pH=5.28).

[c] Stable at temperatures above 100°C.

[d] Always metastable.

[e] Occasionally, CDHA is named as precipitated HA.

[f] In the case $x = 1$ (the boundary condition with Ca/P = 1.5), the chemical formula of CDHA looks as follows: $Ca_9(HPO_4)(PO_4)_5(OH)$.

Moreover, calcium orthophosphate cements can be injected directly into fractures and bone defects, where they intimately adapt to the bone cavity regardless its shape. Besides, they were found to promote development of osteoconductive pathways, possess sufficient compressive strengths, be noncytotoxic, create chemical bonds to the host bones, restore contour and have both the chemical composition and X-ray diffraction patterns similar to those of bone [23]. Finally but yet importantly, they are osteotransductive, *i.e.* after implantation calcium orthophosphate cements are replaced by a new bone tissue [24-26].

The aim of biomimetic bone cements is to disturb bone functions and properties as little as possible and, until a new bone has been grown, to behave temporary in a manner similar to that of bone. From a biological point of view, this term defines cements that can reproduce the composition, structure, morphology and crystallinity of bone crystals [27,28]. Therefore, the discovery of self-setting calcium orthophosphate cements was a significant step forward in the field of bioceramics for bone regeneration, since it established good prospects for minimally invasive surgical techniques that were less aggressive than the classical surgical methods [29]. The cements provide the surgeons with a unique ability of manufacturing, shaping and implanting the bioactive bone substitute material on a patient-specific base in real time in the surgery room. Implanted bone tissues also take benefits from initial setting characteristics of the cements that give, in an acceptable clinical time, a suitable mechanical strength for a shorter tissue functional recovery. The major advantages of the cements include a fast setting time, excellent moldability, outstanding biocompatibility and easy manipulation; therefore, the cements are more versatile in handling characteristics than prefabricated calcium orthophosphate granules or blocks. Besides, like any other bioceramics, calcium orthophosphate cements provide the opportunity for bone grafting using alloplastic materials, which are unlimited in quantity and provide no risk of infectious diseases [30,31].

From the point of view that calcium orthophosphate cements are intended for using as biomaterials for parenteral application, for their chemical composition one might employ all ionic compounds of oligoelements occurring naturally in a human body. The list of possible additives includes (but is not limited to) the following cations: Na^+, K^+, Mg^{2+}, Ca^{2+}, H^+ and anions: PO_4^{3-}, HPO_4^{2-}, $H_2PO_4^-$, CO_3^{2-}, HCO_3^-, SO_4^{2-}, HSO_4^-, Cl^-, F^-, SiO_4^{4-} [24]. Therefore, mixed-type cements consisting of calcium orthophosphates and other calcium salts (*e.g.*, gypsum[2] [35,36], calcium sulfate hemihydrate [37], calcium pyrophosphate [38-40], calcium polyphosphates [41], calcium carbonate [28,42,43], calcium oxide [44-49], calcium hydroxide [50,51], calcium aluminate [52,53], calcium silicate [54,55], strontium orthophosphate [56], *etc.*), as well as cements made of ion substituted calcium orthophosphates (*e.g.*, $Ca_2KNa(PO_4)_2$, $NaCaPO_4$, $Na_3Ca_6(PO_4)_5$, magnesium substituted CDHA, strontium substituted CDHA, *etc.*) [57-62] are available. Moreover, a calcium orthophosphate cement might be prepared in the reaction-setting mixture of $Ca(OH)_2$ – KH_2PO_4 system [63]. A calcium orthophosphate cement possessing magnetic properties due to incorporation of iron oxides is also available [64]. However, with a few important exceptions, such formulations have not been considered in this review.

[2] It is interesting to note that calcium sulfate (gypsum or plaster of Paris) has been implanted into fracture gaps and voids of bones for more than 100 years [32-34].

The purpose of this article is to review the chemistry, physical and mechanical properties of calcium orthophosphate cements with the specific reference to their biomedical applications in dentistry and surgery.

2. Calcium Orthophosphate Cements

According to Wikipedia, the free encyclopedia: "In the most general sense of the word, *cement* is a binder, a substance that sets and hardens independently and can bind other materials together. The name "cement" goes back to the Romans who used the term "*opus caementitium*" to describe masonry, which resembled concrete and was made from crushed rock with burnt lime as binder. The volcanic ash and pulverized brick additives, which were added to the burnt lime to obtain a hydraulic binder, were later referred to as cementum, cimentum, cäment and cement." [65].

The first calcium orthophosphate cement formulation consists of the equimolar mixture of TTCP and dicalcium phosphate (DCPA or DCPD)[3] which is mixed with water at a P/L ratio of 4:1; the paste hardened in about 30 min and formed CDHA [14,15]. This highly viscous, non-injectable paste can be molded and is therefore used mainly as a contouring material in craniofacial surgery. In 1990-s, it was established that there were about 15 different binary combinations of calcium orthophosphates, which gave pastes upon mixing with water or aqueous solutions, so that the pastes set at room or body temperature into a solid cement. The list of these combinations is available in literature [68-70]. From these basic systems, secondary formulations could be derived containing additional or even non-reactive compounds but still setting like cements [24,46,68,71-84]. However, depending upon the pH value of a cement paste, after setting all calcium orthophosphate cements can only form two major end-products: a precipitated poorly crystalline HA or CDHA[4] (under pH>4.2) and DCPD (also called "brushite")[5] (under pH<4.2) [85]. The results of the only study on an ACP cement [82] demonstrated that this end-product was rapidly converted into CDHA. Besides, there is one paper devoted to an OCP cement [86]; however, contrary to reports of early 1990-s, none of the calcium orthophosphate cements synthesized afterwards is of OCP or ACP types. Therefore, all existing formulations of calcium orthophosphate cements have been divided into two major groups: apatite cements and brushite cements.[6] The final sitting product of the cements is of the paramount importance because it determines the solubility and, therefore, *in vivo* bioresorbability. Since the chemical composition of mammalian bones is similar to ion-substituted CDHA, apatite cements have been more

---

[3] There are some differences between TTCP+DCPD and TTCP+DCPA cements. Due to a higher solubility of DCPD (Table 1), a TTCP+DCPD cement sets faster than a TTCP+DCPA cement. Besides, injectability of a TTCP+DCPD cement is better [66,67].

[4] In the vast majority cases, a precipitated poorly crystalline HA and CDHA are undistinguishable and might be considered as synonyms [11].

[5] To honor Prof. George Jarvis Brush (1831–1912), an American mineralogist, Yale University, New Haven, Connecticut, USA [11].

[6] In early 1990-s, depending on the type of calcium orthophosphate formed after setting, five groups of the cement formulations were thought to exist: DCPD, CDHA, HA, ACP and OCP [70,87], while currently only two cement groups remain.

extensively investigated. However, many research papers on brushite cements have been published as well.

All calcium orthophosphate cements are made of an aqueous solution and fine powders of one or several calcium orthophosphate(s). Here, dissolution of the initial calcium orthophosphates (quickly or slowly depending on the chemical composition and solution pH) and mass transport appear to be the primary functions of an aqueous environment, in which the dissolved reactants form a supersaturated (very far away from the equilibrium) microenvironment with regard to precipitation of the final products [88,89]. The relative stability and solubility of various calcium orthophosphates is the major driving force for the setting reactions that occur in these cements. Therefore, mixing of a dry powder with an aqueous solution induces various chemical transformations, where crystals of the initial calcium orthophosphate(s) rapidly dissolve(s) and precipitate(s) into crystals of CDHA or DCPD with possible formation of intermediate precursor phases (*e.g.*, ACP and OCP). The solubility product constant and pH of different calcium orthophosphates determine both viscosity and rheological properties[7] of a cement paste. During precipitation, the newly formed crystals grow and form a web of intermingling microneedles or microplatelets of the final products, thus provide a mechanical rigidity to the hardened cements. In other words, entanglement of the newly formed crystals is the major reason of setting. For the majority of apatite cements, water is not a reactant in the setting reaction. Therefore, the quantity of water, actually needed for setting of apatite cements, is very small [20,88,92]. However, for brushite cements, water always participates in the chemical transformations because it is necessary for DCPD formation. Due to this reason, brushite cements are always hydraulic, while usually this term is not associated with apatite cements.

Setting of calcium orthophosphate cements is a continuous process that always starts with dissolution of the initial compounds in an aqueous system. This process supplies ions of calcium and orthophosphate into the solution, where they chemically interact and precipitate in the form of either the end-products or precursor phases, which causes the cement setting [93,94]. This was confirmed by Ishikawa and Asaoka, who showed that when TTCP and DCPA powders were mixed in double-distilled water, both powders were dissolved. The dissolved calcium and orthophosphate ions in the solution were then precipitated in the form of CDHA on the surface of the powders [95]. The precipitate can be either a gel or a conglomerate of crystals. Therefore, the hardening mechanism is either a sol-gel transition of ACP [82] or entanglement of the precipitated crystals of other calcium orthophosphates [24]. For example, for the classical Brown-Chow cement formulation, after the initial setting, petal or needle-like crystals enlarge epitaxially and are responsible for the adherence and interlocking of the crystalline grains, which result in hardening. After ~2 hours, the newly formed crystals become rod-like, resulting from higher crystallinity with the observation of more material at the inter-particle spaces. During this period, the cement setting reaction proceeded at a near-constant rate, suggesting that the reaction rate was limited by factors that are unrelated to the amounts of the starting materials and the reaction products present in the system. Such factors could be related to the surface area of DCPA or TTCP or to the

[7] The rheological properties of injectable calcium orthophosphate cement slurry are well described elsewhere [90,91].

diffusion distances over which the calcium and orthophosphate ions migrate in order to form CDHA [96-98]. At ~24 hours, the crystals are completely formed, being very compacted in some areas of high density and well separated in areas with more porosity [75,80,81].

The chemical reactions that take place during the setting of calcium orthophosphate cements depend on their chemical composition. However, it can be stated that only two major chemical types of the setting reaction are possible. The first type occurs according to the classical rules of the acid-base interaction, *i.e.* a relatively acidic calcium orthophosphate reacts with a relatively basic one to produce a relatively neutral compound. The first cement by Brown and Chow is a typical example of this type because TTCP (basic) reacts with DCPA (slightly acidic) in an aqueous suspension to form a precipitated poorly crystalline HA[8] (slightly basic) [14,15]:

$$2Ca_4(PO_4)_2O + 2CaHPO_4 \rightarrow Ca_{10}(PO_4)_6(OH)_2 \quad (1)$$

Formation of HA according to equation (1) releases neither acidic nor basic byproducts. Thus, the liquid phase of the cement remains at a near constant pH of ~ 7.5 for the TTCP + DCPD and ~ 8.0 for the TTCP + DCPA formulations, respectively [96-98]. Various deviations from the stoichiometry of chemical equation (1) have been studied in details [101]. The effect of mixing ratio and pH on the reaction between TTCP and DCPA is well described elsewhere [102].

A blend proposed by Lemaitre *et al.* [103,104] is another example of the acid-base interaction where β-TCP (almost neutral) reacts with MCPM (acidic) to form DCPD (slightly acidic):

$$\beta\text{-}Ca_3(PO_4)_2 + Ca(H_2PO_4)_2{\cdot}H_2O + 7H_2O \rightarrow 4CaHPO_4{\cdot}2H_2O \quad (2)$$

In equation (2) MCPM might be substituted by orthophosphoric acid [105] and MCPA, while β-TCP might be replaced by either α-TCP [106,107] or CDHA [108,109]. For example:

$$Ca_9(HPO_4)(PO_4)_5(OH) + 3H_3PO_4 + 17H_2O \rightarrow 9CaHPO_4{\cdot}2H_2O \quad (3)$$

Besides, cement formulations based on mixtures of ACP + α-TCP [110], OCP + TTCP [111] and partially crystallized calcium orthophosphate + DCPA [112] as the initial reagents, are also available.

The second type of the setting reaction might be defined as hydrolysis of a metastable calcium orthophosphate in aqueous media. As the result, both the initial and final compounds have the same Ca/P ionic ratio. Due to the fact, that only one calcium orthophosphate is used; the solid part of such formulations might be called as a single-phase (or single-component) cement powder [113]. Cements made of ACP + an aqueous solution [114], α-TCP + an aqueous solution [115-120], β-TCP + an aqueous solution [119,121], nanocrystalline TTCP +

[8] Earlier, it was believed that DCPA and TTCP reacted upon mixing with water to form the stoichiometric HA [13-16]. However, further investigations have shown that only the first nuclei consist of a nearly stoichiometric HA, whereas further growth of these nuclei occurs in the form of CDHA [99]. Besides, there is a study demonstrating that the initially formed HA further interacts with remaining DCPD to form CDHA [100].

an aqueous solution [122,123] or γ-radiated TTCP + an aqueous solution [124-126] are the typical examples; all of them re-crystallize to CDHA upon contact with water:

$$Ca_xH_y(PO_4)_z{\cdot}nH_2O + H_2O \rightarrow Ca_{10-x}(HPO_4)_x(PO_4)_{6-x}(OH)_{2-x} + nH_2O \quad (4)$$

$$3(\alpha\text{- or }\beta\text{-})Ca_3(PO_4)_2 + H_2O \rightarrow Ca_9(HPO_4)(PO_4)_5(OH) \quad (5)$$

$$3Ca_4(PO_4)_2O + 3H_2O \rightarrow Ca_9(HPO_4)(PO_4)_5(OH) + 3Ca(OH)_2 \quad (6)$$

The experimental details on TTCP hydrolysis under a near-constant composition condition might be found elsewhere [127]. The details on α-TCP hydrolysis are also available. The results indicated that setting of α-TCP was initially controlled by surface dissolution; therefore, it depended on the surface area of the reactants [128-131]. Addition of ~2 wt.% of a precipitated poorly crystalline HA as a seed to α-TCP powder phase might be useful to accelerate the kinetics of reaction (5) [132].

Further, there is a single-phase cement powder consisting of K- and Na- containing CDHA (with the Ca/P ionic ratio of 1.64±0.02) that sets and hardens after mixing with an aqueous solution of sodium citrate and sodium orthophosphate [17]. After setting, this formulation gives rise to formation of a weak cement (the compressive strength of 15 ± 3 MPa) consisting of the ion-substituted CDHA again (presumably, with a different Ca/P ionic ratio), mimicking the bone mineral. Unfortunately, neither the setting reaction nor the setting mechanism of this cement has been disclosed in literature [17]. What's more, a self-setting cement might be prepared from the thermal decomposition product of HA [133].

The hydration process of calcium orthophosphate cements is slightly exothermic (which is beneficial for biomedical applications) and undergoes five periods: initiating period, induction period, accelerating period, decelerating period and terminating period [134]. For the classical Brown-Chow cement formulation, the activation energy of the hydration reaction is 176 kJ/mol [135]. The rate of heat liberation during the solidification of calcium orthophosphate cements is low. The results of adiabatic experiments showed that the temperature rise arrived at the highest value of 37 °C 3 h later, which would cause no harm to surrounding tissues [134]. The results show that the hardening process of this cement is initially controlled by the dissolution of the reactants in a 4 h period and subsequently by diffusion through the product layer of CDHA around the grains [81]. In general, setting of calcium orthophosphate cements occurs mostly within the initial ~6 hours, yielding an ~80% conversion to the final products. The volume of the cements stays almost constant during setting. However, after hardening, calcium orthophosphate cements always form brittle ceramics with the tensile strength of 5 to 20 times lower than the compression strength [136]. Since this material is weak under tensile forces, these cements can only be used either in combination with metal implants or in non-load bearing (*e.g.*, craniofacial) applications [92,137-139]. This is confirmed by the mechanical characterization of a bone defect model filled with ceramic cements [140].

Reactivity of various types of calcium orthophosphate cements has been discussed in details very recently [141]. In that review, the interested reader will find strategies to control the setting reaction of calcium orthophosphate cements and various approaches to modify their reactivity along with a list of compositional effects found to affect the setting time/rate of the cements. The analysis revealed that a better control of the setting rate could probably be achieved by both using fine and monodispersed reagent powders and better controlling the choice of additives, in particular in the mixing liquid of the cement [141].

The United States Food and Drug Administration (FDA) has approved at least three cement formulations for clinical use (Table 2) [20,142]. The same formulations have also received a Conformite Europene (CE) mark for certain maxillofacial indications and for use as a bone-void filler in the specific non-load-bearing orthopedic indications [92]. The major properties of these formulations are available in literature [20]. The list of other commercially available injectable bone cements with their chemical composition (when obtainable) might be found elsewhere [29,98,143], while the various types of bone cements and fillers are listed in another review [144]. Besides, many more cement formulations are in experimental stages.

Table 2. Calcium orthophosphate cement formulations having the 510(k) clearance from the FDA [20,92,142]. The technical data on these cements might be found in literature [20]

Product*	Manufacturer	Applications*
BoneSource™**	Striker Howmedica Osteonics (Rutherford, NJ)	Craniofacial
α-Bone Substitute Material (α-BSM®)***	Etex Corporation (Cambridge, MA)	Filling of bone defects and voids, dental, craniofacial
Skeletal Repair Systems (SRS®)	Norian Corporation (Cupertino, CA)	Skeletal distal radius fractures, craniofacial

* In Europe, other applications may apply, and the materials may be sold with a different commercial name.

** BoneSource™ is the original formulation of calcium orthophosphate cement developed by Brown and Chow.

*** In Europe, it is distributed by Biomet Merck (Zwijndrecht, The Netherlands) as Biobon® [92], while in North America it is marketed by Walter Lorenz Surgical (Jacksonville, FL) as Embarc® [20].

To conclude this chapter, one must stress, that chemical equations (1) – (6) of the cement setting are valid for the *in vitro* conditions only. There are evidences that samples of calcium orthophosphate cement retrieved 12 h after hardening *in vivo* already contained carbonateapatite (type B), even though the initial cement mixture did not contain carbonate as one of the solid components [145]. The mass fraction of carbonate in the 12 h samples was about 1%. The results suggest that under the *in vivo* conditions, carbonate is readily available and this allows formation of carbonateapatite in favor of carbonate-free CDHA [145].

3. Handling

Generally, calcium orthophosphate cements must set slowly enough to provide sufficient time to a surgeon to perform implantation but fast enough to prevent delaying the operation. Ideally, good mechanical properties should be reached within minutes after initial setting

[141]. There are currently 2 standardized methods to study the setting and hardening processes of cements, namely: Gillmore needles method (ASTM C266-89) [146] and Vicat needle method (ASTM C191-92) [147]. The idea of both methods is to examine visually the surface of cement samples to decide whether the cement has already set, *i.e.* if no mark can be seen on the surface after indentation. Besides, the setting process might be monitored in real time by non-destructive methods, *e.g.*, pulse-echo ultrasound technique [148], isothermal differential scanning calorimetry [118,119,149-153] and AC impedance spectroscopy [154]. For example, the very recent calorimetry measurements suggested that in equation (2) the endothermic MCPM dissolution and the highly exothermic β-TCP dissolution occurred simultaneously, followed by the exothermic crystallization of DCPD [153]. Moreover, acid-base reactions (1) – (3) can be and have been analyzed by measuring the pH evolution of a diluted cement paste [141]. Finally, methods of Fourier-transform infrared spectroscopy [155] and X-ray diffraction [40,106] might be applied as well. The latter two techniques proved to be powerful even though they have limitations such as the time required for each measurement (250 s for an X-ray diffraction scan is a problem for fast setting reactions); besides the analysis is located at the surface of the sample where evaporation and thermal effects can modify the reaction rate of the surface compared to that of the bulk [141].

Gillmore needles have been used with success to measure the initial (*I*) and final (*F*) setting times of calcium orthophosphate cements [68]. A light and thick needle is used to measure the initial setting time *I*, while a heavy and thin needle for the final setting time *F* [87]. The clinical meaning is that the cement paste should be implanted before time *I* and that the wound can be closed after time *F* (Figure 1). A cement should not be deformed between times *I* and *F* because in that stage of the setting process any deformation could induce cracks [24]. The following handling requirements (in minutes) have been formulated for calcium orthophosphate cements, as a result [87,156]:

$$3 \leq I < 8$$
$$I - CT \geq 1$$
$$F \leq 15$$

These parameters are represented schematically in Figure 1. The second requirement means, that cohesion time (*CT*)[9] must be at least 1 min before *I*, so that a clinician has at least 1 min to apply and to mold the material. As the mixing in a mortar is about 1 min, the shortest *CT* that can be allowed is about 2 min, so that a clinician has at least 1 min to collect the paste from the mortar and put it on the pallet knife or in the syringe with which it is to be transferred to the wound after *CT* and before *I* [87]. For dental applications, *I* must be close to 3 min, whereas for orthopedic applications it must be close to 8 min. However, in no case it will be tolerable for the clinicians if time *F* becomes greater than 15 min [24,87].

In the clinical situation, calcium orthophosphate cements can be either applied by the fingertips of a surgeon or injected from a syringe to the defect area of a bone. The first type of clinical application requires formulation of a high-viscosity cement paste, which can be

[9] It is the time from which a cement no longer disintegrates when immersed in Ringer's solution [87].

applied manually as dough, while the second type of clinical application requires formulation of a low-viscosity cement paste, which can be applied by injection from a syringe [87].

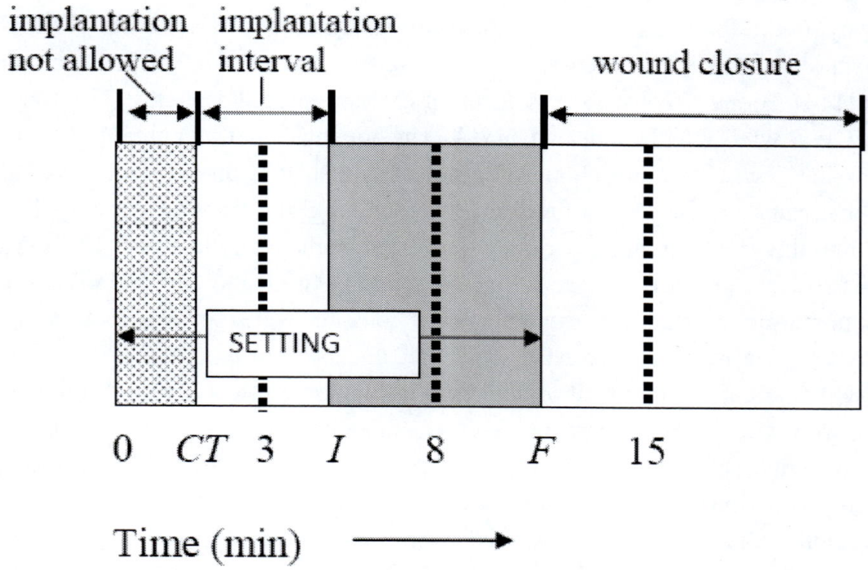

Figure 1. Diagram of the setting parameters relevant for a calcium orthophosphate cement: *CT* – cohesion time; *I* – initial setting time; *F* – final setting time. Adapted from Ref. [24] with permission.

Currently, injection appears to be the preferred method between these two major options. In any case, before using a surgeon needs to have a cement powder and a liquid be mixed properly and thoroughly (to avoid the powder/liquid encapsulation) within the prescribed time and be performed in a sterile environment. Therefore, a mixing procedure is very important because prior to be injected, a cement paste must be transferred from a mixing chamber into a syringe. Ideally, this should be done without trapping air bubbles by the cement paste [157]. Earlier, most calcium orthophosphate cements were manually mixed with aqueous solutions using a mortar and either a pestle or a spatula. That time, some concerns were raised about an insufficient and inhomogeneous mixing thus compromising the implant strength, as well as on inconsistencies between operators causing unpredictable variations in graft performance [137,138]. Mechanical mixing (*e.g.*, by either an electrically powered mixing machine of Norian SRS/CRS® or Mini-malax® mixing system for Cementek® cement, produced by Teknimed S.A.) is the modern approach. It allows mixing the cement paste within 60–80 s and enables a rapid and reliable filling of the application syringe [29]. Besides, a cement powder and an aqueous solution might be placed into a syringe and mixed inside a shaker to produce a consistent cement paste of the desired viscosity [157]. The mechanical mixing was found to decrease both the mean viscosity of the curing cement paste and variability in the viscosity at a given time [158]. However, it did not improve the mechanical strength of the cement [137,138].

Of the cements, listed in Table 2, Norian SRS® is sold as a reactant pack containing two components: a mixture of dry powders (MCPM + α-TCP + $CaCO_3$) and a liquid (aqueous solution of Na_2HPO_4). The components are mixed in the operating room. The paste that is formed is malleable and injectable for ~5 minutes; it hardens within ~10 minutes after injection [20,159]. However, data are available that out of 4.5 ml Norian SRS® cement paste ~3 ml is injectable only, whereas up to 1.5 ml of the cement might remain uninjectable from the syringe [24]. This phenomenon is prescribed to the cement rheology and its interaction with the hydraulic forces of the syringe. α-Bone Substitute Material (α-BSM®) is also a two-component system; it is prepared from a mixture of ACP and DCPD powders and a saline solution [114]. Biopex® consists of 4 different calcium orthophosphates: 75 wt.% α-TCP, 18 wt.% TTCP, 5 wt.% DCPD and 2 wt.% HA. The aqueous solution contains 12 wt.% sodium succinate and 5 wt.% sodium chondroitin sulfate [160]. It is mixed with a spatula inside a syringe that can be opened from the front. After mixing, the front part is closed, a needle is inserted into this front part and the cement paste can be manually injected [137,138].

Some systematic studies on the influence of composition and concentration of the liquids used in preparing of calcium orthophosphate cements were performed as well [21,161]. Unfortunately, the results appeared to be rather unclear. For example, for several cements, mixing with sodium citrate or citric acid resulted in some effects on the initial setting time [21,162], while for other cements the effect was insignificant [161]. Concentration increasing of sodium citrate solution resulted in initial setting time increasing [21,161], although the injectability variations of the cement pastes were inconsistent [21,162].

Injectablity and cohesion are required for the successful *in vivo* introduction of calcium orthophosphate cements. Injectability is the ability to be extruded through a small hole of a long needle (*e.g.*, 2 mm diameter and 10 cm length) [163,164] (other needles are also applied [165]); and for certain applications, injectability is even a prerequisite. It is measured by the weight percentage of the cement paste that could be injected without demixing from a standard syringe by either a hand or a force of 100 N maximum (Figure 2)

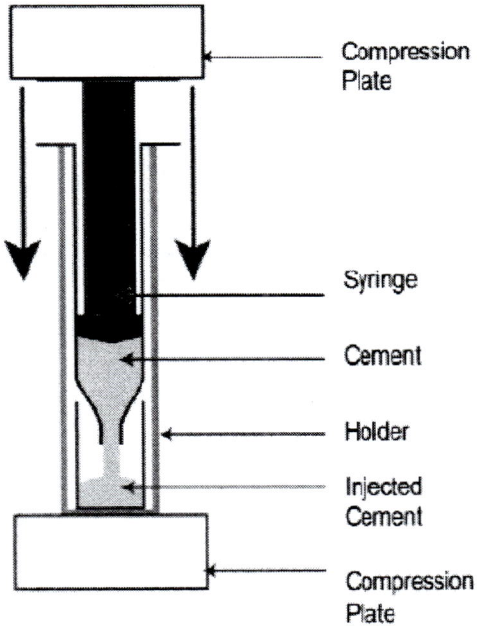

Figure 2. Schematic representation of the experimental setup used to quantify the injectability of the calcium phosphate cements. Reprinted from Ref. [166] with permission.

Usually, injectability of a cement paste varies inversely with its viscosity, the P/L ratio, as well as the time after starting the mixing of liquid and powder [44,164]. When put under pressure, some calcium orthophosphate cements show demixing into a thin paste, which is extruded, and a thick mass, which remains inside the syringe (see the aforementioned example for Norian SRS® [24]). This phenomenon is called filter pressing. In the case of demixing, the exact composition of the extruded part of the paste becomes unknown. Moreover, due to a deviation from the initial P/L ratio, it becomes unclear whether the setting behavior and the mechanical and histological properties of the extruded part are still clinically acceptable. Therefore, a good cohesion of the paste is necessary in order to avoid these problems [24].

An appropriate cohesion was achieved when no disintegration of the cement paste was observed in the fluid. This can be accomplished by keeping a high viscosity for the cement paste [20] or using cohesion promotors (*e.g.*, 1% aqueous solution of sodium alginate [120,167,168] and other chemicals [120,169]). Some calcium orthophosphate cements fulfill both criteria, *e.g.* Norian SRS®, but others fulfill only one or even none of these requirements. For example, BoneSource™ [72] and Cementek® are not injectable and blood must be kept away from the implanting site until setting [137,138]. According to some reports, decohesion of the cement during mixing might lead to inflammatory reactions [170].

Several ways can be adopted to improve both the *in vitro* properties and behavior of calcium orthophosphate cements. The first approach consists of injectability improvement. There are two options for this. Firstly, the injection device can be modified. For example, shorter cannulas with a larger diameter, as well as smaller injection rates favor a good injectability. Secondly, the cement composition can also be adapted. Namely, a decrease of the particle size, the P/L ratio and the plastic limit was found to contribute to a better injectability [163]. For example, injectability was found to be unaffected by P/L ratio within the range of 3.85–4.50 g/ml but drops by nearly 100% between P/L ratio of 4.50 and 5.00 g/ml [21]. However, a decrease in P/L ratio leads to a decrease in the mechanical properties of the cements and the cohesion might be destroyed. Besides, both the initial and final setting times decreased markedly with the P/L ratio increasing [161,171]. Therefore, variations in the P/L ratio appear to be valid to a certain extent only. That is why the manufacturer of Biopex® suggests using a P/L ratio of 2.8 or 3.3 g/ml.

Particle size decreasing of calcium orthophosphate crystals is the second approach for the injectability improvement. For example, α-BSM® is well injectable because it consists of small particles. However, a small particle size requires a large amount of mixing liquid, which decreases cohesion of the paste and leads to a greater porosity and lower mechanical properties [137,138]. An indirect approach is to add calcium orthophosphate particles those act as spacers between other particles. For example, DCPA is added to the formulation of Biocement D® to improve the injectability of the paste [137,138]. Similarly, there is an apatite cement containing spherical particles of TTCP to improve injectability [172].

Using various additives is the second way to improve the physical properties of calcium orthophosphate cements. For example, water demand of calcium orthophosphate cements can be reduced by ionically modifying the liquid component, *e.g.*, by adding nontoxic sodium salts of α-hydroxy di- and tri- acids [173,174]. A list of additives, that have been already studied, includes fluidificants, air-entraining agents, porogens, workability-improvement agents, setting time controllers and reinforcing additives [143]. Besides, radiopacifiers might be used [175]. The main role of a fluidificant is to reduce a mixing time of the cement. Citric acid is an example of this reagent; it retards the dissolution-precipitation reactions in the cement, decreases the compressive strength during initial setting, but increases its strength in the final stages of the cement hardening [162]. Besides, the data are available, that citric acid acts as a setting stimulator and improves the mechanical properties of the hardened cements [176]. Air-entraining agents (*e.g.*, surfactants) are commonly used to induce macroporosity inside calcium orthophosphate cements without affecting their normal setting. For example, crystals of mannitol ($CH_2OH(CHOH)_4CH_2OH$) were tested as an air-entraining agent; however, both loss of workability during the cement mixing and severe depreciation of mechanical properties were discovered simultaneously [177]. Porogenic agents (*e.g.*, oxygen peroxide [178] in the liquid phase and/or iced [179], sucrose granules, $NaHCO_3$ and Na_2HPO_4 crystals of 125-250 μm in size [180], poly(DL-lactic-*co*-glycolic acid) microparticles with the average size of 66±25 μm [181-184], calcium sulfate [37], NaCl crystals varying in size from 420 μm to 1 mm [185], gelatin microspheres [186]) have been also tested to create porosity. These additives could be applied on pre-set cements only. After cement hardening, dissolution of the aforementioned soluble porogens in either water or body fluids produces macropores with the dimensions and shapes of the dissolved crystals. Another method consisting in adding solid $NaHCO_3$ to the starting cement powder and using two different liquids: first, a basic liquid to form the paste and later an acid liquid to obtain CO_2 bubbles to create the porosity is also available [187]. Besides, pore forming CO_2 bubbles appear at hardening of an apatite cement, consisting of an acidic calcium orthophosphate and either $CaCO_3$ [28,42] or $NaHCO_3$ [188,189]. Furthermore, addition of an effervescent porogen formulation comprised from $NaHCO_3$ (54.52%) and citric acid monohydrate (45.48%) has been suggested [190]. Adding of surfactants to calcium orthophosphate cements was found to have two different meanings: they might act as both air-entraining agents by lowering the surface tension [191] and interaction modifiers by shifting the isoelectric point [192].

The major examples of workability-improvement agents, which are added to the cement powders, include water-soluble polymers. Specifically, polysaccharides [66,77,193-196], gelatin [171,197-201] and polyacrylic acid [202,203] are of an interest due to their biocompatibility and good rheological properties. Only small amounts (a few weight %) are needed to dramatically increase the viscosity of the cement pastes. Besides, the cement paste becomes more cohesive and highly resistant to washout immediately after mixing. For example, a 5 % weight sodium chondroitin sulfate solution is used as mixing liquid in Biopex® [137,138]. In the case of gelatin, more than a 50% improvement of the compressive strength was detected [199]. The gelatin-cement after setting was found to exhibit reduced crystallinity, much smaller CDHA crystals and a more compact microstructure; all these phenomena might be accounted for the improved mechanical properties [200]. The use of gelling agents widened a possible application of calcium orthophosphate cements because these cements can be used even when complete homeostasis is difficult. In some cases addition of a gelling agent might cause an increase in hardening time but this was remedied by the use of a sodium orthophosphate solution as the cement liquid [97,98]. Most polysaccharide solutions are thixotropic, *i.e.*, the viscosity of the solution decreases as the shear rate increases. Certain polysaccharides, such as sodium alginate, pectize in contact with calcium ions. This property can be used to make putty-like cement pastes [20]. However, only few polysaccharides are accepted for parenteral use [137,138].

Setting time controllers (accelerators and retardants) include sodium hydrogen pyrophosphate ($Na_2H_2P_2O_7$) and magnesium sulfate (according to another study, ions of citrate, sulfate and pyrophosphate are necessary [204]); they are added in amounts < 1 wt.% [205]. Application of biocompatible α-hydroxylated organic acids (glycolic, lactic, malic, tartaric and citric acids) and their calcium and sodium salts for the modification of both rheological and setting properties of calcium orthophosphate cements is well described elsewhere [206]. Besides, aqueous solutions of sodium orthophosphates are also known as setting time accelerators [66,184,207-211]. An extensive list of the compounds, which might be suitable as accelerators, retarders, additives or reactants in calcium orthophosphate cement formulations, might be found in literature [68].

The subject of the reinforcing additives is discussed in details below in "Reinforced calcium orthophosphate composites and concretes" section.

The factors that significantly influenced the storage stability (shelf life) of initial dry powders of calcium orthophosphate cements were found to be temperature, humidity and the mixing regime of the powders. Various storage conditions appeared to be effective in prolonging the stability of dry brushite cements; in the order of effectiveness, they were ranged: adding solid citric acid retardant > dry argon atmosphere ≈ gentle mixing (minimal mechanical energy input) >> low temperature [208]. Data on sterilization techniques of calcium orthophosphate cements might be found elsewhere [212].

4. Two Major Types of Calcium Orthophosphate Cements

4.1. Apatite Cements

Typically, apatite cement formulations have a precipitated poorly crystalline HA and/or CDHA as the end-product of the setting reaction (see chemical equations (1), (4) – (6)), although traces of the unreacted starting materials can be present [75]. Due to the initial presence of carbonates, such apatite cements as Norian SRS® and Biocement D® form a non-stoichiometric carbonatapatite or dahllite ($Ca_{8.8}(HPO_4)_{0.7}(PO_4)_{4.5}(CO_3)_{0.7}(OH)_{1.3}$) as the end-product [159]. As both CDHA and carbonateapatite are formed in an aqueous environment and have a low crystallinity, they appear to be similar to biological apatite of bones and teeth. These properties are believed to be responsible for the excellent *in vivo* resorption characteristics. Conventional apatite cements contain TCP and/or TTCP phases in their powder components [29], while a single component cement powder consisting of K- and Na-containing CDHA is also available [17]. The reactivity of TCP-based apatite cements varies as a function of TCP crystal phase, crystallinity and particle size. Generally, a higher reactivity is observed with a thermodynamically less stable phase (from β-TCP to α-TCP and ACP) and with a smaller particle size [119]. Nominally, it might be stated that formation of apatites through a cementation reaction is a sort of a biomimetic process because it occurs in physiological environment and at body temperature [31]; however, both the crystallization kinetics and a driving force are very far away from the biomimeticity. A unique feature of the hardened apatite cements is that the force linking the newly formed crystals (of both CDHA and carbonatapatite) is weak; therefore, the crystals can be easily detached from the cement bulk, especially after dissolution has partly occurred. When this happens, osteoclasts and other cells can easily ingest the apatite crystals [219].

Immediately after implantation, any cement becomes exposed to blood and other tissue fluids that delays the setting time. Intrinsic setting time for apatite cements has been extensively studied and it appeared to be rather long. For example, for the original formulation by Brown and Chow it ranged from 15 to 22 min [14,15]. This may result in procedural complications. To remedy this, the amount of liquid might be reduced to a possible minimum. Therefore, all apatite cements are viscous and easily moldable pastes but tend to be difficult to inject. Besides playing with the P/L ratio, the setting time can also be reduced by using additives to the liquid phase (which is distilled water in the Brown-Chow formulation [14,15]). The list of additives includes phosphoric acid, MCPM and other soluble orthophosphates. These additives promote dissolution of the solids by lowering the solution pH. In such cases, a setting time in the range of 10–15 minutes can be obtained [114-121,214]. The influence of soluble orthophosphates (*e.g.*, Na_2HPO_4 or NaH_2PO_4) on the setting time of apatite cements is explained by the fact that dissolution of DCPA and formation of CDHA during setting occur in a linear fashion, thus avoiding early formation of CDHA. This is important because too early formation of CDHA might engulf un-reacted DCPA, which slows down DCPA dissolution and thus the setting kinetics becomes slower, while the presence of sodium orthophosphates prevents DCPA particles from being isolated [211]. Particle size [132,215,216], temperature of the liquid phase and initial presence of HA as a seed in the solid phase are other factors that influence the setting time [14,15,31]; however, *in vitro* studies demonstrated that these parameters did not affect significantly [75]. On the other hand, a reduction in particle size was found to result in a significant decrease in both initial and final setting times [132,215,216], an acceleration of the hardening rate [132] and hydration kinetics of the hardening cement [216]. Besides, the crystallite sizes of the final product can be strongly reduced by increasing the specific surface of the starting powder, which allows developing calcium orthophosphate cements with tailored structures at the micro and nanoscale levels [132]. Unfortunately, an unclear correlation was found between the particle dimensions of the initial calcium orthophosphates and mechanical properties of the hardened cements: namely, a significant increase in compressive strength and storage modulus was reported for some formulations [215,216] but a minor effect on compressive strength was discovered for other ones [132]. Therefore, calcium orthophosphate cements appear to be rather versatile materials and could be adapted to the different clinical requirements of various applications [137,138].

Setting process of the most types of apatite cements occurs according to just one chemical reaction (see chemical equations (1), (4) – (6)) and at near the physiological pH. The latter may additionally contribute to the high biocompatibility observed for these materials [96-98]. For the classical formulation by Brown and Chow, the transmission electron microscopy results suggested the process for early-stage apatite formation as follows: when TTCP and DCPA powders were mixed in an orthophosphate-containing solution, TTCP powder was quickly dissolved due to its higher solubility in acidic media. Then the dissolved ions of calcium and orthophosphate, along with ions already existing in the solution, were precipitated predominantly onto the surface of DCPA particles. Few apatite crystals were observed on the surface of TTCP powder. At a later stage of the reaction, an extensive growth of apatite crystals or whiskers effectively linked DCPA particles together and bridged the larger TTCP particles causing the cement setting [217].

However, Norian SRS® and Cementek® were found to set according to two chemical reactions: precipitation of DCPD, followed by precipitation of either CDHA or carbonatapatite:

$$\alpha\text{-}Ca_3(PO_4)_2 + Ca(H_2PO_4)_2 \cdot H_2O + 7H_2O \rightarrow 4CaHPO_4 \cdot 2H_2O \quad (7)$$

$$5.2CaHPO_4 \cdot 2H_2O + 3.6CaCO_3 \rightarrow Ca_{8.8}(HPO_4)_{0.7}(PO_4)_{4.5}(CO_3)_{0.7}(OH)_{1.3} + \\ +2.9CO_2 + 12H_2O \quad (8)$$

The initial chemical reaction (7) was very fast and provoked DCPD formation and setting of the cement pastes within seconds. The second step was slower: DCDP reacted completely within several hours with remaining $\alpha\text{-}Ca_3(PO_4)_2$ and $CaCO_3$ forming carbonatapatite according to equation (8). The latter step caused the cement hardening. A similar two-step hardening mechanism was established for a cement consisting of MCPM and CaO: in the first step, during the mixing time, MCPM reacted with CaO immediately to give DCPD, which, in the second step, reacted more slowly with the remaining CaO to give CDHA [46].

The aforementioned setting mechanism of an apatite cement was investigated in details for a three component mixture of TTCP, β-TCP and MCPM dry powders in convenient proportions and with the overall atomic Ca/P ratio equal to 1.67. Two liquid phases in a raw were used to damp the cement powder, initially it was water + ethanol (ethanol was added to slow down the hardening) and afterwards orthophosphoric acid and sodium glycerophosphate were added to water to prepare a reactive liquid [88]. At the very beginning, DCPD was found to form according to two chemical reactions:

$$Ca(H_2PO_4)_2 \cdot H_2O + \beta\text{-}Ca_3(PO_4)_2 + 7H_2O \rightarrow 4CaHPO_4 \cdot 2H_2O \quad (9)$$

$$Ca_4(PO_4)_2O + 2H_3PO_4 + 7H_2O \rightarrow 4CaHPO_4 \cdot 2H_2O \quad (10)$$

The formation reactions of DCPD were fast and corresponded to the setting stage. Afterwards, TTCP reacted with the previously formed DCPD and with β-TCP to give CDHA according to the reactions:

$$2Ca_4(PO_4)_2O + 2CaHPO_4 \cdot 2H_2O \rightarrow Ca_{10-x}(HPO_4)_x(PO_4)_{6-x}(OH)_{2-x} + \\ + xCa(OH)_2 + (4-x)H_2O \quad (11)$$

$$2Ca_4(PO_4)_2O + 4\beta\text{-}Ca_3(PO_4)_2 + (2+2x)H_2O \rightarrow \\ 2Ca_{10-x}(HPO_4)_x(PO_4)_{6-x}(OH)_{2-x} + 2xCa(OH)_2 \quad (12)$$

The formation reactions of the CDHA phase were quite slow and corresponded to the hardening stage. Although OCP was not detected in that study, its formation as an intermediate phase was postulated for this cement [88]. A similar suggestion on the intermediate formation of OCP was made for the setting mechanism of Brown-Chow classical cement formulation [70,75]; however, a reliable evidence for its presence is still lacking [116,218]. In both cases, OCP was suggested to appear as an intermediate because it was a faster forming phase than CDHA. This hypothesis is based upon the classical studies performed by Prof. W.E. Brown *et al.* about the precursor phase formation during chemical crystallization of apatites in aqueous solutions [219-221].

Solubility of the hardened apatite cements in aqueous solutions is expected to be rather similar to that of bone mineral. This means that they are relatively insoluble at neutral pH and increasingly soluble as pH drops down; this is an important characteristic of normal bone mineral that facilitates controlled dissolution by osteoclasts [159].

To conclude this part, one should mention, that in 2000 the US bone substitute market for Norian SRS® accounted for ~15% of the total sales, followed by BoneSource™ at ~13%, and α-BSM® at ~8.5% [92].

4.2. Brushite Cements

As indicated by its name, DCPD is the major end-product of the setting reaction of brushite cements (chemical equations (2) and (3)). Mirtchi and Lemaitre introduced this type of the cements in 1987 [103]. Up to now, several formulations have been already proposed, *e.g.* β-TCP + MCPM [103,104], β-TCP + H_3PO_4 [222-224] and TTCP + MCPM + CaO [225]. All brushite cements are set by the acid-base interaction only. As DCPD can only precipitate at the solution pH < 6, the paste of brushite cement is acidic during setting [224,226]. For example, during setting of a β-TCP + MCPM cement, the cement pH varies from very acidic pH values of ~2.5, to almost neutral pH values of ~6 [224]. Replacing MCPM by orthophosphoric acid renders the cement paste very acidic for the initial ~30 s but then the pH profile follows that obtained with MCPM. It is important to notice, that β-TCP + H_3PO_4 formulations have several advantages over β-TCP + MCPM formulations, namely: (i) easier and faster preparation, (ii) a better control of the chemical composition and reactivity, (iii) improved physico-chemical properties, such as longer setting times and larger tensile strengths due to a higher homogeneity. However, the use of orthophosphoric acid might impair the biocompatibility of the cement formulation, due to low pH values during setting [224]. If a cement paste contains an excess of a basic phase, the equilibrium pH will be given by the intersection of the solubility isotherms of the basic phase with that of DCPD. For example, the equilibrium pH values of β-TCP + MCPM, HA + MCPM and TTCP + MCPM mixtures are 5.9, 4.2 and 7.6, respectively [137,138].

As the solubility of calcium orthophosphates decreases with increasing of their basicity (Table 1), the setting time of brushite cements much depends on the solubility of a basic phase: the higher its solubility, the faster the setting time. Therefore, the setting time of the cements made of MCPM + a basic calcium orthophosphate increases in the order: HA > β-TCP > α-TCP [137,138]. For example, HA + MCPM mixtures have a setting time of several minutes, β-TCP + MCPM mixtures – of 30 to 60 seconds and α-TCP + MCPM mixtures – of a few seconds [103,104]. Despite this initial high reactivity, the hardening reaction of brushite cements typically lasts one day until completion [141]. Additives that inhibit the crystal growth of DCPD have successfully been used to increase the setting time of β-TCP + MCPM mixtures [204]. In contrast to apatite cements, brushite cements can be initially liquid and still set within a short period of time [137,138].

Brushite cements are remarkably biocompatible and bioresorbable. Due to both a better solubility of DCPD if compared to that of CDHA (Table 1) and metastability of DCPD under physiological conditions [227], brushite cements are faster degradable than apatite cements [228,229]. They are quickly resorbed *in vivo* and suffered from a rapid decrease in strength (although the mechanical properties of the healing bone increase as bone ingrowth occurs [230]). However, short setting times, low mechanical strength and limited injectability prevent brushite cements from a broader clinical application. Use of sodium citrate or citric acid as setting retardants is an option to get more workable and less viscous pastes of brushite cements [21,161,162,231]. Similar effect might be achieved by addition of chondroitin 4-sulfate [232] and glycolic acid [233]. For the cement formulations with orthophosphoric acid as the initial reactant (see chemical equation (3)), acid deficient formulations were also found to improve the workability. In this case, the setting reaction might be described by the following chemical equation [231]:

$$3.7\beta\text{-}Ca_3(PO_4)_2 + H_3PO_4 + 27.8H_2O \rightarrow 3CaHPO_4{\cdot}2H_2O + \\ +2.7\beta\text{-}Ca_3(PO_4)_2 + 21H_2O \qquad (13)$$

Occasionally, when large quantities of brushite cements were used, a certain degree of tissue inflammation during the first weeks of *in vivo* implantation were reported [229,231,234]. Further investigations indicated that the inflammatory could be due to a partial transformation of DCPD into CDHA with release of orthophosphoric acid [137,138]:

$$(10-x)CaHPO_4{\cdot}2H_2O \rightarrow Ca_{10-x}(HPO_4)_x(PO_4)_{6-x}(OH)_{2-x} + \\ +(4-x)H_3PO_4 + (18-x)H_2O \qquad (14)$$

Transformation of DCPD into CDHA occurs via two processes: dissolution and precipitation [235] and can be retarded by adding magnesium ions to the cement paste, thus reducing the possibility of inflammation [137,138]. The aforementioned case of acid deficient formulations of brushite cements (chemical equation (13)) is an alternative, because it reduces the amount of unreacted acid in the cement [231] with an option to consume liberating in chemical equation (14) orthophosphoric acid by the excess of β-TCP. Implantation of previously set brushite cement might be the third option, because a solid material was found to be better tolerated than paste implants. Besides, more bone was formed at the solid implant contact and the solid material degraded not so rapidly [236]. For brushite cements, a linear degradation rate of 0.25 mm/week was reported [237]. This rapid degradation rate might lead to formation of an immature bone. Adding β-TCP granules to the cement paste could solve this problem because β-TCP granules might act as bone anchors and encourage formation of a mature bone [237,238].

5. Bioresorption and Replacement of the Cements by Bones

Due to the excellent bioresorbability of DCPD and CDHA, a newly forming woven bone might substitute the hardened calcium orthophosphate cements. For example, the implants made of BoneSource™ were partly resorbed and replaced by natural bone, depending upon the size of the cranial defect [72]. α-BSM® was evaluated in a canine femoral slot model. New bone was found to form in 3 weeks via an osteoconductive pathway. After 4 weeks, only 1.7% of the implanted material was observed. The hybrid bone possessed the strength of normal, unoperated bone after 12 weeks. In 26 weeks, the boundary between old and new bone was virtually indistinguishable, with only 0.36% of the implant recognizable [114]. Norian SRS® was evaluated in canine tibial and femoral metaphyseal defects. The cement appeared to be gradually remodeled over time, with blood vessels penetrating through it. However, some amounts of Norian SRS® were detected in the medullary area as long as 78 weeks after being implanted in dog femurs [27]. An interesting study on the *in vitro* resorption of three apatite cements (conventional, fast-setting and anti-washout) by osteoclasts if compared with similar resorption of sintered HA and a cortical bone revealed an intermediate behavior of the cements: they were resorbed slower than bone but faster than HA [239]. Evidences of the direct contact of bone and a calcium orthophosphate cement without soft tissue interposition might be found in literature [240].

Different studies reported on both cement bioresorption and the progress of bone formation around calcium orthophosphate cements which in certain cases demonstrated both osteoconductive and osteoinductive properties. However, some studies did not confirm the osteoinductive properties of calcium orthophosphate cements [241]. Some inflammatory reactions were noticed when the cement did not set [170]. As solubility of CDHA is higher than that of stoichiometric HA (Table 1), the biodegradability of apatite cements is always better than that of dense bioceramics made of sintered HA; however, still it is rather poor. For example, histologically, at 2 weeks, spicules of living bone with normal bone marrow and osteocytes in lacunae could be seen in the cement. At 8 weeks, the cement was almost totally surrounded by mature bone. At this stage, no resorption of the cement was observed [242]. Only 30% decrease of the implanted amount of Norian SRS® was reported after 24 months in a rabbit femur [243]. Moreover, several differences can be expected depending on the cement type. For example, as the end-product of BoneSource™ and Teknimed® is a very crystalline CDHA, BoneSource™ and Teknimed® are expected to resorb slower than other apatite cements. Indeed no resorption of BoneSource™ was observed after several years implantation; though some resorption of Biobone® was detected. However, as Biobone® is more porous than BoneSource™, the discovered diversity could be due to the differences in the cement porosity [137,138]. The latter conclusion is confirmed by the results of other studies: a positive influence of the cement porosity on the resorption rate was found [168]. The interested readers are referred to the study on the suitability of porous calcium orthophosphate cements as scaffold material for bone regeneration, using a rabbit model [244].

The resorption properties of bioceramics are generally believed to relate to the solubility of their constitutive phases. The implanted calcium orthophosphates might be resorbed by two possible mechanisms, namely: an active resorption, mediated by the cellular activity of macrophages, osteoclasts and other types of living cells (so called phagocytosis or literally "cell-eating") [245,247] and a passive resorption due to either chemical dissolution [11] or chemical hydrolysis (brushite cements only) [231] in the body fluids. Unfortunately, the factors concerning the biodegradation of calcium orthophosphate biomaterials have not been completely elucidated yet. The chemical composition, physical characteristics and crystal structures certainly play an important role in the biological behavior of calcium orthophosphates. In addition to this, the biodegradation may be influenced by the experimental conditions: experimental models, implantation sites and animal species [246].

The data are available that macrophages and giant cells decompose quickly resorbed calcium orthophosphate cements (*e.g.*, brushite cements) [229,248], while slowly (from months to years) resorbed apatite cements are decomposed by osteoclast-type cells [25,213,248]. Clearly, a fast resorption of brushite cements can only be achieved if the cement resorption occurs before its conversion to CDHA according to equation (14). Both types of the resorption mechanisms (active + passive) might occur almost simultaneously, if a hardened cement consists of two different calcium orthophosphates, *e.g.*, from DCPD and β-TCP. For example, the biphasic brushite cement ChronOS™ Inject was found to resorb by dissolution with cement disintegration and particle formation followed by the phagocytosis of the cement particles through macrophages [249]. A similar cement was found to be degraded through a dissolution process associated with a cellular process [246]. The interested readers are referred to a very interesting review on the cellular mechanisms of calcium orthophosphate ceramic degradation [250].

The summary (as of 2003) of brushite cement implantation studies in various animal models and defect locations is available in literature [231]. Generally, in the same animal model, a degradation rate decreases with a sample size increases, as does DCPD to HA conversion time. The compositional changes of a brushite cement after implantation in sheep is well described elsewhere [205].

The kinetics of passive resorption depends on porosity of the samples, ionic substitutions, crystallinity and pH of the cement-tissue interface. The active resorption is due to cellular activity; however, it is also related to the passive one. Solution pH near macrophages and osteoclasts can drop to ~ 5 by the excretion of lactic acid, whereas near osteoblasts (bone forming cells) solution pH can become as high as 8.5 by the excretion of ammonia [24]. Dissolution chemistry of CDHA (therefore, of the hardened apatite cements) in acidic media (calcium orthophosphates are almost insoluble in alkaline solutions [10,11,226]) might be described as a sequence of four successive chemical equations [251,252]:

$$Ca_{10-x}(HPO_4)_x(PO_4)_{6-x}(OH)_{2-x} + (2-x)H^+ \rightarrow Ca_{10-x}(HPO_4)_x(PO_4)_{6-x}(H_2O)_{2-x}^{(2-x)+} \quad (15)$$

$$Ca_{10-x}(HPO_4)_x(PO_4)_{6-x}(H_2O)_{2-x}^{(2-x)+} \rightarrow 3Ca_3(PO_4)_2 + (1-x)Ca^{2+} + (2-x)H_2O \quad (16)$$

$$Ca_3(PO_4)_2 + 2H^+ \rightarrow Ca^{2+} + 2CaHPO_4 \quad (17)$$

$$CaHPO_4 + H^+ \rightarrow Ca^{2+} + H_2PO_4^- \quad (18)$$

Obviously, the dissolution chemistry of DCPD[10] (therefore, of the hardened brushite cements) in acidic media is described by equation (18).

The mechanism of bone healing caused by calcium orthophosphate cements is very multifactorial because the surface of the cements is rapidly colonized by cells. Several types of these cells degrade calcium orthophosphates by either phagocytotic mechanisms (fibroblasts, osteoblasts, monocytes/macrophages) or an acidic mechanism with a proton pump to reduce the pH of the microenvironment and resorb the hardened bioceramics (osteoclasts) [250,253]. Various mesenchymal cells located at the implantation sites can induce solubilization of calcium orthophosphates. Upon the cells arrival, various active enzymes, such as acid phosphatase, are secreted that causes dissolution of the hardened cements [254-256]. Much more biology, than chemistry and material science altogether, is involved into this very complex process and many specific details still remain unknown. Due to a lack of the necessary experimental data for calcium orthophosphates, the major bone healing steps caused by the cements might be schematically described by a modified scheme for the bioactivity mechanism of bioactive glasses – the concept introduced by Prof. Larry Hench [257,258]. The mechanism of bonding of bioactive glasses to living tissue involves a sequence of 11 successive reaction steps. The initial 5 steps occurred on the surface of bioactive glasses are "chemistry" only, while the remaining 6 steps belong to "biology" because the latter include colonization by osteoblasts, followed by proliferation and differentiation of the cells to form a new bone that had a mechanically strong bond to the implant surface (Figure 3).

It is well known that various polypeptides and growth factors present in bone matrix might be adsorbed onto HA and modulate the local milieu of cells. This is supported by many purification protocols of growth factors and bone morphogenetic proteins/osteogenins involving HA chromatography [260,261]. However, osteoblasts are not found in direct contact with calcium orthophosphates. A complex proteinaceous layer, usually osteoid, directly contacts the osteoblasts. After implantation of calcium orthophosphate cements, mitogenic events could occur either during the initial mesenchymal cell contact or after osteoid degradation by osteoblast collagenase. In a dense, mineralized material such as calcium orthophosphate cements, which provides a barrier to the free diffusion of circulating hormones, growth factors, and cytokines, it is questionable whether the local responses at the periphery of the material regulate osteoconduction [20]. The tissue response to injectable calcium orthophosphate cements is well described in literature [188,234,248,262,263]. Very recent histological and mechanical evaluation of self-setting calcium orthophosphate cements in a sheep vertebral bone void model is available elsewhere [264]. The interested readers are also advised to get through a recent paper on the *in vitro* biodegradation of brushite cements by a macrophage cell-line [85].

To conclude this part, one should note that calcium orthophosphate cements are able to provide short-term biologically desirable properties and then be replaced by a new bone, which is very important.

[10] Water is omitted for simplicity. Therefore, dissolution of DCPA is written instead.

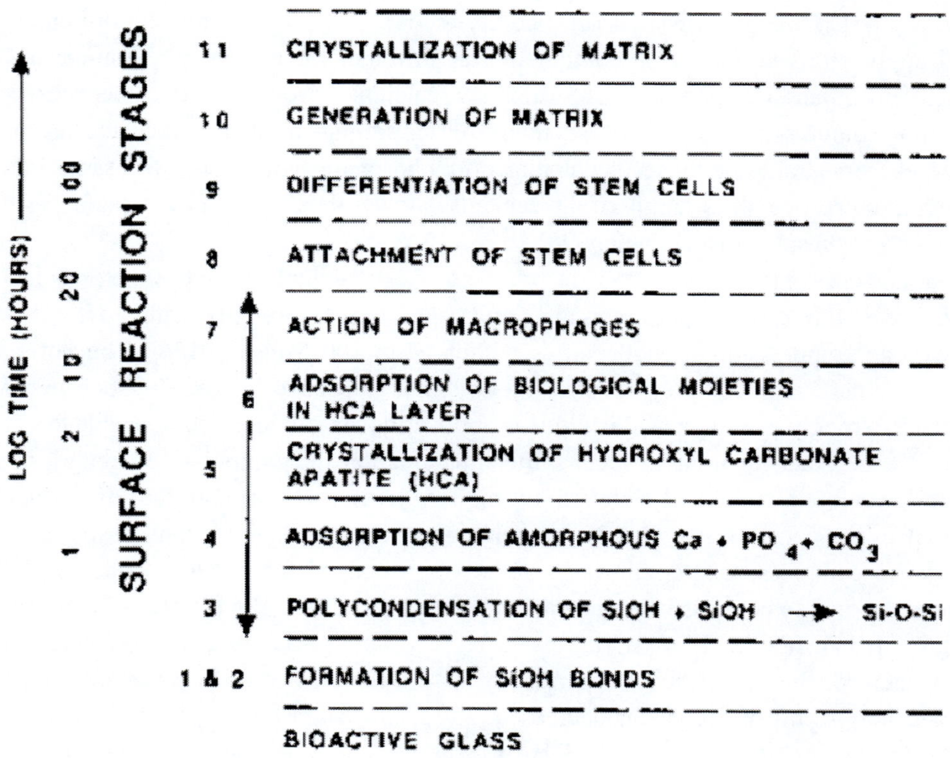

Figure 3.. The sequence of interfacial reactions involved in forming a bond between tissue and bioactive glasses. The border between "dead" and "alive" occurs approximately at stage 6. For want of anything better, the bioactivity mechanism of calcium orthophosphate cements should also be described by this scheme with omitting of several initial stages, as it was made for HA in Ref. [259], where 3 initial chemical stages of the Hench's mechanism were replaced by partial dissolution of HA. Reprinted from Ref. [258] with permission.

The growth rate of a newly forming bone depends on age, sex and general metabolic health of the recipient as well as on the anatomic site, porosity, bulk site, crystallinity, chemical composition (brushite or apatite), particle sizes and P/L ratio of the cements. Considering all these factors, it might take from 3 to 36 months for different calcium orthophosphate cements to be completely resorbed and replaced by bone [142]. However, additional sound scientific data to determine the exact degree of biodegradability for calcium orthophosphate cements are still needed, viz. animal studies performed in a critical-size defect model. One must stress that the rate of cement resorption should be balanced with the rate of new bone formation to avoid collapse at the fracture site, which might occur if the resorption is too fast.

6. The Mechanical Properties

As in most clinical applications calcium orthophosphate cements are applied in direct contact with human trabecular bones, it may be stated as a mechanical requirement that the strength of the cements must be at least as high as that of trabecular bones, which is close to

10 MPa [265]. Three-dimensional (3D) complex load is applied during the orthopedic and dental applications because of a combination of different forces that may include bending, torsion, tension and compression. Unfortunately, calcium orthophosphate cements are strong enough at compression only [136]. In theory, after setting, they can reach the mechanical properties comparable to those of calcium orthophosphate blocks with the same porosity. However, in practice, the strength of the cements is lower than that of bones, teeth or sintered calcium orthophosphate bioceramics [98].

Having the ceramic origin, the set products of all calcium orthophosphate cements are brittle, have both a low impact resistance and a low tensile strength (within 1 to 10 MPa), whereas the compression strength varies within 10 to 100 MPa [95,136]. The latter value exceeds the maximum compression strength of human trabecular bones. The poor mechanical properties strongly reduce a wider clinical application of calcium orthophosphate cements [266]. On the other hand, at 12 weeks after implantation the compressive strength of these cements was found to be still significantly higher (60 to 70 MPa) than that of normal bone [230]. Brushite cements are slightly weaker than apatite cements. A tensile strength of 10 MPa and a compressive strength of 60 MPa were obtained for brushite cements [267]. In comparison, apatite cements can reach a tensile strength of 16 MPa [268] and a compressive strength of 83 MPa [269]. *In vivo*, the difference between apatite and brushite cements boosts: namely, the mechanical properties of apatite cements were found to increase [210], whereas those of brushite cements decreased [230]. This is attributed to a higher solubility of DCPD when compared with that of CDHA (Table 1). After a few weeks of implantation, the mechanical properties of brushite cements began to increase due to bone ingrowth [230]. The interested readers are suggested to get through the mechanical characterization of a bone defect model filled with ceramic cements [140].

To improve the mechanical properties of calcium orthophosphate cements, addition of water-soluble polymers might be considered. For example, in early 1990-s, Miyazaki *et al.* [270,271] used a number of polymers, including polyacrylic acid and polyvinyl alcohol to improve the properties of a TTCP-DCPD cement. They noted marked increases (up to threefold) in mechanical properties, but with an unacceptable reduction of workability and setting time. Later, another research group reported similar results using sodium alginate and sodium polyacrylate [272]. Afterwards, other researchers added several polyelectrolytes, polyethylene oxide and a protein bovine serum albumin into α-BSM™ cement paste to create calcium phosphate–polymer composites [273]. Composites of α-BSM™ with polycations (polyethylenimine and polyallylamine hydrochloride) exhibited compressive strengths up to six times greater than that of pure α-BSM™ material. Composites of α-BSM™ with bovine serum albumin developed compressive strengths twice that of the original α-BSM™ cement. This effect was explained by an inhibiting effect of the aforementioned additives on the crystal growth kinetics of newly forming crystals of calcium orthophosphates, which resulted in smaller crystallites and, hence, a denser and more interdigitated microstructure. However, the increased strength was attributed mainly to the polymer's capacity to bridge between multiple crystallites (thus forming a more cohesive composite) and to absorb energy through a plastic flow [273].

As presence of pores simplifies for cracks to run throughout the hardened mass, the mechanical properties of the hardened cements were found to decrease exponentially with the porosity increase. In theory, calcium orthophosphate cements can be made with almost any porosity. However, for most commercial cements, the pores are of 8 – 12 μm in diameter and, after the cement is set, about 40 – 50% of its volume is the porosity [274]. Pressure can be applied to reduce the porosity of calcium orthophosphate cements [95,275,276]. The pore dimensions in hardened cements are too small to allow fast bone ingrowth. Besides, unless the special efforts have been performed, the pores are not interconnected. Due to these reasons, after injection, osteoclastic cells are able to degrade the hardened cements layer-by-layer only, starting at the bone-cement interface throughout its inner part (in other words, from the outside to the inside). This is the main drawback of the classical cement formulations when compared to calcium orthophosphate ceramic scaffolds with an open porosity [137,138].

Since the compression strength is reciprocally proportional to porosity, the former might be adjusted by varying the P/L ratio in the hardening mixture. Elevated compression strength would be applicable in cranioplasty for regions requiring significant soft-tissue support. For smaller bone defects, such as root canal fillings, low-compression cements might be used [92]. Concerning the tensile strength of calcium orthophosphate cements, as a rule of thumb, it appears to increase two-fold with each 10 vol. % decrease of the porosity, *i.e.* 5, 10, 20, 40 and 80 MPa for 80, 70, 60, 50 and 40% porosity, respectively [137,138]. The effect of porosity on the compressive modulus of calcium orthophosphate cements is available as Figure 4 in Ref. [276]. Ishikawa and Asaoka showed a linear relation (R^2=0.94) between ln diametral tensile strength and porosity of a calcium orthophosphate cement where porosity was controlled by compaction pressure (up to 173 MPa) [95]. Besides, an empirical relationship between strength, S, and porosity, P is also available [277]:

$$S = S_0 e^{-bP}$$

where: S_0 is the theoretical strength at P = 0 (fully dense), and b is an empirical constant.

Because the porosity is mainly due to an excess of water used in the cement compositions, attempts were made to reduce the amount of water. Besides, the amount of water determines the rheological properties of the cement paste: a decrease in water content leads to a large increase in viscosity, eventually leading to non-flowable pastes. As calcium orthophosphate cements set at an almost constant volume, the final porosity can be predicted from the initial composition [137,138]. A shrinkage degree of ~ 1% causes no restrictions on clinical use [134]. Very recent studies on the *in vivo* evaluation of an injectable macroporous calcium orthophosphate cements revealed a higher bioresorption rate due to both a higher surface contact with body fluids (which increases dissolution) and enhancing cellular activity due to particle degradation [168,188].

As was stated by Bohner [137], it appeared to be difficult to compare the mechanical properties of different cement formulations. For example, the following numeric values of the compression strength and setting time were obtained for Norian SRS®: 33±5 MPa and 8.5±0.5 min (≈ 50% porosity),[11] Cementek®: 8±2 MPa and 17±1 min, Biocement D®: 83±4

[11] Further details on the major properties of Norian SRS® are available elsewhere [143,278].

MPa and 6.5±0.5 min (≈ 40% porosity) and α-BSM®: 4±1 MPa and 19±1 min (≈ 80% porosity), respectively [269]. Among them, Biocement D® has the highest compressive strength but the lowest porosity. A high compressive strength does not necessarily mean that Biocement D® is the least breakable implant. *In vivo*, shear and tensile forces indeed play a very important role. Therefore, the tensile strength of the cements should also be considered, for example, using the Mohr circle approach [279]. Finally, it should be kept in mind that the initial mechanical properties of calcium orthophosphate cements may vary with implantation time. Animal studies indicated that the mechanical properties of apatite cements tended to increase continually [210], in contrast to those of brushite cements, which initially decreased and again increased when bone was growing [230].

The porosity level of calcium orthophosphate cements might be controlled to a certain extent by adjusting particle sizes and P/L ratio. When the P/L ratio is high, the porosity of the apatite cement is low [137,138]. Besides, successful attempts have been made to introduce macroporosity into calcium orthophosphate cements by using soluble particles (porogens) [177,180,196,277,280], resorbable polymers [281,282], fast resorptive phases [178,225] or foaming agents (*e.g.*, dehydrated albumen) [168,178]. According to calculations, the tensile strength of the cements with zero porosity could be as high as 103 MPa [95]. However, a high density and a lack of pores decreases cement bioresorbability because a newly forming bone appears to be unable to grow into the pores; it might grow only simultaneously with dissolution of the cement. Thus, the porosity of calcium orthophosphate cements is a very important factor for the cement degradability [137,138]. Other factors affecting strength are the materials used in the solid phase, particle sizes, incorporation of fillers into the solid phase, P/L ratio and various liquid phases [75].

The strength of the cement-prosthesis interface might be studied by a pullout test. The details are available elsewhere [52].

7. Reinforced Calcium Orthophosphate Composites and Concrete

Being aware of the excellent bioresorbability of DCPD and CDHA, researchers are focused on attempts to overcome the mechanical weakness of calcium orthophosphate cements by using different fillers, fibers and reinforcing additives that give rise to formation of various multiphasic composites [73,74,78,139,160,169,274,277,283-288]. Even carbon nanotubes have been successfully tested to reinforce calcium orthophosphate cements [289]. Although the biomaterials community does not use this term, a substantial amount of such formulations might be defined as calcium orthophosphate concretes.[12] The idea behind the concretes is simple: if a strong filler is present in the matrix, it might stop crack propagation. However, adding fillers always reduced the porosity that negatively influenced the ability of the concretes to allow bone ingrowth into pores. Hence, a denser cement has a slower

[12] According to Wikipedia, the free encyclopedia: "*Concrete* is a construction material that consists of a cement (commonly Portland cement), aggregates (generally gravel and sand) and water. It solidifies and hardens after mixing and placement due to a chemical process known as hydration. The water reacts with the cement, which bonds the other components together, eventually creating a stone-like material." [290].

resorption rate and thus a slower bone substitution [95]. Moreover, due to the presence of fillers, the rheological properties and injectability of calcium orthophosphate concretes frequently appear to be worse than those properties of calcium orthophosphate cements. Thus, it is difficult to increase strength of the cements without having a negative influence on the other properties.

Calcium orthophosphate concretes can be prepared from both apatite and brushite cement formulations. For example, in an attempt to improve the mechanical properties of calcium orthophosphate cements, a group of investigators prepared concretes by adding human cadaveric femur bone chips in amounts of 25, 50 and 75% (w/w) to α-BSM® cement [284]. The mechanical tests revealed that the specimens of pure cement exhibited a relatively high stiffness but a low ductility. However, for the cement-bone concretes an increasing of bone content was found to result in the elastic modulus decreasing and the ductility increasing; however, the ultimate strength showed only small changes with no apparent trend [284]. A concrete of Biopex® cement with allografts taken from femurs and tibiae of rabbits is also available. Unfortunately, nothing is written on the mechanical properties improvement but, surprisingly, by the addition of allografts, the hydrolysis process of Biopex® was significantly changed [160]. By adding polymers and composites, other researchers succeeded in improving the mechanical strength of the cements up to 30 MPa; however, the kinetics of CDHA formation and thus the bioactivity of the material were decreased [79,291]. Xu *et al.* reported that incorporation of long carbon fibers at a volume fraction of 5.7% increased the flexural strength about 4 times and work of fracture 100 times, if compared to un-reinforced calcium orthophosphate cements [292]. The reinforcement mechanisms were found to be crack bridging and fiber pullout, while fiber length and volume fraction were key microstructural parameters that determined the concrete properties [292]. Although addition of polypropylene, nylon and carbon fibers was found to reduce the compression strength of a double-setting calcium orthophosphate cement because of increased porosity, it strongly increased the cement's fracture toughness and tensile strength, relative to the values for the un-reinforced variant of this cement [285]. A knitted two-dimensionally oriented polyglactin fiber-mesh was found to be effective in improving load-bearing behavior of a calcium orthophosphate cement for potential structural repair of bone defects [139]. To make the material stronger, fast setting and anti-washout, chitosan was added to the cements [270,293-298]. Calcium orthophosphate cements doped by SiO_2, and TiO_2 particles showed a significant (~ 80-100 MPa) increase in the compressive strength, whilst no change in the mechanical behavior of the cements was observed when ZrO_2 particles were added [286]. Besides, calcium orthophosphate cements might be successfully reinforced by addition of calcium silicates [54], polypeptide copolymers [299] and collagen [300,301].

Yet another team examined the effects of varying fiber type, fiber length and volume fraction of fiber-reinforced concretes [293,302]. Four fibers were studied: aramid, carbon, E-glass and polyglactin. Fiber length ranged from 3–200 mm and fiber volume fraction ranged from 1.9–9.5%. The results indicated that a self-setting calcium orthophosphate cement was substantially strengthened via fiber reinforcement. Aramid contributed to the largest increase in composite strength, followed by carbon, E-glass and polyglactin. Fiber length, fiber volume fraction and fiber strength were found to be key microstructural parameters that controlled the mechanical properties of calcium orthophosphate concretes [293,302]. Fiber reinforcement of porous cements (mannitol was used as a porogen) was discovered as well [303]. Namely, reinforcement by aramid fibers (volume fraction of 6%) was found to improve the properties of a calcium orthophosphate cement with the strength increasing threefold at 0% mannitol, sevenfold at 30% mannitol and nearly fourfold at 40% mannitol. Simultaneously, the work of fracture increased by nearly 200 times, however the modulus was not changed as a result of fiber reinforcement [303]. Addition of 20 wt% of acrylamide and 1 wt% ammonium polyacrylate to the liquid increased the compressive and tensile strength of α-TCP bone cement by 149 and 69% (55 and 21 MPa), respectively [304]. A positive influence of polyamide fibers is also known [305].

In the cases, when bioresorbable reinforcement fibers are used, strength augmentation is attained at the initial stages [281,306-309]. For example, the initial strength of a concrete was threefold higher than that of the unreinforced cement control [306]. The work of fracture (toughness) was found to increase by two orders of magnitude for other composites of calcium orthophosphate / resorbable fiber (namely, Vicryl polyglactin 910, Ethicon, Somerville, NJ [307] and a mesh of copolymer of polyglycolic and polylactic acids [281]). When implanted *in vivo*, bioresorbable fibers would provide initial strength and then dissolve to form interconnecting macroscopic channels which could facilitate bone ingrowth into the implant [97,98,281,306]. For example, interconnected macropores were formed in a calcium orthophosphate cement at 84 days' immersion in a physiological solution [281]. One should note that, apart from the mechanical properties of the reinforcing material, the structure of the incorporated fibres, regular or random, appears to be crucial for the resulting flexural strength and modulus of elasticity [309]. A higher strength might help extending the use of calcium orthophosphate cements to larger stress-bearing repairs, while the macropores might facilitate tissue ingrowth and integration of the cement with an adjacent bone. To extend this idea further, several types of fibers with different rates of bioresorbability might be simultaneously incorporated into a cement formulation.

Besides the aforementioned, it is important to mention on concretes, after hardening consisting of calcium orthophosphates only [237,249,310-312]. The first biphasic composition consisting of a hardened DCPD matrix filled with β-TCP granules was introduced in 1992 [311]. Further development of this formulation might be found in other papers [237,249]; unfortunately, neither the mechanical nor the rheological properties of this concrete have been disclosed. At physiologic pH, the *in vitro* solubility of DCPD is approximately 8 times higher than β-TCP; the same order of magnitude applies for the *in vivo* resorption of these calcium orthophosphates. A new bone forms in the space left after resorption of the DCPD matrix, while β -TCP granules act as guiding structures. This feature of the cement can be considered an inverse scaffolding effect [313]. Another group of investigators invented a formulation that incorporated as major powder components α-TCP, ACP and biphasic calcium phosphate (BCP; consisting of an intimate mixture of HA and β-TCP in various HA/β-TCP ratios) [283]. It was believed that after setting such a formulation could provide a porous ceramics *in vivo* due to preferential dissolution of a better soluble ACP component compared to the other calcium orthophosphates in the matrix. Further, this combination was extended to a multiphase concrete composition consisting of 70% w/w settable matrix (mixture of 45% α-TCP, 5% MCPM and 25% ACP[13]) with the average particle dimensions of 15 μm and 30% BCP granules (ranging between 80 and 200 μm) as a filler [310]. The role of BCP granules is quite interesting: after implantation of a cement without BCP granules, the quality of newly formed bone was not identical to the host bone, while implantation of a concrete with BCP granules resulted in formation of a new bone identical to the host bone. The reason of this phenomenon is not clear yet; but, perhaps, it correlates with similar results for β-TCP granules, which act as bone anchors and encourage formation of a mature bone [237,238]. A strength improvement was found when DCPA and TiO_2 crystals were used as fillers for mechanically activated α-TCP cements [314]. Calcium orthophosphate concretes reinforced by whiskers made of calcium carbonate [43] and HA [312] have been also developed.

To conclude this part, one should briefly mention on the reverse situation: there are bone concretes made of acrylic cements, reinforced by calcium orthophosphate powders or granules [315-321]. The calcium orthophosphates presented in these formulations act as fillers, which are necessary to improve the mechanical properties and to impart bioactivity; they do not participate in the hardening mechanisms. Polymerization of monomers is primarily responsible for setting of such composites. However, that is another story.

8. Clinical and Medical Applications

Injectable osteoconductive calcium orthophosphate cements have been introduced as an adjunct to internal fixation for treating selected fractures. Different studies have already shown that they are highly biocompatible and osteoconductive materials, which can stimulate tissue regeneration [20,322]. The main purpose of calcium orthophosphate cements is to fill voids in metaphyseal bone, thereby reducing the need for bone graft, although the cements also might improve the holding strength around metal devices in osteoporotic bone. The combination of a self-setting nature, moldability, biocompatibility, lack of any by-products and a great potential for being replaced by bone make calcium orthophosphate cements very promising materials for clinical applications: they can easily be used by bone remodeling cells for reconstruction of damaged parts of bones [71,72,229,263,323,324]. The ability to be molded in place also is a very important property, because a cement can easily be delivered into the desired place and can be fitted perfectly with bone defects [72]. Besides, some formulations were found to possess an antimicrobial activity [44,47,49,55,325], as well as promote osteoblast cell adhesion and gene expression *in vitro* [326].

Recent studies reported optimistic results in relation to the clinical application of calcium orthophosphate cements. For example, the recent data on cytocompatibility and early osteogenic characteristics are available in literature [327]. The ratio of the cases determined to be “effective” or “better” among the 74 cases we found to be 97.3% [328]. Besides, the results of intra-articular degradation and resorption kinetics of these cements revealed no signs of pronounced acute or chronic inflammation [329]. Injected Norian SRS® cement was mainly found as a single particle, anterior to the cruciate ligaments. The cement became

[13] Ion-substituted ACPs contained other ions (carbonates, Mg, Zn, F) were used in that study [310].

surrounded by synovial tissues within 4 weeks and showed signs of superficial resorption [329]. Unfortunately, disintegration or washout of calcium orthophosphate cements has been reported as a potential clinical problem [95,214]. Perhaps, this problem could be solved by putting pressure on the paste during the setting period. In addition, sodium alginate might be added; however, the mechanical properties (strength) of this formulation are still poor [77].

According to the available information, the first animal study of calcium orthophosphate cements was performed in 1991: a cement consisting of TTCP and DCPA was investigated histologically by implanting disks made of this cement within the heads of nine cats [330]. Simultaneously, another research group evaluated the tissue reaction to this cement in the teeth of monkeys [331]. The important examples of the most significant directions of current medical applications of calcium orthophosphate cements and concretes are given below.

8.1. Dental Applications

A group of investigators extracted all mandibular premolar teeth from beagles [332]. After one month of healing, alveolar bone was reduced to make space for a previously fabricated calcium orthophosphate cement block. One more month later, 8-mm HA implants were placed in such a manner that the apical half was embedded into alveolar bone and the coronal half in the calcium orthophosphate cement block. The investigators observed that the cement block was gradually replaced by bone and histopathologic features of the cement area were similar to that of natural bone. Moreover, the coronal half of the implants, previously surrounded by the calcium orthophosphate cement, was firmly attached by natural bone [332]. In another study, the same researchers used fluorescent labeling analysis and electron microanalysis to measure the extent of new bone formation and elemental (Ca, P, Mg) distribution [333]. The results indicated the presence of newly formed bone at 1 month after surgery and similar elemental distributions in the calcium orthophosphate cement and natural bone areas at 6 months after surgery [142]. Besides, calcium orthophosphate cements were tried as root canal fillers [47,334,335] and for pulp capping [336].

A hydraulic calcium orthophosphate cement was injected as a bone filler for gaps around oral implants placed on the medial femoral condyles of six goats and found excellent bone formation around the graft material. Unfortunately, the degradation rate of the cement appeared to be very slow and no resorption was observed [337]. In another study, a cement was placed on artificially created periodontal defects but no significant difference was found between the cement and control. However, the cement acted as a scaffold for bone formation and provided histocompatible healing of periodontal tissues [338]. Still other investigators used a cement for direct pulp capping and compared it to calcium hydroxide. Both materials were found to be equally capable of producing a secondary dentin at 24 weeks [339].

8.2. Craniofacial and Maxillofacial Applications

The use of calcium orthophosphate cements for craniofacial applications seems logical, as there is little or no stress generated under these conditions. Moreover, the ability to mold the material at placement is an enormous advantage from a cosmetics standpoint [142]. For example, BoneSource™ is indicated for the repair of neurosurgical burr holes, contiguous craniotomy cuts and other cranial defects with a surface area no larger than 25 cm^2 per a defect. In addition, it may be used in the sinus region for facial augmentation and the cement can be supported by metal hardware [72]. In dogs, BoneSource™ was employed to supplement the supraorbital ridge and to augment skull base defects [340]. Another group performed trials to ascertain the inflammation around the site and the degree of loss of the implanted BoneSource™. The material was found to be osteoconductive with both periosteal and endosteal bone formation [341]. One more group presented excellent results using the material combined with an underlying resorbable mesh in calvarian defects of Yorkshire pigs. They found progressive bone ingrowths in all defects at 180 days, with nearly complete replacement by host bone [282]. Besides, excellent results for over 100 human patients were reported when a calcium orthophosphate cement was used in cranial defects. The success rate of the cement after 6 years was 97% [64]. The results of still other medical trials are available elsewhere [274,342-346].

8.3. Orthopedic Applications

Calcium orthophosphate cements have successfully been used for treatment of the distal radius fracture [159,347,348]. Besides, other successful attempts have been made to use the cements for calcaneal fractures [349], hip fractures [350,351], augmentation of osteoporotic vertebral bodies [352], tibial plateau fractures [27,353-356], restoration of pedicle screw fixation [357], reinforcement of both thoracolumbar burst fractures [358], cancellous bone screws [359], in wrist arthrodesis [360] and for fixation of titanium implants [361]. A very recent study on a cement augmentation of the femoral neck defect might be found elsewhere [362]. Considering their properties, calcium orthophosphate cements might potentially be applied to reinforce osteoporotic vertebral bodies [352,363]. Further details are available elsewhere [364,365]. Besides, calcium orthophosphate cements appear to be a reliable subchondral replacement material when the bone defect is adjacent to the articular cartilage [366].

8.4. Vertebroplasty and Kyphoplasty Applications

Vertebroplasty and kyphoplasty are two surgical procedures that recently have been introduced to medically manage of osteoporosis-induced vertebral compression fractures. Particularly, both procedures aim to augment the weakened vertebral body, stabilize it and/or restore it to as much of its normal height and functional state as possible. Both procedures involve injection of a self-setting paste of a calcium orthophosphate cement into the fractured vertebral body, which resulted in a faster healing [143,367-371].

8.5. Drug Delivery Applications

In general, a potential substrate to be used as a drug carrier must have the ability to incorporate a drug, retain it in a specific target site and deliver it progressively with time in the surrounding tissues. Additional advantages are provided if the material is injectable, biodegradable, sets at ambient temperature, has near neutral pHs and a large surface area [30,31]. These properties make calcium orthophosphate cements to be very attractive candidates as drug carriers for therapeutic peptides [372], antibiotics [373-375], anticancer drugs [376], anti-inflammatory drugs [377], hormones [378] and bone morphogenetic proteins [298,379-381]. For example, a "growth factor cement (GFC)" has been reported [382]. In that study, a combination of bone morphogenetic protein-2, transforming growth factor-beta, platelet-derived growth factor and basic fibroblast growth factor was used in a calcium orthophosphate cement for treatment of peri-implant defects in a dog model. The findings indicated a significant effect of GFC on increased bone-to-implant contact and amount of bone per surface area if compared with both the cement-only and no-cement treatment groups [382].

In principle, drugs might be incorporated into both a liquid and a powder phase of the cements. After setting, the drugs are slowly released through the cement pores. For example, a group of investigators added flomoxef sodium to a cement formulation and found that the release of antibiotic could be easily controlled *in vivo* by adjusting the content of sodium alginate in the formula [214]. *In vitro* elution of vancomycin from calcium orthophosphate cement has been studied as well [383]. The possibility of using calcium orthophosphate cements as a drug-delivery system offers an attractive and efficient solution for the treatment of various bone diseases, *e.g.*, tumours, osteoporosis and osteomyelitis, which normally require long and painful therapies.

The laboratory studies on drugs incorporation into the cements cover different aspects. Firstly, it is necessary to verify that addition of a drug does not influence the setting reaction not only in terms of the setting and hardening mechanisms but also with respect to the rheological behavior and injectability. Secondly, it is necessary to determine the *in vitro* kinetics of drug release. Thirdly, the drug delivery properties of the cement must be studied *in vivo*. Finally, but still importantly, the clinical performance of the drug delivery system must be evaluated as well [30,31]. For example, recombinant human transforming growth factor $\beta 1$ (rhTGF-$\beta 1$) was added to a calcium orthophosphate cement [384-386]. This resulted in formation of a bioactivated cement that could be used as a bone filler and for the replacement of bone [384]. It appeared that after 8 weeks the addition of growth factors stimulated and increased bone formation (50% volume) and bone contact (65%) in comparison to control calvarian defects in an animal study. Besides, the growth factor group reduced the remaining volume of the cement by 20% [385]. An example of bone morphogenetic protein rhBMP-2 release from a loaded porous calcium orthophosphate cement might be found elsewhere [387], while an experimental study on calcium orthophosphate cement impregnated with dideoxy-kanamycin B is also available [388].

Further details and additional examples of the drug delivery application of calcium orthophosphate cements are well described elsewhere [24,30,31].

8.6. Brief Conclusions on the Medical Applications

To conclude this part, one should stress that despite several encouraging results, not every surgeon' expectation has been met yet. First of all, calcium orthophosphate cements and concretes are not superior to autografts, despite offering primary stability against compressive loading [389]. One of the main concerns of clinicians is to reach higher rates of bioresorption, an improvement of bone reconstruction and to a lesser extent, higher mechanical resistance [28]. Besides, clinical application of the cements in comminuted fractures revealed penetration of the viscous paste into the joint space [390-392]. The interested readers are suggested to read a paper on cement leakage during vertebroplasty [393]. To date, cadaveric studies have already shown that using calcium orthophosphate cements with conventional metal fixation in certain fractures of the distal radius, tibial plateau, proximal femur and calcaneus can produce better stability, stiffness and strength than metal fixation alone. Early clinical results have revealed a reduced time to full load bearing when the cements were used for augmentation of tibial plateau and calcaneal fractures, more rapid gain of strength and range of motion when used in distal radius fractures and improved stability in certain hip fractures [324,347]. However, surgeons reported on difficulties in filling the vertebral bodies (a bad injectability of present formulations) and other problems, such as filter-pressing and cement decohesion, observed during vertebral body injection that resulted in bone instability due to low mechanical strength as well as long setting times of the cements [394]. This happens due to not only low mechanical properties of calcium orthophosphate cements but also some difficulties of filling vertebral bodies. In order to maintain good cohesion, calcium orthophosphate cements need to be more viscous (hence, less injectable) [137,138]. For example, calcium orthophosphate cements might be modified by addition of polyacrylic acid [202,203], polysaccharides [66,77,193-196] and gelatin [171,197-201].

Another type of concerns has been raised that the use of calcium orthophosphate cements for the augmentation of fractured and osteoporotic bones might aggravate cardiovascular deterioration in the event of pulmonary cement embolism by stimulating coagulation [395]. To investigate these potential problems, 2.0 ml of either calcium orthophosphate or polymethylmethacrylate (PMMA) cement were injected intravenously in 14 sheep. Intravenous injection of calcium orthophosphate cement resulted in a more severe increase in pulmonary arterial pressure and decrease in arterial blood pressure compared to the PMMA cement. Disintegration of the calcium orthophosphate cement seemed to be the reason for more severe reaction that represents a risk of cardiovascular complications. The authors concluded that further research efforts should aim at improving cohesion of calcium orthophosphate cements in an aqueous environment for future clinical applications such as vertebral body augmentation [395].

To conclude the medical part of this review, currently there are no doubts concerning a very great potential of the clinical applications of calcium orthophosphate cements and concretes for healing of bone and dental defects. As this manuscript is intended to be read mainly by chemists and materials researchers, the biological, medical and clinical aspects of calcium orthophosphate cement applications have not been discussed in many details. For further clinical and biomedical particulars, the interested readers are referred to other papers and reviews [20,24,30,31,92,324,328,389].

9. Future Developments

As calcium orthophosphate cements and concretes represent an intriguing group of new materials for bone augmentation and reconstruction, there is a great potential for further improvement of their properties, in which the ideal characteristics (see Table 3) should be achieved by manipulations with the chemical composition, powder particle size and distribution, as well as by means of various additives. Only a few commercial apatite cements are currently approved for clinical use [92,159,330,342]. New formulations of both apatite and brushite cements are expected to appear in the market soon. The forthcoming commercial formulations will need to be improved in order to take the advantage of a variety of possibilities offered by calcium orthophosphate cements [137,138]. New formulations will include (i) injectable and open macroporous formulations to optimize their osteoconduction [171], (ii) formulations containing only one calcium orthophosphate (single-phase cement powders) [17] and (iii) drug-loaded and hormone-loaded cements for the treatment of bone diseases [24,30,31]. Obviously, the former two directions deal with both chemistry and material science, while the last direction is more related to tissue engineering and medicine.

Two innovative approaches of injectable formulations of calcium orthophosphate cements have been introduced rather recently. The researches combined a water-reactive cement such as a mixture of TTCP and DCPD powders with a nonaqueous but water-miscible liquid (*e.g.*, glycerol, polyethylene glycol) + a gelling agent (*e.g.*, hydroxypropylmethylcellulose, carboxymethylcellulose, chitosan) + a hardening accelerator (*e.g.*, tartaric acid, malic acid, malonic acid, citric acid or glycolic acid) to form a stable paste that can be directly injected into a bone defect [396-398]. In literature, this type of cement pastes is called "premixed calcium phosphate cements" (occasionally referred to as PCPC) in which the paste remains stable during storage and hardens only after placement into the defect. Setting occurs upon contact with body fluids or in a physiological solution and results in CDHA formation. This approach eliminates the powder-liquid mixing stage during surgery and might improve the cement performance. Besides, it allows shortening the surgical time. The first formulation of premixed calcium phosphate cements had a setting time of longer than 1 h and a low mechanical strength [396]. More recently, an improved formulation has been developed; it exhibits a rapid setting when immersed in a physiological solution, yielding a hardened cement with a higher mechanical strength, approached the reported strengths of sintered porous HA implants and cancellous bone [397,398]. Creation of premixed macroporous calcium orthophosphate cement scaffolds reinforced by slow-dissolving fibers (in other words, premixed macroporous concrete scaffolds) is the latest achievement of this approach [280]. Other researchers invented cements in the form of two injectable pastes that can be mixed together and injected at the time of implantation (with a static mixer incorporated in the injection cannula) [399]. However, the latter approach is limited to acid-base cement formulations only [29].

Table 3. Major advantages and disadvantages of the calcium orthophosphate cements [30,31,142].

Advantages	Disadvantages
1. Self-setting ability *in vivo*. 2. Good injectability that allows cement implantation by minimally invasive surgical techniques, which are less damageable than the traditional surgical techniques. 3. Good osteoconductivity and occasional osteoinductivity: the initial biological properties of the hardened cements are similar to those of CDHA or brushite. 4. Can be replaced by newly formed bone after a period of time (osteotransductivity). 5. Moldability: the perfect fit to the implant site, which assures good bone-material contact, even in geometrically complex defects. 6. Excellent biocompatibility and bioactivity. 7. No toxicity. 8. Low cost. 9. Ease of preparation and handling. 10. Setting at body temperature. 11. Form chemical bonds to the host bone. 12. Clinically safe materials in their powder components. 13. Can be used to deliver antibiotics, anti-inflammatory drugs, growth factors, morphogenic proteins, *etc.* at local sites, which are able to stimulate certain biological responses.*	1. Mechanical weakness: limited use due to potential collapse of material followed by soft tissue formation instead of bone formation (loaded areas). Until cements with adequate shear strength are available, most complex fractures that can be repaired with cement also will require metal supports. 2. Can be washed out from surgical defect if excess of blood. 3. Lack of macroporosity (especially interconnected pores), which prevents fast bone ingrowth and the cements degrade layer-by-layer from the outside to the inside only. 4. The *in vivo* biodegradation of many formulations is slower than the growth rate of a newly forming bone.

*Further studies are necessary.

A lack of macropores is a substantial disadvantage of many current formulations of calcium orthophosphate cements [168]. As a result, biodegradation takes place layer-by-layer on the surface, from outside to inside. To solve this problem, either soluble particles, such as sugar [400], mannitol [277,280], NaCl [185] and calcite [225], or resorbable fibers [281,306-308] might be incorporated into the cement.

After the cement is implanted, the particles are dissolved, leaving pores in the cement matrix; however, such pores are not always interconnected. Using a hydrophobic liquid instead of soluble particles could be an alternative. At the turn of the millennium, an open macroporous structure was obtained using a mixture of oil and a cement paste [401]; however, since than no research papers on this subject have been published. Besides, by means of surfactants, air bubbles might be created in the bulk of the cements [191]. Finally, addition of carbonates to the cement formulation is able to create pores [28,42,187,188]. Unfortunately, the mechanical strength and porosity are conflicting requirements. As the porosity in calcium orthophosphate cements appears to be of paramount importance to achieve the excellent bioresorbability, other experimental approaches have to be developed [402].

A layered structure was designed very recently by combining a macroporous layer of calcium orthophosphate cement with a strong fiber-reinforced calcium orthophosphate cement layer. The rationale for such construction was for the macroporous layer to accept tissue ingrowth, while the fiber-reinforced strong layer would provide the needed early-strength [403].

In the case of calcium orthophosphate concretes, future studies could combine in one formulation porogens and biodegradable fibers of different shapes and dissolution rates to form after *in vivo* hardening calcium orthophosphate scaffolds with sustained strength. In such a system, one porogen quickly dissolves and creates macropores to start a bone ingrowth process, while the second type of fibers provides the required strength to the implant. After significant bone ingrowth into the initial pores increased the implant strength, the second set of fibers would then dissolve to create additional macropores for bone ingrowth [306]. Such complicated compositions already exist. For example, chitosan, sodium orthophosphate and hydroxypropylmethylcellulose were used to render calcium orthophosphate cement fast setting and resistant to washout, while absorbable fibers and mannitol porogen were incorporated for strength and macropores, respectively. Both the strength and fracture resistance of this concrete were substantially increased and approached those values for sintered porous HA implants [404]. Turning on a bit of imagination, one might predict development of polymeric drugs [166], hormones, growth factors, *etc.* (*e.g.*, by either incorporation into or crosslinking with either water-soluble or bioresorbable polymers). Coupled with reinforcing biodegradable fibers and porogens, such types of "healing fibers" might be added to calcium orthophosphate concretes, which not only accelerate the remedial process, but also allow simultaneous improvement in both their strength and injectability.

Stability (insolubility) in normal physiological fluid environment and resorbability under acidic conditions produced by osteoclasts appears to be among the most important *in vivo* characteristics of modern calcium orthophosphate cements. For some clinical applications, such as cranioplasty, a relatively slow resorption and replacement by bone is quite acceptable, whereas in other applications, such as periodontal bone defects repair, sinus lift, *etc.*, the ability of the hardened cement to be replaced quickly by bone is crucial. Experimental results suggest that a number of parameters of calcium orthophosphate cements, such as Ca/P ionic ratio, carbonate content, ionic substitution, crystallinity, *etc.* might affect the dissolution characteristics of the cements in slightly acidic solutions. This gives an opportunity to formulate cements, possessing different resorption rates, which is suited for different applications [97,98].

The discovery of calcium orthophosphate cements has already opened up new perspectives in synthesis of bioceramic scaffolds, possessing sufficient mechanical properties [178,179,196,277]. In the past, such scaffolds could only be manufactured by the sintering route at elevated temperatures. Therefore, until recently it was impossible to produce resorbable preset low-temperature hydrated 3D ceramics for various applications, *e.g.*, scaffolds and granules, from low-temperature calcium orthophosphate phases, such as ACP, DCPA, DCPD, OCP and CDHA. Now, using the appropriate techniques, open macroporous 3D scaffolds consisting of the aforementioned low-temperature phases (currently, excluding ACP and OCP) can be produced via a cementitious reaction [405], thus dramatically widening the application of these calcium orthophosphates as biomaterials and bioceramics. This type of materials could be very promising for tissue engineering applications. Among them, CDHA is of a special interest due to its chemical similarity to bone material and a large specific surface area.

To conclude this part, one should stress, that the most promising direction of the future developments of calcium orthophosphate cements is obviously seen in their functionalization by incorporation or impregnation of various hormones, growth factors, drugs, other bioorganic compounds, as well as incorporation of living cells and other tiny biological objects [406-410]. The initial attempts have already been performed but without a great success yet. For example, researchers have already found that unset calcium orthophosphate cements might have toxic effects when placed on cell monolayers, while the set cements are biocompartible for the same type of cells (MC3T3-E1 osteoblast-like cells were tested). A gel encapsulation in alginate beads was found to be a possible solution to protect living cells for seeding into calcium orthophosphate cement pastes [411]. *In vitro* cytotoxic effect of a calcium orthophosphate cement based on α-TCP was also observed [412]. In light of these results, the encapsulation approach could potentially be used to seed a patient's *ex vivo* expanded stem cells into a cement to create an osteoinductive bone graft substitute that could be used to treat that patient. However, this becomes more related to tissue engineering and biology, rather than to chemistry and material science.

Finally, besides the aforementioned chemical, material and biomedical improvements of calcium orthophosphate cements, one should not forget on a better design of both the mixing equipment and delivery (injection) techniques. As an example, the interested readers are referred to a new cannula to ease cement injection during vertebroplasty [413]; however, this subject is beyond the scope of current review.

Conclusions

Thus, among the diverse range of bone replacing biomaterials, calcium orthophosphate cements undoubtedly represent a distinct group because they are relatively simple materials formed by combining a calcium orthophosphate mixture with an aqueous solution. However, they symbolize an important breakthrough in the field of bone repair biomaterials, since they offer the possibility of obtaining thermally unstable calcium orthophosphates in a monolithic form at room or body temperature by means of a cementation reaction. This particular fabrication technique implies that the cements are mouldable and therefore can adapt easily to the bone cavity providing a good fixation and the optimum tissue-biomaterial contact, necessary for stimulating bone ingrowth into them and their subsequent osteotransduction [24].

Unfortunately, the perfect grafting material does not exist. Calcium orthophosphate cements and concretes are not an exception to this statement. While possessing excellent biological properties (osteoconduction and, occasionally, osteoinduction), adequate setting time, excellent moldability and the capability to deliver different bone-enhancing proteins/antibiotics at a local level, unfortunately, the material lacks adequate mechanical properties for applications other than non-loaded surgical sites. Nevertheless, even in its present state calcium orthophosphate cements appear to be suitable for a number of applications. They can be injected into osteoporotic bone to reinforce it or can be used to make granules and blocks out of low-temperature calcium orthophosphates. Several types of calcium orthophosphate cements are now on the market, while scaffolds made of low-temperature calcium orthophosphates are being tested. The use of slightly different chemical compositions and various dopants affects both the setting time and tensile strength that enables further improvements. In addition, new trials are conducted with the reinforced compositions and concretes, which represent additional attempts to improve the existing products.

It is anticipated that the use of calcium orthophosphate cements will enable a faster and more aggressive rehabilitation, as the strength of the cement makes it possible to allow full weight-bearing earlier than when bone graft is used. Although, preliminary clinical trials have already confirmed the great potential of this novel therapeutic product, calcium orthophosphate cements need to be improved further; in particular, their bioresorption needs to be accelerated as well as their injectability and mechanical properties need to get better. Besides, extra clinical studies are required to define the most appropriate indications and limitations of calcium orthophosphate cements for fracture repair.

In the author's humble opinion, the best way to conclude this review would be using Prof. James M. Anderson's opinion on the history of biomaterials field. According to Prof. Anderson, within 1950–1975 researchers studied bioMATERIALS, within 1975–2000 researchers studied BIOMATERIALS and since 2000, the time for BIOmaterials has been coming [414]. Here, the capital letters emphasis the major direction of the research efforts in the complex subject of biomaterials. As the history of calcium orthophosphate cements started only in 1983, the aforementioned periods appeared to be shifted along the time scale. Certainly, the bioMATERIALS-epoch for calcium orthophosphate cements is almost over (all possible combinations of calcium orthophosphates have been already tested), while the

BIOmaterials-era (where cells act as the key factor) either has not started yet or is just at the very initial stage. Most likely, the current state-of-art of calcium orthophosphate cements and concretes corresponds to BIOMATERIALS-phase with approximately equal contribution of biological and materials directions; therefore, still there is much room for versatile ideas and approaches.

References

[1] Albee F, Morrison H. Studies in bone growth. *Annals Surg*. 1920;71:32-38.

[2] Haldeman K, Moore J. Influence of a local excess of calcium and phosphorus on the healing of fractures. *Arch. Surg*. 1934;29:385-396.

[3] Ray R, Degge J, Gloyd P, Mooney G. Bone regeneration. *J. Bone Joint Surg*. 1952;34A:638-647.

[4] Getter L, Bhaskar S, Cutright D, Perez B, Brady J, Driskell T, O'Hara M. Three biodegradable calcium orthophosphate slurry implants in bone. *J. Oral Surg*. 1972;30:263-268.

[5] Roy D, Linnehan S. Hydroxyapatite formed from coral skeletal carbonate by hydrothermal exchange. *Nature* 1974;247:220-222.

[6] Koster K, Karbe E, Kramer H, Heide H, Konig R. Experimenteller Knochenersatz durch resorbierbare Calciumphosphat-Keramik. *Langenbecks Arch. Chir*. 1976;341:77-86.

[7] Peelen J, Rejda B, Vermeiden J, de Groot K. Sintered tri-calcium orthophosphate as bioceramic. *Science of Ceramics*. 1977;9:226-236.

[8] Jarcho M, Kay J, Gumaer K, Doremus R, Drobeck H. Tissue, cellular and subcellular events at a bone-ceramic hydroxyapatite interface. *J. Bioengineering* 1977;1:79-92.

[9] Jarcho M. Calcium phosphate ceramics as hard tissue prosthetics. *Clin. Orthop*. 1981;157:259-278.

[10] LeGeros RZ. *Calcium phosphates in oral biology and medicine*. Karger, Basel, 1991.

[11] Dorozhkin SV. *Calcium orthophosphates as biomaterials and bioceramics*. (this book).

[12] LeGeros RZ, Chohayeb A, Shulman A. Apatitic calcium phosphates: possible dental restorative materials. *J. Dent. Res*. 1982;61(Special issue):343.

[13] Brown WE, Chow LC. A new calcium phosphate setting cement. *J. Dent. Res*. 1983;62(Special issue):672.

[14] Brown WE, Chow LC. A new calcium phosphate water setting cement. In: Brown PW, ed. *Cements Research Progress*. Westerville, OH, American Ceramic Society, 1986, pp. 352-379.

[15] Brown WE, Chow LC. Dental restorative cement pastes. US Patent No. 4518430. May 21, 1985.

[16] Gruninger SE, Siew C, Chow LC, O'Young A, Ts'ao NK, Brown WE. Evaluation of the biocompatibility of a new calcium phosphate setting cement. *J. Dent. Res*. 1984;63(Special issue):200.

[17] Tas AC. Porous, biphasic $CaCO_3$-calcium phosphate biomedical cement scaffolds from calcite ($CaCO_3$) powder. *Int. J. Appl. Ceram. Technol*. 2007;4:152–163.

[18] Driskell TD, Heller AL, Koenigs JF. *Dental treatments*. US Patent No. 3913229. October 21, 1975.

[19] Driessens FCM, Planell JA, Gil FJ. in: *Encyclopedic Handbook of Biomaterials and Bioengineering,* Part B, Applications, Vol. 2, edited by Wise DL, Trantolo DJ, Altobelli DE, Yaszemski MJ, Gresser JD, Schwarz ER. Marcel Dekker, New York, 1995, pp. 855-877.

[20] Schmitz JP, Hollinger JO, Milan SB. Reconstruction of bone using calcium phosphate bone cements: A critical review. *J. Oral Maxillofac. Surg*. 1999;57:1122-1126.

[21] Gbureck U, Barralet JE, Spatz K, Grover LM, Thull R. Ionic modification of calcium phosphate cement viscosity. Part I: Hypodermic injection and strength improvement of apatite cement. *Biomaterials* 2004;25:2187–2195.

[22] Tagaya M, Goto H, Iinuma M, Wakamatsu N, Tamura Y, Doi Y. Development of self-setting Te-Cp/alpha-TCP cement for pulpotomy. *Dent Mater J.* 2005;24:555-561.

[23] Driessens FCM, Boltong MG, Khairoun I, De Maeyer EAP, Ginebra MP, Wenz R, Planell JA, Verbeeck RMH. Applied aspects of calcium phosphate bone cement, in: Wise DL, Trantolo DJ, Lewandrowski KU, Gresser JD, Cattaneo MV (Eds.), *Biomaterials Engineering and Devices: Human Applications*. Vol. 2: Orthopaedic, Dental and Bone Graft Applications, Humana Press, Totowa, NJ, 2000, pp. 253–260.

[24] Driessens FCM, Planell JA, Boltong M, Khairoun I, Ginebra MP. Osteotransductive bone cements. *Proc. Instn. Mech. Engrs. Part H: J. Engin. Med.* 1998;212:427-435.

[25] Frankenburg EP, Goldstein SA, Bauer TW, Harris SA, Poser RD. Biomechanical and histological evaluation of a calcium phosphate cement. *J. Bone Joint Surg. Am.* 1998;80:1112–1124.

[26] Frayssinet P, Gineste L, Conte P, Fages J, Rouquet N. Short-term implantation effects of a DCPD-based calcium phosphate cement. Biomaterials 1998;19:971–977.

[27] Rey C, Tofighi A, Mounic S, Combes C, Lee D. Biomimetism and calcium phosphate cements. In: Mainard D, Louis JP, editors. *Actualités en Biomatériaux*, Vol. 6. Paris: Editions Romillat; 2002. pp. 27–37.

[28] Combes C, Bareille R, Rey C. Calcium carbonate-calcium phosphate mixed cement compositions for bone reconstruction. *J. Biomed. Mater. Res. Part A* 2006;79A:318–328.

[29] Bohner M, Gbureck U, Barralet JE. Technological issues for the development of more efficient calcium phosphate bone cements: a critical assessment. *Biomaterials* 2005;26:6423–6429.

[30] Ginebra MP, Traykova T, Planell JA. Calcium phosphate cements: Competitive drug carriers for the musculoskeletal system? *Biomaterials* 2006;27:2171–2177.

[31] Ginebra MP, Traykova T, Planell JA. Calcium phosphate cements as bone drug delivery systems: A review. *J. Controlled Release* 2006;113:102–110.

[32] Dreesmann H. Knochenplombierung bei Hohlenforigen Defekten des Knochens. Beitr. *Klin. Chir*. 1892;9:804–810.

[33] Peltier LF. The use of plaster of Paris to fill defects in bone. *Clin. Orthop*. 1961;21:1–29.

[34] Kelly CM, Wilkins RM, Gitelis S, Hartjen C, Watson JT, Kim PT. The use of a surgical grade calcium sulfate as a bone graft substitute: Results of a multicenter trial. *Clin. Orthop.* 2001;382:42–50.

[35] Bohner M. New hydraulic cements based on α-tricalcium phosphate – calcium sulfate dihydrate mixtures. *Biomaterials* 2004;25:741-749.

[36] Fernandez E, Vlad MD, Gel MM, Lopez J, Torres R, Cauich JV, Bohner M. Modulation of porosity in apatitic cements by the use of α-tricalcium phosphate – calcium sulphate dihydrate mixtures. *Biomaterials* 2005;26:3395-3404.

[37] Nilsson M, Fernandez E, Sarda S, Lidgren L, Planell JA. Characterization of a novel calcium phosphate/sulphate bone cement. *J. Biomed. Mater. Res.* 2002;61:600–607.

[38] Grover LM, Gbureck U, Wrightc AJ, Tremaynec M, Barralet JE. Biologically mediated resorption of brushite cement *in vitro*. *Biomaterials* 2006;27:2178–2185.

[39] Grover LM, Gbureck U, Wright AJ, Barralet JE. Cement formulations in the calcium phosphate H_2O–H_3PO_4–$H_4P_2O_7$ system. *J. Amer. Ceram. Soc.* 2005;88:3096-3103.

[40] Grover LM, Gbureck U, Young AM, Wright AJ, Barralet JE. Temperature dependent setting kinetics and mechanical properties of β-TCP–pyrophosphoric acid bone cement. *J. Mater. Chem.* 2005;46:4955-4962.

[41] Lilley KJ, Gbureck U, Wright AJ, Knowles JC, Farrar DF, Barralet JE. Brushite cements from polyphosphoric acid, calcium phosphate systems. *J. Amer. Ceram. Soc.* 2007;90:1892–1898.

[42] Calafiori AR, di Marco G, Martino G, Marotta M. Preparation and characterization of calcium phosphate biomaterials. *J. Mater. Sci. Mater. Med.* 2007;18:2331-2338.

[43] Kon M, Hirakata LM, Miyamoto Y, Kasahara H, Asaoka K. Strengthening of calcium phosphate cement by compounding calcium carbonate whiskers. *Dent. Mater. J.* 2005;24:104-110.

[44] Serraj S, Michailesco P, Margerit J, Bernard B, Boudeville P. Study of a hydraulic calcium phosphate cement for dental applications. *J. Mater. Sci. Mater. Med.* 2002;13:125-131.

[45] Nurit L, Margerit J, Terol A, Boudeville P. pH-metric study of the setting reaction of monocalcium phosphate monohydrate/calcium oxide-based cements. *J. Mater. Sci. Mater. Med.* 2002;13:1007-1014.

[46] Boudeville P, Serraj S, Leloup JM, Margerit J, Pauvert B, Terol A. Physical properties and self-setting mechanism of calcium phosphate cements from calcium bis-dihydrogenophosphate monohydrate and calcium oxide. *J. Mater. Sci. Mater. Med.* 1999;10:99-109.

[47] Michaïlesco P, Kouassi M, Briak HE, Armynot A, Boudeville P. Antimicrobial activity and tightness of a DCPD–CaO-based hydraulic calcium phosphate cement for root canal filling. *J. Biomed. Mater. Res. Part B: Appl. Biomater.* 2005;74B:760–767.

[48] Briak HE, Durand D, Nurit J, Munier S, Pauvert B, Boudeville P. Study of a hydraulic dicalcium phosphate dihydrate/calcium oxide-based cement for dental applications. *J. Biomed. Mater. Res.* (Appl. Biomater.) 2002;63:447–453.

[49] El Briak H, Durand D, Boudeville P. Study of a hydraulic DCPA/CaO-based cement for dental applications. *J. Mater. Sci. Mater. Med.* 2008;19:737-744.

[50] Takagi S, Chow LC, Ishikawa K. Formation of hydroxyapatite in new calcium phosphate cements. *Biomaterials* 1998;19:1593–1599.

[51] Yang Q, Troczynski T, Liu DM. Influence of apatite seeds on the synthesis of calcium phosphate cement. *Biomaterials* 2002;23:2751-2760.

[52] Roemhildt ML, McGee TD, Wagner SD. Novel calcium phosphate composite bone cement: strength and bonding properties. *J. Mater. Sci. Mater. Med.* 2003;14:137-141.

[53] Roemhildt ML, Wagner SD, McGee TD. Characterization of a novel calcium phosphate composite bone cement: Flow, setting, and aging properties. *J. Mater. Sci. Mater. Med.* 2006;17:1127–1132.

[54] Wang X, Ye J, Wang Y, Chen L. Self-setting properties of a β-dicalcium silicate reinforced calcium phosphate cement. *J. Biomed. Mater. Res. Part B: Appl. Biomater.* 2007;82B:93–99.

[55] Huan Z, Chang J. Novel tricalcium silicate/monocalcium phosphate monohydrate composite bone cement. *J. Biomed. Mater. Res. Part B: Appl. Biomater.* 2007;82B:352–359.

[56] Wang X, Ye J. Variation of crystal structure of hydroxyapatite in calcium phosphate cement by the substitution of strontium ions. *J. Mater. Sci. Mater. Med.* 2008;19:1183-1186.

[57] Gbureck U, Knappe O, Grover LM, Barralet JE. Antimicrobial potency of alkali ion substituted calcium phosphate cements. *Biomaterials* 2005;26:6880–6886.

[58] Driessens FCM, Boltong MG, de Mayer EAP, Wenz R, Nies B, Planell JA. The Ca/P range of nanoapatitic calcium phosphate cements. *Biomaterials* 2002;23:4011–4017.

[59] Gbureck U, Thull R, Barralet JE. Alkali ion substituted calcium phosphate cement formation from mechanically activated reactants. *J. Mater. Sci. Mater. Med.* 2005;16:423–427.

[60] Doi Y, Shimizu Y, Moriwaki Y, Aga M, Iwanaga H, Shibutani T, Yamamoto K, Iwayama Y. Development of a new calcium phosphate cement that contains sodium calcium phosphate. *Biomaterials* 2001;22:847-854.

[61] Lilley J, Gbureck U, Knowles JC, Farrar DF, Barralet JE. Cement from magnesium substituted hydroxyapatite. *J. Mater. Sci. Mater. Med.* 2005;16:455–460.

[62] Ni GX, Lu WW, Tang B, Ngan AHW, Chiu KY, Cheung KMC, Li ZY, Luk KDK. Effect of weight-bearing on bone-bonding behavior of strontium-containing hydroxyapatite bone cement. *J. Biomed. Mater. Res. Part A* 2007;83A:570-576.

[63] Fadeeva IV, Barinov SM, Komlev VS, Fedotov DA, Durisin J, Medvecky L. Apatite formation in the reaction-setting mixture of $Ca(OH)_2$ – KH_2PO_4 system. *J. Biomed. Mater. Res. Part A* 2004;70A:303-308.

[64] Fernandez E, Vlad MD, Hamcerencu M, Darie A, Torres R, Lopez J. Effect of iron on the setting properties of α-TCP bone cements. *J. Mater. Sci.* 2005;40:3677–3682.

[65] http://en.wikipedia.org/wiki/Cement (accessed in January 2008).

[66] Burguera EF, Xu HHK, Weir MD. Injectable and rapid-setting calcium phosphate bone cement with dicalcium phosphate dihydrate. *J. Biomed. Mater. Res. Part B: Appl. Biomater.* 2006;77B:126–134.

[67] Burguera EF, Guitian F, Chow LC. A water setting tetracalcium phosphate – dicalcium phosphate dihydrate cement. *J. Biomed. Mater. Res. Part A* 2004;71A:275–282.

[68] Driessens FCM, Boltong MG, Bermudez O, Planell JA. Formulation and setting times of some calcium orthophosphate cements: a pilot study. *J. Mater. Sci. Mater. Med.* 1993;4:503-508.

[69] Chow LC, Markovic M, Takagi S. Calcium phosphate cements. *Cements Res. Prog.* 1996;215–238.

[70] Driessens FCM, Boltong MG, Bermudez O, Planell JA, Ginebra MP, Fernández E. Effective formulations for the preparation of calcium phosphate bone cements. *J. Mater. Sci. Mater. Med.* 1994;5:164-170.

[71] Kurashina K, Hirano M, Kotani A, Klein CPAT, de Groot K. *In vivo* study of calcium phosphate cements: implantation of an α-tricalcium phosphate / dicalcium phosphate dibasic / tetracalcium phosphate monoxide cement paste. *Biomaterials* 1997;18:539-543.

[72] Friedman CD, Costantino PD, Takagi S, Chow LC. BoneSource^{TM} hydroxyapatite cement: a novel biomaterial for craniofacial skeletal tissue engineering and reconstruction. *J. Biomed. Mater. Res.* (Appl. Biomater.) 1998;43:428-432.

[73] Khairoun I, Boltong MG, Driessens FCM, Planel JA. Effect of calcium carbonate on the compliance of apatitic calcium phosphate bone cement. *Biomaterials* 1997;18:1535-1539.

[74] Fernández E, Gil FJ, Best SM, Ginebra MP, Driessens FCM, Planell JA. Improvement of the mechanical properties of new calcium phosphate bone cements in the $CaHPO_4$ – α-$Ca_3(PO_4)_2$ system: compressive strength and microstructural development. *J. Biomed. Mater. Res.* 1998;41:560-567.

[75] Fukase Y, Eanes ED, Takagi S, Chow LC, Brown WE. Setting reactions and compressive strengths of calcium phosphate cements. *J. Dent. Res.* 1990;69:1852-1856.

[76] Xie L, Monroe EA. Calcium phosphate dental cements. *Mat. Res. Soc. Symp. Proc.* 1991;179:25-39.

[77] Ishikawa K, Miyamoto Y, Kon M, Nagayama M, Asaoka K. Non-decay type fast-setting calcium orthophosphate cement: composite with sodium alginate. *Biomaterials* 1995;16:527-532.

[78] Xu HHK, Quinn JB, Takagi S, Chow LC. Processing and properties of strong and non-rigid calcium phosphate cement. *J. Dent. Res.* 2002;81:219-224.

[79] Lee YK, Lim BS, Kim CW. Mechanical properties of calcium phosphate based dental filling and regeneration materials. *J. Oral Rehabil.* 2003;30:418-425.

[80] Ginebra MP, Fernández E, de Mayer EAP, Verbeeck RM, Boltong MG, Ginebra J, Driessens FCM, Planell JA. Setting reaction and hardening of an apatitic calcium phosphate cement. *J. Dent. Res.* 1997;76:905-912.

[81] Liu C, Shen W, Gu Y, Hu L. Mechanism of the hardening process for a hydroxyapatite cement. *J. Biomed. Mater .Res.* 1997;35:75-80.

[82] Driessens FCM, de Mayer EAP, Fernández E, Boltong MG, Berger G, Verbeeck RMH, Ginebra MP, Planell JA. Amorphous calcium phosphate cements and their transformation into calcium deficient hydroxyapatite. *Bioceramics* 1996;9:231-234.

[83] Driessens FCM, Planell JA, Gil F. Calcium phosphate bone cements. In: Wise DL, Trantolo DJ, Altobelli DE, Yaszemski MJ, Cresser JD, Schwartz ER. eds.

Encyclopedic handbook of biomaterials and bioengineering, Part B, vol 2. New York: Marcel Dekker, 1995.

[84] Lemaitre J. Injectable calcium phosphate hydraulic cements: new developments and potential applications. *Inn. Tech. Biol. Med.* 1995;16:109-120.

[85] Xia Z, Grover LM, Huang Y, Adamopoulos IE, Gbureck U, Triffitt JT, Shelton RM, Barralet JE. *In vitro* biodegradation of three brushite calcium phosphate cements by a macrophage cell-line. *Biomaterials* 2006;27:4557–4565.

[86] Bermudez O, Boltong MG, Driessens FCM, Planell JA. Development of an octocalcium phosphate cement. *J. Mater. Sci. Mater. Med.* 1994;5:144-146.

[87] Khairoun I, Boltong MG, Driessens FCM, Planell JA. Limited compliance of some apatitic calcium phosphate bone cements with clinical requirements. *J. Mater. Sci. Mater. Med.* 1998;9:667-671.

[88] Lacout J, Mejdoubi E, Hamad M. Crystallization mechanisms of calcium orthophosphate cement for biological uses. *J. Mater. Sci. Mater. Med.* 1996;7:371-374.

[89] Song Y, Feng Z, Wang T. *In situ* study on the curing process of calcium phosphate bone cement. J. Mater. Sci. Mater. Med. 2007;18:1185–1193.

[90] Liu C, Shao H, Chen F, Zheng H. Rheological properties of concentrated aqueous injectable calcium phosphate cement slurry. *Biomaterials* 2006;27:5003–5013.

[91] Sarda S, Fernandez E, Llorens J, Martinez S, Nilsson M, Planell JA. Rheological properties of an apatitic bone cement during initial setting. *J. Mater. Sci. Mater. Med.* 2001;12:905-909.

[92] Weiss DD, Sachs MA, Woodard CR. Calcium phosphate bone cements: a comprehensive review. *J. Long Term Effects Med. Implants* 2003;13:41-47.

[93] Brown WE, Chow LC. A new calcium phosphate water-setting cement. In: *Cements Research Progress*. Brown PW. Ed., Westerville, OH: American Ceramic Society, 1986, pp. 351–379.

[94] Hatim Z, Freche M, Keribech A, Lacout JL. The setting mechanism of a phosphocalcium biological cement. *Ann. Chim. Sci. Mat.* 1998;23:65–68.

[95] Ishikawa K, Asaoka K. Estimation of ideal mechanical strength and critical porosity of calcium phosphate cement. *J. Biomed. Mater. Res*. 1995;29:1537–1543.

[96] Chow LC. Development of self-setting calcium phosphate cements. *J. Ceram. Soc. Japan* 1991;99:954–964.

[97] Chow LC. Calcium phosphate cements: chemistry, properties, and applications. Mat. Res. Soc. Syrnp. Proc. 2000;599:27–37.

[98] Chow LC. Calcium phosphate cements. In: Chow LC, Eanes ED. (Eds.) *Octacalcium Phosphate. Monographs in Oral Science*. Basel, Karger, 2001, vol. 18, pp. 148-163.

[99] Brown PW, Fulmer M. Kinetics of hydroxyapatite formation at low temperature. *J. Amer. Ceram. Soc*. 1991;74:934–940.

[100] TenHuisen KS, Brown PW. The formation of hydroxyapatite-ionomer cements at 38°C. J. Dent. Res. 1994;3:598–606.

[101] Ishikawa K, Takagi S, Chow LC, Suzuki K. Reaction of calcium phosphate cements with different amounts of tetracalcium phosphate and dicalcium phosphate anhydrous. *J. Biomed. Mater. Res.* 1999;46:504–510.

[102] Matsuya S, Takagi S, Chow LC. Effect of mixing ratio and pH on the reaction between $Ca_4(PO_4)_2O$ and $CaHPO_4$. *J. Mater. Sci. Mater. Med.* 2000;11:305-311.

[103] Lemaitre J, Mirtchi AA, Mortier A. Calcium phosphate cements for medical use: state of the art and perspectives of development. *Silicates Industriels* 1987;9-10:141-146.

[104] Mirtchi AA, Lemaitre J, Terao N. Calcium phosphate cements: study of the β-tricalcium phosphate - monocalcium phosphate system. *Biomaterials* 1989;10:475-480.

[105] Bohner M, Lemaitre J, Ring TA. Effects of sulphate, pyrophosphate and citrate ions on the physiochemical properties of cements made of β-tricalcium phosphate – phosphoric acid – water mixtures. *J. Amer. Ceram. Soc.* 1996;79:1427–1434.

[106] Fernandez E, Gil FJ, Best SM, Ginebra MP, Driessens FCM, Planell JA. The cement setting reaction in the $CaHPO_4$–α-$Ca_3(PO_4)_2$ system: an X-ray diffraction study. *J. Biomed. Mater. Res.* 1998;42:403–406.

[107] Fernandez E, Gil FJ, Ginebra MP, Driesens FCM, Planell JA, Best SM. Production and characterisation of new calcium phosphate bone cements in the $CaHPO_4$–α-$Ca_3(PO_4)_2$ system: pH, workability and setting times. *J. Mater. Sci. Mater. Med.* 1999;10:223–230.

[108] Barralet JE, Lilley KJ, Grover LM, Farrar DF, Ansell C, Gbureck U. Cements from nanocrystalline hydroxyapatite, *J. Mater. Sci. Mater. Med.* 2004;15:407–411.

[109] Lilley KJ, Gbureck U, Wright AJ, Farrar DF, Barralet JE. Cement from nanocrystalline hydroxyapatite: Effect of calcium phosphate ratio. *J. Mater. Sci. Mater. Med.* 2005;16:1185–1190.

[110] Wang X, Ye J, Wang Y, Wu X, Bai B. Control of crystallinity of hydrated products in a calcium phosphate bone cement. *J. Biomed. Mater. Res. Part A* 2007;81A:781–790.

[111] de Maeyer EAP, Verbeeck RMH, Vercruysse CWJ. Conversion of octacalcium phosphate in calcium phosphate cements. *J. Biomed. Mater. Res.* 2000;52:95–106.

[112] Wang X, Ye J, Wang Y. Hydration mechanism of a novel PCCP + DCPA cement system. *J. Mater. Sci. Mater. Med.* 2008;19:813-816.

[113] Zoulgami M, Lucas A, Briard P, Gaudé J. A self-setting single-component calcium phosphate cement. *Biomaterials* 2001;22:1933-1937.

[114] Knaack D, Goad ME, Aiolova M, Rey C, Tofighi A, Chakravarthy P, Lee DD. Resorbable calcium phosphate bone substitute. *J. Biomed. Mater. Res.* 1998;43:399–409.

[115] Monma H, Kanazawa T. The hydration of α-tricalcium phosphate. *Yogyo-Kyokai-Shi* 1976;84:209–213.

[116] Fernandez E, Ginebra MP, Boltong MG, Driessens FCM, Ginebra J, De Maeyer EAP, Verbeeck RMH, Planell JA. Kinetic study of the setting reaction of a calcium phosphate bone cement. *J. Biomed. Mater. Res.* 1996;32:367–374.

[117] Gbureck U, Barralet JE, Radu L, Klinger HG, Thull R. Amorphous α-tricalcium phosphate: preparation and aqueous setting reaction. *J. Amer. Ceram. Soc.* 2004;87:1126–1132.

[118] Bohner M. Malsy AK, Camire CL, Gbureck U. Combining particle size distribution and isothermal calorimetry data to determine the reaction kinetics of α-tricalcium phosphate-water mixtures. *Acta Biomater.* 2006;2:343–348.

[119] Brunner TJ, Grass RN, Bohner M, Stark WJ. Effect of particle size, crystal phase and crystallinity on the reactivity of tricalcium phosphate cements for bone reconstruction. *J. Mater. Chem*. 2007;38:4072-4078.

[120] Alves HLR, dos Santos LA, Bergmann CP. Injectability evaluation of tricalcium phosphate bone cement. *J. Mater. Sci. Mater. Med.* 2008;19:2241-2246.

[121] Gbureck U, Grolms O, Barralet JE, Grover LM, Thull R. Mechanical activation and cement formation of β-tricalcium phosphate. *Biomaterials* 2003;24:4123–4131.

[122] Gbureck U, Barralet JE, Hofmann MP, Thull R. Nanocrystalline tetracalcium phosphate cement. *J. Dent. Res*. 2004;83:425-428.

[123] Gbureck U, Barralet JE, Hofmann MP, Thull R. Mechanical activation of tetracalcium phosphate. *J. Amer. Ceram. Soc*. 2004;87:311–313.

[124] Tsai CH, Ju CP, Lin JHC. Morphology and mechanical behavior of TTCP-derived calcium phosphate cement subcutaneously implanted in rats. *J. Mater. Sci. Mater. Med.* 2008;19:2407-2415.

[125] Tsai CH, Lin RM, Ju CP, Lin JHC. Bioresorption behavior of tetracalcium phosphate-derived calcium phosphate cement implanted in femur of rabbits. *Biomaterials* 2008;29:984-993.

[126] Tsai CH, Lin JHC, Ju CP. γ-radiation-induced changes in structure and properties of tetracalcium phosphate and its derived calcium phosphate cement. *J. Biomed. Mater. Res. Part B: Appl. Biomater*. 2007;80B:244–252.

[127] Chow LC, Markovic M, Frukhtbeyn SA, Takagi S. Hydrolysis of tetracalcium phosphate under a near-constant composition condition – effects of pH and particle size. *Biomaterials* 2005;26;393-401.

[128] TenHuisen KS, Brown PW. Formation of calcium-deficient hydroxyapatite from α-tricalcium phosphate. *Biomaterials* 1998;19:2209–2217.

[129] Ginebra MP, Fernandez E, Driessens FCM, Planell JA. Modeling of the hydrolysis of α-TCP. *J. Amer. Ceram. Soc*. 1999;82:2808–2812.

[130] Durucan C, Brown PW. α-tricalcium phosphate hydrolysis to hydroxyapatite at and near physiological temperature. *J. Mater. Sci. Mater. Med.* 2000;11:365–371.

[131] Durucan C, Brown PW. Kinetic model for α-tricalcium phosphate hydrolysis. *J. Amer. Ceram. Soc.* 2002;85:2013–2018.

[132] Ginebra MP, Driessens FCM, Planell JA. Effect of the particle size on the micro and nanostructural features of a calcium phosphate cement: a kinetic analysis. *Biomaterials* 2004;25:3453–3462.

[133] Koshino T, Kubota W, Morii T. Bone formation as a reaction to hydraulic hydroxyapatite thermal decomposition product used as bone cement in rabbits. *Biomaterials* 1995;16:125-128.

[134] Liu C, Huang Y, Chen J. The physicochemical properties of the solidification of calcium phosphate cement. *J. Biomed. Mater. Res. Part B: Appl. Biomater*. 2004;69B:73–78.

[135] Liu C, Gai W, Pan S, Liu Z. The exothermal behavior in the hydration process of calcium phosphate cement. *Biomaterials* 2003;24:2995–3003.

[136] Charrière E, Terrazzoni S, Pittet C, Mordasini P, Dutoit M, Lemaitre J, Zysset P. Mechanical characterization of brushite and hydroxyapatite cements. *Biomaterials* 2001;22:2937-2945.

[137] Bohner M. Calcium orthophosphates in medicine: from ceramics to calcium phosphate cements. *Injury* 2000;31;Suppl.4:S-D37-S-D47.

[138] Bohner M. Physical and chemical aspects of calcium phosphates used in spinal surgery. *Eur. Spine J.* 2001;10:S114–S121.

[139] von Gonten AS, Kelly JR, Antonucci JM. Load-bearing behavior of a simulated craniofacial structure fabricated from a hydroxyapatite cement and bioresorbable fiber-mesh. *J. Mater. Sci. Mater. Med.* 2000;11:95-100.

[140] Gisep A, Kugler S, Wahl D, Rahn B. The mechanical characterization of a bone defect model filled with ceramic cements. *J. Mater. Sci. Mater. Med.* 2004;15:1065-1071.

[141] Bohner M. Reactivity of calcium phosphate cements. *J. Mater. Chem.* 2007;38:3980-3986.

[142] Ambard AJ, Mueninghoff L. Calcium phosphate cement: review of mechanical and biological properties. *J. Prosthodont.* 2006;15:321-328.

[143] Lewis G. Injectable bone cements for use in vertebroplasty and kyphoplasty: state-of-the-art review. *J. Biomed. Mater. Res. B: Appl. Biomater.* 2006;76B:456–468.

[144] Kenny SM, Buggy M. Bone cements and fillers: A review. *J. Mater. Sci. Mater. Med.* 2003;14:923-938.

[145] Takagi S, Chow LC, Markovic M, Friedman CD, Costantino PD. Morphological and phase characterizations of retrieved calcium phosphate cement implants. *J. Biomed. Mater. Res.* (Appl. Biomater.) 2001;58:36–41.

[146] Standard test method for time of setting of hydraulic cement paste by Gillmore needles. ASTM C266-89. In: *Annual Book of ASTM Standards*, Vol. 04.01, Cement, Lime, Gypsum. American Society for Testing and Materials, Philadelphia, 1993:189-191.

[147] Standard test method for time of setting of hydraulic cement paste by Vicat needle. ASTM C191-92. In: *Annual Book of ASTM Standards*, Vol. 04.01, Cement, Lime, Gypsum. American Society for Testing and Materials, Philadelphia, 1993:158-160.

[148] Nilsson M, Carlson J, Fernandez E, Planell JA. Monitoring the setting of calcium-based bone cements using pulse-echo ultrasound. *J. Mater. Sci. Mater. Med.* 2002;13:1135-1141.

[149] Hofmann MP, Nazhat SN, Gbureck U, Barralet JE. Real-time monitoring of the setting reaction of brushite-forming cement using isothermal differential scanning calorimetry. *J. Biomed. Mater. Res. Part B: Appl. Biomater.* 2006;79B:360–364.

[150] Martin RI, Brown PW. The effects of magnesium on hydroxyapatite formation in vitro from $CaHPO_4$ and $Ca_4(PO_4)_2O$ at 37.4°C. *Calcif. Tissue Int.* 1997;60:538–546.

[151] Brunner TJ, Bohner M, Dora C, Gerber C, Stark WJ. Comparison of amorphous TCP nanoparticles to micron-sized α-TCP as starting materials for calcium phosphate cements. *J. Biomed. Mater. Res. B: Appl. Biomater.* 2007;83B:400-407.

[152] Gao WY, Wang YW, Dong LM, Yu ZW. Thermokinetic analysis of the hydration process of calcium phosphate cement. *J. Therm. Anal. Cal.* 2006;85:785–789.

[153] Bohner M, Gbureck U. Thermal reactions of brushite cements. *J. Biomed. Mater. Res. B: Appl. Biomater.* 2008;84B:375-385.

[154] Liu C, Huang Y, Zheng H. Study of the hydration process of calcium phosphate cement by AC impedance spectroscopy. *J. Amer. Ceram. Soc.* 1999;82:1052–1057.

[155] Hofmann MP, Young AM, Gbureck U, Nazhat SN Barralet JE. FTIR-monitoring of a fast setting brushite bone cement: effect of intermediate phases. *J. Mater. Chem.* 2006;16:3199–3206.

[156] Ginebra MP, Fernandez E, Driessens FCM, Boltong MG, Muntasell J, Font J, Planell JA. The effects of temperature on the behaviour of an apatitic calcium phosphate cement. *J. Mater. Sci. Mater. Med.* 1995;6:857–860.

[157] Leung KS, Siu WS, Li SF, Qin L, Cheung WH, Tam KF, Po P, Lui Y. An *in vitro* optimized injectable calcium phosphate cement for augmenting screw fixation in osteopenic goats. *J. Biomed. Mater. Res. Part B: Appl. Biomater.* 2006;78B:153–160.

[158] Baroud G, Matsushita C, Samara M, Beckman L, Steffen T. Influence of oscillatory mixing on the injectability of three acrylic and two calcium phosphate bone cements for vertebroplasty. *J. Biomed. Mater. Res. B: Appl. Biomater.* 2004;68B:105–111.

[159] Constantz BR, Ison IC, Fulmer MT, Poser RD, Smith ST, van Wagoner M, Ross J, Goldstein SA, Jupiter JB, Rosenthal DI. Skeletal repair by *in situ* formation of the mineral phase of bone. *Science* 1995;267:1796-1799.

[160] Nomoto T, Haraguchi K, Yamaguchi S, Sugano N, Nakayama H, Sekino T, Niihara K. Hydrolyses of calcium phosphates-allografts composite in physiological solutions. *J. Mater. Sci. Mater. Med.* 2006;17: 379–385.

[161] Barralet JE, Grover LM, Gbureck U. Ionic modification of calcium phosphate cement viscosity. Part II: Hypodermic injection and strength improvement of brushite cement. *Biomaterials* 2004;25:2197–2203.

[162] Sarda S, Fernández E, Nilsson M, Balcells M, Planell JA. Kinetic study of citric acid influence on calcium phosphate bone cements as water-reducing agent. *J. Biomed. Mater.* Res. 2002;61:653–659.

[163] Bohner M, Baroud G. Injectability of calcium phosphate pastes. *Biomaterials* 2005;26:1553–1563.

[164] Khairoun I, Boltong MG, Driessens FCM, Planell JA. Some factors controlling the injectability of calcium phosphate bone cements. *J. Mater. Sci. Mater. Med.* 1998;9:425-428.

[165] Burguera EF, Xu HHK, Sun L. Injectable calcium phosphate cement: effects of powder-to-liquid ratio and needle size. *J. Biomed. Mater. Res. B: Appl. Biomater.* 2008:84B:493-502.

[166] Ginebra MP, Rilliard A, Fernandez E, Elvira C, San Roman J, Planell JA. Mechanical and rheological improvement of a calcium phosphate cement by the addition of a polymeric drug. *J. Biomed. Mater. Res.* 2001;57:113–118.

[167] Bermudez O, Boltong MG, Driessens FCM, Planell JA. Compressive strength and diametral tensile strength of some calcium-orthophosphate cements: a pilot study. *J. Mater. Sci. Mater. Med.* 1993;4:389–393.

[168] del Valle S, Miño N, Muñoz F, González A, Planell JA, Ginebra MP. *In vivo* evaluation of an injectable macroporous calcium phosphate cement. *J. Mater. Sci. Mater. Med.* 2007;18:353–361.

[169] Khairoun I, Driessens FCM, Boltong MG, Planell JA, Wenz R. Addition of cohesion promotors to calcium orthophosphate cements. *Biomaterials* 1999;20:393-398.

[170] Miyamoto Y, Ishikawa K, Takechi M, Toh T, Yuasa T, Nagayama M, Suzuki K. Histological and compositional evaluations of three types of calcium orthophosphate cements when implanted in subcutaneous tissue immediately after mixing. *J. Biomed. Mater. Res. (Appl. Biomater.)* 1999;48:36-42.

[171] Bigi A, Bracci B, Panzavolta S. Effect of added gelatin on the properties of calcium phosphate cement. *Biomaterials* 2004;25:2893–2899.

[172] Ishikawa K, Matsuya S, Nakagawa M, Udoh K, Suzuki K. Basic properties of apatite cement containing spherical tetracalcium phosphate made with plasma melting method. *J. Mater. Sci. Mater. Med.* 2004;15:13-17.

[173] Barralet JE, Hofmann M, Grover LM, Gbureck U. High strength apatitic cement by modification with α-hydroxy acid salts. *Adv. Mater.* 2003;15:2091–2095.

[174] Barralet JE, Duncan CO, Dover MS, Bassett DC, Nishikawa H, Monaghan A, Gbureck U. Cortical bone screw fixation in ionically modified apatite cements. *J. Biomed. Mater. Res. Part B: Appl. Biomater.* 2005;73B:238–243.

[175] Wang X, Ye J, Wang Y. Influence of a novel radiopacifier on the properties of an injectable calcium phosphate cement. *Acta Biomater.* 2007;3:757-763.

[176] Watanabe M, Tanaka M, Sakurai M, Maeda M. Development of calcium phosphate cement. *J. Europ. Ceram. Soc.* 2006;26:549–552.

[177] Markovic M, Takagi S, Chow LC. Formation of macropores in calcium phosphate cements through the use of mannitol crystals. *Key Eng. Mater.* 2001;192–195:773–776.

[178] Almirall A, Larrecq G, Delgado JA, Martínez S, Planell JA, Ginebra MP. Fabrication of low temperature macroporous hydroxyapatite scaffolds by foaming and hydrolysis of an α-TCP paste. *Biomaterials* 2004;25:3671-3680.

[179] Barralet JE, Grover L, Gaunt T, Wright AJ, Gibson IR. Preparation of macroporous calcium phosphate cement tissue engineering scaffold. *Biomaterials* 2002;23:3063–3072.

[180] Takagi S, Chow LC. Formation of macropores in calcium phosphate cement implants. *J. Mater. Sci. Mater. Med.* 2001;10:135-139.

[181] Simon CG Jr, Khatri CA, Wight SA, Wang FW. Preliminary report on the biocompatibility of a moldable, resorbable, composite bone graft consisting of calcium phosphate cement and poly(lactide-*co*-glycolide) microspheres. *J. Orthop. Res.* 2002;20:473–482.

[182] Ruhe PQ, Hedberg EL, Padron NT, Spauwen PHM, Jansen JA, Mikos AG. Biocompatibility and degradation of poly(DL-lactic-*co*-glycolic acid)/calcium phosphate cement composites. *J. Biomed. Mater. Res. Part A* 2005;74A:533–544.

[183] Habraken WJ, Wolke JGC, Mikos AG, Jansen JA. Injectable PLGA microsphere/calcium phosphate cements: physical properties and degradation characteristics. *J. Biomater. Sci. Polym.* Ed. 2006;17:1057-1074.

[184] Link DP, van den Dolder J, van den Beucken JJJP, Cuijpers VM, Wolke JGC, Mikos AG, Jansen JA. Evaluation of the biocompatibility of calcium phosphate cement/PLGA microparticle composites. *J. Biomed. Mater. Res. Part A* 2008;87A:760-769.

[185] Tas AC. Preparation of porous apatite granules from calcium phosphate cement. *J. Mater. Sci. Mater. Med.* 2008;19:2231-2239.

[186] Habraken WJEM, de Jonge LT, Wolke JGC, Yubao L, Mikos AG, Jansen JA. Introduction of gelatin microspheres into an injectable calcium phosphate cement. *J. Biomed. Mater. Res. Part A* 2008;87A:643-655.

[187] del Real RP, Wolke JGC, Vallet-Regi M, Jansen JA. A new method to produce macropores in calcium phosphate cements. *Biomaterials* 2002;23:3673–3680.

[188] del Real RP, Ooms E, Wolke JGC, Vallet-Regi M, Jansen JA. *In vivo* bone response to porous calcium phosphate cement. *J. Biomed. Mater. Res. Part A* 2003;65A:30–36.

[189] Hesaraki S, Moztarzadeh F, Sharifi D. Formation of interconnected macropores in apatitic calcium phosphate bone cement with the use of an effervescent additive. *J. Biomed. Mater. Res. Part A* 2007;83A:80-87.

[190] Hesaraki S, Moztarzadeh F, Solati-Hashjin M. Phase evaluation of an effervescent-added apatitic calcium phosphate bone cement. *J. Biomed. Mater. Res. Part B: Appl. Biomater.* 2006;79B:203–209.

[191] Sarda S, Nilsson M, Balcells M, Fernández E. Influence of surfactant molecules as air-entraining agent for bone cement macroporosity. *J. Biomed. Mater. Res. Part A* 2003;65A:215–221.

[192] Friberg J, Fernández E, Sarda S, Nilsson M, Ginebra MP, Martinez S, Planell JA. An experimental approach to the study of the rheology behavior of synthetic bone calcium phosphate cements. *Key Eng. Mater.* 2001;192–195:777–780.

[193] Andrianjatovo H, Lemaître J. Effects of polysaccharides on the cement properties in the monocalcium phosphate/β-tricalcium phosphate system. *Innov. Tech. Biol. Med.* 1995;16:140–147.

[194] Cherng A, Takagi S, Chow LC. Effects of hydroxypropylmethylcellulose and other gelling agents on the handling properties of calcium phosphate cement. *J. Biomed. Mater. Res.* 1997;35:273–277.

[195] Yokoyama A, Matsuno H, Yamamoto S, Kawasaki T, Kohgo T, Uo M, Watari F, Nakasu M. Tissue response to a newly developed calcium phosphate cement containing succinic acid and carboxymethyl-chitin. *J. Biomed. Mater. Res. Part A* 2003;64A:491–501.

[196] Xu HHK, Weir MD, Burguera EF, Fraser AM. Injectable and macroporous calcium phosphate cement scaffold. *Biomaterials* 2006;27:4279–4287.

[197] Bigi A, Torricelli P, Fini M, Bracci B, Panzavolta S, Sturba L, Giardino R. A biomimetic gelatin-calcium phosphate bone cement. *Int. J. Artif. Organs* 2004;27:664-673.

[198] Bigi A, Panzavolta S, Sturba L, Torricelli P, Fini M, Giardino R. Normal and osteopenic bone-derived osteoblast response to a biomimetic gelatin – calcium phosphate bone cement. *J. Biomed. Mater. Res. Part A* 2006;78A:739–745.

[199] Fujishiro Y, Takahashi K, Sato T. Preparation and compressive strength of α-tricalcium phosphate/gelatin gel composite cement. *J. Biomed. Mater. Res.* 2001;54:525–530.

[200] Bigi A, Panzavolta S, Rubini K. Setting mechanism of a biomimetic bone cement. *Chem. Mater.* 2004;16:3740 -3745.

[201] Panzavolta S, Torricelli P, Sturba L, Bracci B, Giardino R, Bigi A. Setting properties and *in vitro* bioactivity of strontium-enriched gelatin-calcium phosphate bone cements. *J. Biomed. Mater. Res. Part A* 2008;84A:965-972.

[202] Majekodunmi AO, Deb S, Nicholson JW. Effect of molecular weight and concentration of poly(acrylic acid) on the formation of a polymeric calcium phosphate cement. *J. Mater. Sci. Mater. Med.* 2003;14:747-752.

[203] Majekodunmi AO, Deb S. Poly(acrylic acid) modified calcium phosphate cements: the effect of the composition of the cement powder and of the molecular weight and concentration of the polymeric acid. *J. Mater. Sci. Mater. Med.* 2007;18:1883-1888.

[204] Bohner M, Merkle HP, van Landuyt P, Trophardy G, Lemaitre J. Effect of several additives and their admixtures on the physico-chemical properties of a calcium phosphate cement. *J. Mater. Sci. Mater. Med.* 2000;11:111-116.

[205] Bohner M, Theiss F, Apelt D, Hirsiger W, Houriet R, Rizzoli G, Gnos E, Frei C, Auer JA, von Rechenberg B. Compositional changes of a dicalcium phosphate dihydrate cement after implantation in sheep. *Biomaterials* 2003;24:3463–3474.

[206] Barralet JE, Tremayne MJ, Lilley KJ, Gbureck U. Chemical modification of calcium phosphate cements with α-hydroxy acids and their salts. *Chem. Mater.* 2005;17:1313–1319.

[207] Driessens FCM, Boltong MG, de Maeyer EAP, Verbeeck RMH, Wenz R. Effect of temperature and immersion on the setting of some calcium phosphate cements. *J. Mater. Sci. Mater. Med.* 2000;11:453-457.

[208] Gbureck U, Dembski S, Thull R, Barralet JE. Factors influencing calcium phosphate cement shelf life. *Biomaterials* 2005;26:3691–3697.

[209] Ishikawa K, Takagi S, Chow LC, Ishikawa Y. Properties and mechanisms of fast-setting calcium phosphate cements. *J. Mater. Sci. Mater. Med.* 1995;6:528–533.

[210] Miyamoto Y, Ishikawa K, Fukao K, Sawada M, Nagayama M, Kon M, Asaoka K. *In vivo* setting behavior of fast-setting calcium phosphate cement. *Biomaterials* 1995;16:855–860.

[211] Fulmer MT, Brown PW. Effects of Na_2HPO_4 and NaH_2PO_4 on hydroxyapatite formation. *J. Biomed. Mater. Res.* 1993;27:1095-1102.

[212] Takechi M, Miyamoto Y, Momota Y, Yuasa T, Tatehara S, Nagayama M, Ishikawa K. Effects of various sterilization methods on the setting and mechanical properties of apatite cement. *J. Biomed. Mater. Res. Part B: Appl. Biomater.* 2004;69B:58–63.

[213] Yuan H, Li Y, de Bruijn JD, de Groot K, Zhang X. Tissue responses of calcium phosphate cement: a study in dogs. *Biomaterials* 2000;21:1283-1290.

[214] Takechi M, Miyamoto Y, Ishikawa K, Toh T, Yuasa T, Nagayama M, Suzuki K. Initial histological evaluation of anti-washout type fast-setting calcium phosphate cement following subcutaneous implantation. *Biomaterials* 1998;19:2057-2063.

[215] Otsuka M, Matsuda Y, Suwa Y, Fox JL, Higuchi WI. Effect of particle size of metastable calcium phosphates on mechanical strength of a novel self-setting bioactive calcium phosphate cement. *J. Biomed. Mater. Res.* 1995;29:25–32.

[216] Liu C, Shao H, Chen F, Zheng H. Effects of granularity of raw materials on the hydration and hardening process of calcium phosphate cement. *Biomaterials* 2003;24:4103– 4113.

[217] Chen WC, Lin JHC, Ju CP. Transmission electron microscopic study on setting mechanism of tetracalcium phosphate / dicalcium phosphate anhydrous-based calcium phosphate cement. *J. Biomed. Mater. Res.* 2003;64:664–671.

[218] Fernandez E, Gil FJ, Ginebra MP, Driessens FCM, Planell JA, Best SM. Calcium phosphate bone cements for clinical applications. Part II: Precipitate formation during setting reactions. *J. Mater. Sci. Mater. Med.* 1999;10:177–183.

[219] Brown WE. Crystal growth of bone mineral. Clin. Orthop. Rel. Res. 1966;44:205-220.

[220] Tung MS, Brown WE. An intermediate state in hydrolysis of amorphous calcium phosphate. *Calcif. Tissue Int.* 1983;35:783-790.

[221] Brown WE, Eidelman N, Tomazic BB. Octacalcium phosphate as a precursor in biomineral formation. *Adv. Dent. Res.* 1987, 1, 306-313.

[222] Bohner M, Lemaitre J, Ring T. Hydraulic properties of tri-calcium orthophosphate – phosphoric acid – water mixtures. In: Duran P, Fernandez JF. Eds. *Third Euro-Ceramics*. Castellon de la Plana, Spain: Faenza Editrice Iberica S.L., 1993.

[223] Bajpai P, Fuchs C, McCullum D. Development of tricalcium orthophosphate ceramic cement. In: Lemons J. ed. *Quantitative characterization and performance of porous implants for hard tissue applications*, ASTM STP 953. American Society for Testing and Materials, Philadelphia, 1987:377-388.

[224] Bohner M, van Landuyt P, Merkle H, Lemaitre J. Composition effects on the pH of a hydraulic calcium orthophosphate cement. *J. Mater. Sci. Mater. Med.* 1997;8:675-681.

[225] Constantz BR, Barr BM, Ison IC, Fulmer MT, Baker J, McKinney LA, Goodman SB, Gunasekaren S, Delaney DC, Ross J, Poser RD. Histological, chemical, and crystallographic analysis of four calcium orthophosphate cements in different rabbit osseous sites. *J. Biomed. .Mater. Res. (Appl. Biomater.)* 1998;43:451-461.

[226] Elliott JC. *Structure and chemistry of the apatites and other calcium orthophosphates*. Amsterdam: Elsevier, 1994.

[227] Vereecke G, Lemaitre J. Calculation of the solubility diagrams in the system $Ca(OH)_2$–H_3PO_4–KOH–HNO_3–CO_2–H_2O. *J. Crystal Growth* 1990;104:820-832.

[228] Klein CP, de Groot K, Driessen AA, van der Lubbe HB. Interaction of biodegradable β-whitlockite ceramics with bone tissue: an *in vivo* study. *Biomaterials* 1985;6:189–192.

[229] Apelt D, Theiss F, El-Warrak AO, Zlinszky K, Bettschart-Wolfisberger R, Bohner M, Matter S, Auer JA, von Rechenberg B. *In vivo* behavior of three different injectable hydraulic calcium phosphate cements. *Biomaterials* 2004;25:1439–1451.

[230] Ikenaga M, Hardouin P, Lemaitre J, Andrianjatovo H, Flautre B. Biomechanical characterization of a biodegradable calcium orthophosphate hydraulic cement: a comparison with porous biphasic calcium orthophosphate ceramics. *J. Biomed. Mater. Res.* 1998;40:139-144.

[231] Grover LM, Knowles JC, Fleming GJP, Barralet JE. *In vitro* ageing of brushite calcium phosphate cement. *Biomaterials* 2003;24:4133–4141.

[232] Mariño FT, Mastio J, Rueda C, Blanco L, Cabarcos EL. Increase of the final setting time of brushite cements by using chondroitin 4-sulfate and silica gel. *J. Mater. Sci. Mater. Med.* 2007;18:1195–1201.

[233] Mariño FT, Torres J, Hamdan M, Rodríguez CR, Cabarcos EL. *Advantages of using glycolic acid as a retardant in a brushite forming cement*. 2007;83B:571-579.

[234] Flautre B, Delecourt C, Blary M, van Landuyt P, Lemaitre J, Hardouin P. Volume effect on biological properties of a calcium phosphate hydraulic cement: Experimental study on sheep. *Bone* 1999;25:S35–S39.

[235] Xie J, Riley C, Chittur K. Effect of albumin on brushite transformation to hydroxyapatite. *J. Biomed. Mater. Res*. 2001;57:357–365.

[236] Frayssinet P, Roudier M, Lerch A, Ceolin JL, Depres E, Rouquet N. Tissue reaction against a self-setting calcium phosphate cement set in bone or outside the organism. *J.* Mater. Sci. Mater. Med. 2000;11:811-815.

[237] Ohura K, Bohner M, Hardouin P, Lemaitre J, Pasquier G, Flautre B. Resorption of, and bone formation from, new β-tricalcium orthophosphate – monocalcium orthophosphate cements: an *in vivo* study. *J. Biomed. Mater. Res*. 1996;30:193-200.

[238] Flautre B, Maynou C, Lemaitre J, van Landuyt P, Hardouin P. Bone colonization of β-TCP granules incorporated in brushite cements. *J. Biomed. Mater. Res. (Appl. Biomater.)* 2002;63:413–417.

[239] Yuasa T, Miyamoto Y, Ishikawa K, Takechi M, Nagayama M, Suzuki K. *In vitro* resorption of three apatite cements with osteoclasts. *J. Biomed. Mater. Res.* 2001;54:344–350.

[240] Khairoun I, Magne D, Gauthier O. Bouler JM, Aguado E, Daculsi G, Weiss P. *In vitro* characterization and *in vivo* properties of a carbonated apatite bone cement. *J. Biomed. Mater. Res*. 2002;60:633–642.

[241] Bodde EWH, Cammaert CTR, Wolke JGC, Spauwen PHM, Jansen JA. Investigation as to the osteoinductivity of macroporous calcium phosphate cement in goats. *J. Biomed. Mater. Res. Part B: Appl. Biomater.* 2007;83B:161-168.

[242] Miyamoto Y, Ishikawa K, Takeshi M, Toh T, Yoshida Y, Nagayama M, Kon M, Asaoka K. Tissue response to fast-setting calcium phosphate cement in bone. *J. Biomed. Mater. Res.* 1997;37:457-464.

[243] Young S, Holde M, Gunasekaran S, Poser R, Constantz BR. The correlation of radiographic, MRI, and histological evaluations over two years of a carbonated apatite cement in a rabbit model. *Proceedings of the 44th Annual Meeting,* Orthopaedic Research Society, New Orleans, USA, March 16-19, 1998:846.

[244] Kroese-Deutman HC, Wolke JGC, Spauwen PHM, Jansen JA. Closing capacity of cranial bone defects using porous calcium phosphate cement implants in a rabbit animal model. *J. Biomed. Mater. Res. Part A* 2006;79A:503–511.

[245] Bourgeois B, Laboux O, Obadia L, Gauthier O, Betti E, Aguado E, Daculsi G, Bouler JM. Calcium-deficient apatite: A first *in vivo* study concerning bone ingrowth. *J. Biomed. Mater. Res. Part A* 2003;65A:402-408.

[246] Lu JX, Descamps M, Dejou J, Koubi G, Hardouin P, Lemaitre J, Proust JP. The biodegradation mechanism of calcium phosphate biomaterials in bone. *J. Biomed. Mater. Res. (Appl. Biomater.)* 2002;63:408–412.

[247] Wenisch S, Stahl JP, Horas U, Heiss C, Kilian O, Trinkaus K, Hild A, Schnettler R. *In vivo* mechanisms of hydroxyapatite ceramic degradation by osteoclasts: Fine structural microscopy. *J. Biomed. Mater. Res. Part A* 2003;67A:713–718.

[248] Ooms EM, Wolke JG, van der Waerden JP, Jansen JA. Trabecular bone response to injectable calcium phosphate (Ca-P) cement. *J. Biomed. Mater. Res.* 2002;61:9–18.
[249] Theiss F, Apelt D, Brand B, Kutter A, Zlinszky K, Bohner M, Matter S, Frei C, Auer JA, von Rechenberg B. Biocompatibility and resorption of a brushite calcium phosphate cement. *Biomaterials 2005*;26:4383–4394.
[250] Heymann D, Pradal G, Benahmad M. Cellular mechanisms of calcium phosphate degradation. *Histol Histopathol* 1999;14:871–877.
[251] Dorozhkin SV. Inorganic chemistry of the dissolution phenomenon: the dissolution mechanism of calcium apatites at the atomic (ionic) level. *Comments Inorg. Chem.* 1999;20:285–299.
[252] Dorozhkin SV. A review on the dissolution models of calcium apatites. *Prog. Crystal Growth Charact.* 2002;44:45–61.
[253] Knabe C, Driessens FCM, Planell JA, Gildenhaar R, Berger G, Reif D, Fitzner R, Radlanski RJ, Gross U. Evaluation of calcium phosphates and experimental calcium phosphate bone cements using osteogenic cultures. *J. Biomed. Mater. Res.* 2000;52:498–508.
[254] Teitelbaum SL. Bone resorption by osteoclasts. *Science* 2000;289:1504-1508.
[255] Mostov K, Werb Z. Journey across the osteoclast. *Science* 1997;276:219 –220.
[256] Rodan GA, Martin TJ. Therapeutic approaches to bone diseases. *Science* 2000;289:1508-1514.
[257] Hench LL. Bioceramics: from concept to clinic. *J. Amer. Ceram. Soc.* 1991;74:1487–1510.
[258] Hench LL. Bioceramics. *J. Amer. Ceram. Soc.* 1998;81:1705–1728.
[259] Sun L, Berndt CC, Gross KA, Kucuk A. Material fundamentals and clinical performance of plasma-sprayed hydroxyapatite coatings: A review. *J. Biomed. Mater. Res. Part B: Appl. Biomater.* 2001;58:570–592.
[260] Renault F, Chabriere E, Andrieu JP, Dublet B, Masson P, Rochu D. Tandem purification of two HDL-associated partner proteins in human plasma, paraoxonase (PON1) and phosphate binding protein (HPBP) using hydroxyapatite chromatography. *J. Chromatography B* 2006;836:15-21.
[261] Yoshitake T, Kobayashi S, Ogawa T, Okuyama T. Hydroxyapatite chromatography of guanidine denatured proteins: 1. Guanidine containing phosphate buffer system. *Chromatography* 2006;27:19-26.
[262] Ooms EM, Egglezos EA, Wolke JGC, Jansen JA. Soft-tissue response to injectable calcium phosphate cements. *Biomaterials* 2003;24:749–757.
[263] Ooms EM, Wolke JGC, van de Heuvel MT, Jeschke B, Jansen JA. Histological evaluation of the bone response to calcium phosphate cement implanted in cortical bone. *Biomaterials* 2003;24:989–1000.
[264] Kobayashi N, Ong K, Villarraga M, Schwardt J, Wenz R, Togawa D, Fujishiro T, Turner AS, Seim III HB, Bauer TW. Histological and mechanical evaluation of self-setting calcium phosphate cements in a sheep vertebral bone void model. *J. Biomed. Mater. Res. Part A* 2007;81A:838–846.

[265] Fernandez E, Ginebra MP, Bermudez O, Boltong MG, Driessens FCM, Planell JA. Dimensional and thermal behaviour of calcium phosphate cements during setting compared to PMMA bone cements. *J. Mater. Sci. Lett.* 1995;14:4–5.

[266] Yamamoto H, Niwa S, Hori M, Hattori T, Sawai K, Aoki S, Hirano M, Takeuchi H. Mechanical strength of calcium phosphate cement *in vivo* and *in vitro*. *Biomaterials* 1998;19: 1587-1591.

[267] Andrianjatovo H, Jose F, Lemaitre J. Effect of β-TCP granulometry on setting time and strength of calcium orthophosphate hydraulic cements. *J. Mater. Sci. Mater. Med.* 1996;7:34-39.

[268] Ishikawa K, Takagi S, Chow LC, Ishikawa Y, Eanes E, Asaoka K. Behavior of a calcium orthophosphate cement in simulated blood plasma *in vitro*. *Dent. Mater.* 1994;10:26-32.

[269] Driessens FCM. *Chemistry and applied aspects of calcium orthophosphate bone cements*. Concepts and clinical applications of ionic cements. Sept. 8, Arcachon, France, 1999.

[270] Miyazaki K, Horibe T, Antonucci JM, Takagi S, Chow LC. Polymeric calcium phosphate cements: Analysis of reaction products and properties. *Dent. Mater.* 1993;9:41–45.

[271] Miyazaki K, Horibe T, Antonucci JM, Takagi S, Chow LC. Polymeric calcium phosphate cements: Setting reaction modifiers. *Dent. Mater*. 1993;9:46–50.

[272] dos Santos LA, de Oliveira LC, Rigo ECS, Carrodeguas RG, Boschi AO, de Arruda ACF. Influence of polymeric additives on the mechanical properties of α-tricalcium phosphate cement. *Bone* 1999;25:99S–102S.

[273] Mickiewicz RA, Mayes AM, Knaack D. Polymer–calcium phosphate cement composites for bone substitutes. *J. Biomed. Mater. Res.* 2002;61:581–592.

[274] Costantino PD, Friedman CD, Jones K, Chow LC, Sisson GA. Experimental hydroxyapatite cement cranioplasty. *Plast. Reconstr. Surg*. 1992;90:174-185.

[275] Chow LC, Hirayama S, Takagi S, Parry E. Diametral tensile strength and compressive strength of a calcium phosphate cement: Effect of applied pressure. *J. Biomed. Mater. Res. (Appl. Biomater.)* 2000;53:511–517.

[276] Barralet JE, Gaunt T, Wright AJ, Gibson IR, Knowles JC. Effect of porosity reduction by compaction on compressive strength and microstructure of calcium phosphate cement. *J. Biomed. Mater. Res. (Appl. Biomater.)* 2002;63:1–9.

[277] Zhang Y, Xu HHK, Takagi S, Chow LC. *In situ* hardening hydroxyapatite-based scaffold for bone repair. *J. Mater. Sci. Mater. Med.* 2006;17:437–445.

[278] Morgan EF, Yetkinler DN, Constantz BR, Dauskardt RH. Mechanical properties of carbonated apatite bone mineral substitute: Strength, fracture and fatigue behaviour. *J. Mater. Sci. Mater. Med.* 1997;8:559–570.

[279] Pittet C, Lemaitre J. Mechanical characterization of brushite cements: A Mohr circles approach. *J. Biomed. Mater. Res. (Appl. Biomater.)* 2000;53:769-780.

[280] Xu HHK, Carey LE, Simon CG Jr. Premixed macroporous calcium phosphate cement scaffold. *J. Mater. Sci. Mater. Med.* 2007;18:1345–1353.

[281] Xu HHK, Simon CG Jr. Self-hardening calcium phosphate cement-mesh composite: Reinforcement, macropores, and cell response. *J. Biomed. Mater. Res. Part A* 2004;69A:267–278.

[282] Losee JE, Karmacharya J, Gannon FH, Slemp AE, Ong G, Hunenko O, Gorden AD, Bartlett SP, Kirschner RE. Reconstruction of the immature craniofacial skeleton with a carbonated calcium phosphate bone cement: interaction with bioresorbable mesh. *J. Craniofacial Surg.* 2003;14:117-124.

[283] Khairoun I, LeGeros RZ, Daculsi G, Bouler JM, Gauthier O, Guicheux J. Macroporous, resorbable and injectable calcium phosphate-based cements (MCPC) for bone repair, augmentation, regeneration, and osteoporosis treatment. Patent No. WO/2005/077049. August 25, 2005.

[284] Speirs AD, Oxland TR, Masri BA, Poursartip A, Duncan CP. Calcium phosphate cement composites in revision hip arthroplasty. *Biomaterials*, 2005;26:7310-7318.

[285] dos Santos LA, Carrodeguas RG, Boschi AO, de Arruda ACF. Fiber-enriched double-setting calcium phosphate bone cement. *J. Biomed. Mater. Res. Part A* 2003;65A:244–250.

[286] Gbureck U, Spatz K, Thull R. Improvement of mechanical properties of self-setting calcium phosphate bone cements mixed with different metal oxides. *Materialwissenschaft und Werkstofftechnik* 2003;34:1036–1040.

[287] Zhang Y, Xu HHK. Effects of synergistic reinforcement and absorbable fiber strength on hydroxyapatite bone cement. *J. Biomed. Mater. Res. Part A* 2005;75A:832–840.

[288] Buchanan F, Gallagher L, Jack V, Dunne N. Short-fibre reinforcement of calcium phosphate bone cement. Proc. Instn. Mech. Engrs H: *J. Engin. Med.* 2007;221:203-212.

[289] Wang X, Ye J, Wang Y, Chen L. Reinforcement of calcium phosphate cement by bio-mineralized carbon nanotube. *J. Amer. Ceram. Soc.* 2007;90:962-964.

[290] http://en.wikipedia.org/wiki/Concrete (accessed in January 2008).

[291] Dickens-Venz SH, Takagi S, Chow LC, Bowen RL, Johnston AD, Dickens B. Physical and chemical properties of resin-reinforced calcium phosphate cements. *Dent. Mater.* 1994;10:100–106.

[292] Xu HHK, Eichmiller FC, Barndt PR. Effects of fiber length and volume fraction on the reinforcement of calcium phosphate cement. *J. Mater. Sci. Mater. Med.* 2001;12:57-65.

[293] Xu HHK, Quinn JB, Takagi S, Chow LC. Synergistic reinforcement of *in situ* hardening calcium phosphate composite scaffold for bone tissue engineering. *Biomaterials* 2004;25:1029–1037.

[294] Sun L, Xu HHK, Takagi S, Chow LC. Fast setting calcium phosphate cement – chitosan composite: mechanical properties and dissolution rates. *J. Biomaterials Applications* 2007;21:299-316.

[295] Pan ZH, Jiang PP, Fan QY, Ma B, Cai HP. Mechanical and biocompatible influences of chitosan fiber and gelatin on calcium phosphate cement. *J. Biomed. Mater. Res. Part B: Appl. Biomater.* 2007;82B:246–252.

[296] Liu H, Li H, Cheng W, Yang Y, Zhu M, Zhou C. Novel injectable calcium phosphate/chitosan composites for bone substitute materials. *Acta Biomater.* 2006;2:557-565.

[297] Pan ZH, Cai HP, Jiang PP, Fan QY. Properties of a calcium phosphate cement synergistically reinforced by chitosan fiber and gelatin. *J. Polymer Res*. 2006;13:323-327.

[298] Weir MD, Xu HHK. High-strength, *in situ*-setting calcium phosphate composite with protein release. *J. Biomed. Mater. Res. Part A* 2008;85A:388-396.

[299] Lin J, Zhang S, Chen T, Liu C, Lin S, Tian X. Calcium phosphate cement reinforced by polypeptide copolymers. *J. Biomed. Mater. Res. Part B: Appl. Biomater*. 2006;76B:432–439.

[300] Miyamoto Y, Ishikawa K, Takechi M, Toh T, Yuasa T, Nagayama M, Suzuki K. Basic properties of calcium phosphate cement containing atelocollagen in its liquid or powder phases. *Biomaterials* 1998;19:707–715.

[301] Otsuka M, Kuninaga T, Otsuka K, Higuchi WI. Effect of nanostructure on biodegradation behaviors of self-setting apatite/collagen composite cements containing vitamin K_2 in rats. *J. Biomed. Mater. Res. Part B: Appl. Biomater*. 2006;79B:176–184.

[302] Xu HHK, Eichmiller FC, Giuseppetti AA. Reinforcement of a self-setting calcium phosphate cement with different fibers. *J. Biomed. Mater. Res*. 2000;52:107–114.

[303] Xu HHK, Quinn JB, Takagi S, Chow LC, Eichmiller FC. Strong and macroporous calcium phosphate cement, effects of porosity and fiber reinforcement on mechanical properties. *J. Biomed. Mater. Res*. 2001;57:457–466.

[304] dos Santos LA, Carrodeguas RG, Boschi AO, de Arruda ACF. Dual-setting calcium phosphate cement modified with ammonium polyacrylate. *Artif. Organs* 2003;27:412-418.

[305] dos Santos LA, de Oliveira LC, da Silva Rigo EC, Carrodéguas RG, Boschi AO, de Arruda ACF. Fiber reinforced calcium phosphate cement. *Artif. Organs* 2000;24:212–216.

[306] Xu HHK, Simon CG Jr. Self-hardening calcium phosphate composite scaffold for bone tissue engineering. *J. Orthop. Res*. 2004;22:535-543.

[307] Burguera EF, Xu HHK, Takagi S, Chow LC. High early strength calcium phosphate bone cement: Effects of dicalcium phosphate dihydrate and absorbable fibers. *J. Biomed. Mater. Res. Part A* 2005;75A:966–975.

[308] Xu HHK, Quinn JB. Calcium phosphate cement containing resorbable fibers for short-term reinforcement and macroporosity. *Biomaterials* 2002;23:193–202.

[309] Gorst NJS, Perrie Y, Gbureck U, Hutton AL, Hofmann MP, Grover LM, Barralet JE. Effects of fibre reinforcement on the mechanical properties of brushite cement. *Acta Biomater*. 2006;2:95-102.

[310] Julien M, Khairoun I, LeGeros RZ, Delplace S, Pilet P, Weiss P, Daculsi G, Bouler JM, Guicheux J. Physico-chemical–mechanical and *in vitro* biological properties of calcium phosphate cements with doped amorphous calcium phosphates. *Biomaterials* 2007;28:956–965.

[311] Lemaitre J, Munting E, Mirtchi AA. Setting, hardening and resorption of calcium phosphate hydraulic cements. *Rev. Stomatol. Chir. Maxillofac*. 1992;93:163–165.

[312] Müller FA, Gbureck U, Kasuga T, Mizutani Y, Barralet JE, Lohbauer U. Whisker-reinforced calcium phosphate cements. *J. Amer. Ceram. Soc*. 2007;90:3694-3697.

[313] Gisep A, Wieling R, Bohner M, Matter S, Schneider E, Rahn B. Resorption patterns of calcium-phosphate cements in bone. *J. Biomed. Mater. Res. Part A* 2003;66A:532–540.

[314] Gbureck U, Spatz K, Thull R, Barralet JE. Rheological enhancement of mechanically activated α-tricalcium phosphate cements. *J. Biomed. Mater. Res. Part B: Appl. Biomater.* 2005;73B:1–6.

[315] Castaldini A, Cavallini A. Setting properties of bone cement with added synthetic hydroxyapatite. *Biomaterials* 1985;6:55–60.

[316] Sogal A, Hulbert SF. Mechanical properties of a composite bone cement: polymethylmethacrylate and hydroxyapatite. Proceedings of the 5th International Symposium on Ceramics in Medicine, *Bioceramics*, 1992, Vol. 5, pp. 213–224.

[317] Harper EJ, Behiri JC, Bonfield W. Flexural and fatigue properties of a bone cement based upon polyethylmethacrylate and hydroxyapatite. *J. Mater. Sci. Mater. Med.* 1995;6:799–803.

[318] Harper EJ. Bioactive bone cements. *Proc. Instn. Mech. Engrs. Part H: J. Engin. Med.* 1998;212:113–120.

[319] Shinzato S, Kobayashi M, Mousa WF, Kamimura M, Neo M, Kitamura Y, Kokubo T, Nakamura T. Bioactive polymethylmethacrylate-based bone cement: Comparison of glass beads, apatite- and wollastonite-containing glass-ceramic, and hydroxyapatite fillers on mechanical and biological properties. *J. Biomed. Mater. Res.* 2000;51:258–272.

[320] Harper EJ, Braden M, Bonfield W. Mechanical properties of hydroxyapatite reinforced poly(ethylmethacrylate) bone cement after immersion in a physiological solution: Influence of a silane coupling agent. *J. Mater. Sci. Mater. Med.* 2000;11:491–497.

[321] Xu HHK, Quinn JB. Whisker-reinforced bioactive composites containing calcium phosphate cement fillers: Effects of filler ratio and surface treatments on mechanical properties. *J. Biomed. Mater. Res.* 2001;57:165–174.

[322] Claes L, Höllen I, Ignatius A. Resorbable bone cements. *Orthopäde* 1997;26:459–462.

[323] Jansen JA, de Ruijter JE, Schaeken HG, van der Waerden JPC, Planell JA, Driessens FCM. Evaluation of tricalciumphosphate/hydroxyapatite cement for tooth replacement: an experimental animal study. *J. Mater. Sci. Mater. Med.* 1995;6:653–657.

[324] Larsson S, Bauer TW. Use of injectable calcium phosphate cement for fracture fixation: a review. *Clin. Orthop. Relat. Res.* 2002;395:23–32.

[325] Gbureck U, Knappe O, Hofmann N, Barralet JE. Antimicrobial properties of nanocrystalline tetracalcium phosphate cements. *J. Biomed. Mater. Res. Part B: Appl. Biomater.* 2007;83B:132-137.

[326] Sethuraman S, Nair LS, El-Amin S, Nguyen MTN, Greish YE, Bender JD, Brown PW, Allcock HR, Laurencin CT. Novel low temperature setting nanocrystalline calcium phosphate cements for bone repair: osteoblast cellular response and gene expression studies. *J. Biomed. Mater. Res. Part A* 2007;82A:884 – 891.

[327] Link DP, van den Dolder J, Wolke JG, Jansen JA. The cytocompatibility and early osteogenic characteristics of an injectable calcium phosphate cement. *Tissue Eng.* 2007;13:493-500.

[328] Oda H, Nakamura K, Matsushita T, Yamamoto S, Ishibashi H, Yamazaki T, Morimoto S. Clinical use of a newly developed calcium phosphate cement (XSB-671D). *J. Orthop. Sci.* 2006;11:167–174.

[329] Braun C, Rahn B, Fulmer M, Steiner A, Gisep A. Intra-articular calcium Phosphate cement: its fate and impact on joint tissues in a rabbit model. *J. Biomed. Mater. Res. Part B: Appl. Biomater.* 2006;79B:151-158.

[330] Costantino P, Friedman C, Jones K, Chow LC, Pelzer H, Sisson G. Hydroxyapatite cement. I. Basic chemistry and histologic properties. *Arch. Otolaryngol. Head Neck* Surg. 1991;117:379–384.

[331] Hong YC, Wang JT, Hong CY, Brown WE, Chow CY. The periapical tissue reactions to a calcium phosphate cement in the teeth of monkeys. J. Biomed. Mater. Res. 1991;25:485–498.

[332] Sugawara A, Fujikawa K, Kusama K, Nishiyama M, Murai S, Takagi S, Chow LC. Histopathologic reaction of calcium phosphate cement for alveolar ridge augmentation. *J. Biomed. Mater. Res.* 2002;61:47-52.

[333] Fujikawa K, Sugawara A, Kusama K, Nishiyama M, Murai S, Takagi S, Chow LC. Fluorescent labeling analysis and electron probe microanalysis for alveolar ridge augmentation using calcium phosphate cement. *Dent. Mater. J.* 2002;21:296-305.

[334] Sugawara A, Chow LC, Takagi S, Chohayeb H. *In vitro* evaluation of the sealing ability of a calcium phosphate cement when used as a root canal sealer-filler. *J. Endod.* 1990;16:162–165.

[335] Noetzel J, Özer K, Reisshauer BH, Anil A, Rössler R, Neumann K, Kielbassa AM. Tissue responses to an experimental calcium phosphate cement and mineral trioxide aggregate as materials for furcation perforation repair: a histological study in dogs. *Clin. Oral Invest.* 2006;10:77–83.

[336] Zhang W, Walboomers XF, Jansen JA. The formation of tertiary dentin after pulp capping with a calcium phosphate cement, loaded with PLGA microparticles containing TGF-β1. *J. Biomed. Mater. Res. Part A* 2008;85A:439-444.

[337] Comuzzi L, Ooms E, Jansen JA. Injectable calcium phosphate cement as a filler for bone defects around oral implants: an experimental study in goats. *Clin. Oral Implants Res.* 2002;13:304-311.

[338] Shirakata Y, Oda S, Kinoshita A, Kikuchi S, Tsuchioka H, Ishikawa I. Histocompatible healing of periodontal defects after application of injectable calcium phosphate bone cement. A preliminary study in dogs. *J. Periodontol.* 2002;73:1043-1053.

[339] Chaung HM, Hong CH, Chiang CP, Lin SK, Kuo YS, Lan WH, Hsieh CC. Comparison of calcium phosphate cement mixture and pure calcium hydroxide as direct pulp-capping agents. *J. Formos Med. Assoc.* 1996;95:545-550.

[340] Sliindo ML, Costantino PD, Friedman CD, Chow LC. Facial skeletal augmentation using hydroxyapatite cement cranioplasty. *Arch. Otolaryngol. Head Neck Surg.* 1993;119:185-190.

[341] Bifano CA, Edgin WA, Colleton C, Bifano SL, Constantino PD. Preliminary evaluation of hydroxyapatite cement as an augmentation device in the edentulous atrophic canine mandible. *Oral Surg.* 1998;85:512-516.

[342] Friedman C, Costantino P, Jones K, Chow LC, Pelzer H, Sisson G. Hydroxyapatite cement. II. Obliteration and reconstruction of the cat frontal sinus. *Arch. Otolaryngol. Head Neck Surg*. 1991;117:385-389.

[343] Sinikovic B, Kramer FJ, Swennen G, Lubbers HT, Dempf R. Reconstruction of orbital wall defects with calcium phosphate cement: clinical and histological findings in a sheep model. *Int. J. Oral Maxillofac. Surg*. 2007;36:54-61.

[344] Smartt JM, Karmacharya J, Gannon FH, Ong G, Jackson O, Bartlett SP, Poser RD, Kirschner RE. Repair of the immature and mature craniofacial skeleton with a carbonated calcium phosphate cement: assessment of biocompatibility, osteoconductivity, and remodeling capacity. *Plast. Reconstr. Surg*. 2005;115:1642-1650.

[345] Reddi SP, Stevens MR, Kline SN, Villanueva P. Hydroxyapatite cement in craniofacial trauma surgery: Indications and early experience. *J. Craniomaxillofac. Trauma* 1999;5:7–12.

[346] Friedman CD, Costantino PD, Synderman CH, Chow LC, Takagi S. Reconstruction of the frontal sinus and frontofacial skeleton with hydroxyapatite cement. *Arch. Facial Plast. Surg*. 2000;2:124 –129.

[347] Liverneaux P. Osteoporotic distal radius curettage–filling with an injectable calcium phosphate cement. *A cadaveric study. Eur. J. Orthop. Surg. Traumatol*. 2005;15:1–6.

[348] Liverneaux P, Vernet P, Robert C, Diacono P. Cement pinning of osteoporotic distal radius fractures with an injectable calcium phosphate bone substitute: report of 6 cases. *Eur. J. Orthop. Surg. Traumatol*. 2006;16:10–16.

[349] Thordarson D, Hedman T, Yetkinler D, Eskander E, Lawrence T, Poser R. Superior compressive strength of a calcaneal fracture construct augmented with remodelable cancellous bone cement. *J. Bone Joint Surg*. 1999;81A:239-246.

[350] Stankewich C, Swiontkowski M, Tencer A, Yetkinler D, Poser R. Augmentation of femoral neck fracture fixation with an injectable calcium-phosphate bone mineral cement. *J. Orthopaedic Res*. 1996;14:786-793.

[351] Goodman S, Bauer T, Carter D, Casteleyn PP, Goldstein SA, Kyle RF, Larsson S, Stankewich CJ, Swiontkowski MF, Tencer AF, Yetkinler DN, Poser RD. Norian SRS cement augmentation in hip fracture treatment. *Clin. Orthop. Rel. Res*. 1998;348:42-50.

[352] Bai B, Jazrawi L, Kummer F, Spivak J. The use of an injectable, biodegradable calcium orthophosphate bone substitute for the prophylactic augmentation of osteoporotic vertebrae and the management of vertebral compression fractures. *Spine* 1999;24:1521-1526.

[353] Horstmann WG, Verheyen CCPM, Leemans R. An injectable calcium phosphate cement as a bone-graft substitute in the treatment of displaced lateral tibial plateau fractures. *Injury* 2003;34:141–144.

[354] Simpson D, Keating JF. Outcome of tibial plateau fractures managed with calcium phosphate cement. *Injury* 2004;35:913–918.

[355] Welch RD, Zhang H, Bronson DG. Experimental tibial plateau fractures augmented with calcium phosphate cement or autologous bone graft. *J. Bone Joint Surg. Am*. 2003;85:222–231.

[356] Keating JF, Hajducka CL, Harper J. Minimal internal fixation and calcium phosphate cement in the treatment of fractures of the tibial plateau: A pilot study. *J. Bone Joint Surg. Br.* 2003;85:68–73.

[357] Moore D, Maitra R, Farjo L, Graziano G, Goldstein S. Restoration of pedicle screw fixation with an *in situ* setting calcium orthophosphate cement. *Spine* 1997;22:1696¬1705.

[358] Mermelstein LE, McLain RF, Yerby SA. Reinforcement of thoracolumbar burst fractures with calcium phosphate cement. *Spine* 1998;23:664–671.

[359] Mermelstein L, Chow LC, Friedman C, Crisco J. The reinforcement of cancellous bone screws with calcium orthophosphate cement. *J. Orthop. Trauma* 1996;10:15-20.

[360] Liverneaux P, Khallouk R. Calcium phosphate cement in wrist arthrodesis: three cases. *J. Orthop. Sci.* 2006;11:289–293.

[361] Ooms EM, Wolke JGC, van der Waerden JPCM, Jansen JA. Use of injectable calcium phosphate cement for the fixation of titanium implants: an experimental study in goats. *J. Biomed. Mater. Res. Part B: Appl. Biomater.* 2003;66B:447–456.

[362] Strauss EJ, Pahk B, Kummer FJ, Egol K. Calcium phosphate cement augmentation of the femoral neck defect created after dynamic hip screw removal. *J. Orthop. Trauma* 2007;21:295-300.

[363] Schildhauer TA, Bennett AP, Wright TM, Lane JM, O'Leary PF. Intravertebral body reconstruction with an injectable *in situ*-setting carbonated apatite: biomechanical evaluation of a minimally invasive technique. *J. Bone Joint Surg.* 1999;17:67–72.

[364] Jansen J, Ooms E, Verdonschot N, Wolke J. Injectable calcium phosphate cement for bone repair and implant fixation. *Orthop. Clin. North Am.* 2005;36:89–95.

[365] Maestretti G, Cremer C, Otten P, Jakob RP. Prospective study of standalone balloon kyphoplasty with calcium phosphate cement augmentation in traumatic fractures. *Eur. Spine J.* 2007;16:601–610.

[366] Hisatome T, Yasunaga Y, Ikuta Y, Fujimoto Y. Effects on articular cartilage of subchondral replacement with polymethylmethacrylate and calcium phosphate cement. *J. Biomed. Mater. Res.* 2002;59:490–498.

[367] Lim TH, Brebach GT, Renner SM, Kim WJ, Kim JG, Lee RE, Andersson GB, An HS. Biomechanical evaluation of an injectable calcium phosphate cement for vertebroplasty. *Spine* 2002;27:1297-1302.

[368] Belkoff SM, Mathis JM, Jasper LE, Deramond H. An *ex vivo* biomechanical evaluation of a hydroxyapatite cement for use with vertebroplasty. *Spine* 2001;26:1542–1546.

[369] Heini PF, Berlemann U, Kaufmann M, Lippuner K, Fankhauser C, van Landuyt P. Augmentation of mechanical properties in osteoporotic vertebral bones – a biomechanical investigation of vertebroplasty efficacy with different bone cements. Eur. *Spine J.* 2001;10:164-171.

[370] Tomita S, Kin A, Yazu M, Abe M. Biomechanical evaluation of kyphoplasty and vertebroplasty with calcium phosphate cement in a simulated osteoporotic compression fracture. *J. Orthop. Sci.* 2003;8:192–197.

[371] Libicher M, Hillmeier J, Liegibel U, Sommer U, Pyerin W, Vetter M, Meinzer HP, Grafe I, Meeder P, Nöldge G, Nawroth P, Kasperk C. Osseous integration of calcium

phosphate in osteoporotic vertebral fractures after kyphoplasty: initial results from a clinical and experimental pilot study. *Osteoporos Int.* 2006;17:1208–1215.

[372] Otsuka M, Matsuda Y, Suwa Y, Fox JL, Higuchi WI. A novel skeletal drug-delivery system using a self-setting calcium orthophosphate cement. 3. Physicochemical properties and drug-release rate of bovine insulin and bovine albumin. *J. Pharm. Sci.* 1994;83:255-258.

[373] Yu D, Wong J, Matsuda Y, Fox JL, Higuchi WI, Otsuka M. Self-setting hydroxyapatite cement: a novel skeletal drug-delivery system for antibiotics. *J. Pharm. Sci.* 1992; 81:529-531.

[374] Bohner M, Lemaitre J, van Landuyt P, Zambelli P, Merkle H, Gander B. Gentamicin-loaded hydraulic calcium orthophosphate bone cement as antibiotic delivery system. *J. Pharm. Sci.* 1997;86:565-572.

[375] Kisanuki O, Yajima H, Umeda T, Takakura Y. Experimental study of calcium phosphate cement impregnated with dideoxy-kanamycin B. *J. Orthop. Sci.* 2007;12:281-288.

[376] Otsuka M, Matsuda Y, Suwa Y, Fox JL, Higuchi WI. A novel skeletal drug delivery system using a self-setting calcium orthophosphate cement. 5. Drug release behavior from a heterogeneous drug-loaded cement containing an anticancer drug. *J. Pharm. Sci.* 1994;83:1565-1568.

[377] Otsuka M, Matsuda Y, Suwa Y, Fox JL, Higuchi WI. A novel skeletal drug delivery system using a self-setting calcium orthophosphate cement. 2. Physicochemical properties and drug release rate of the cement-containing indomethacin. *J. Pharm. Sci.* 1994;83:611-615.

[378] Li DX, Fan HS, Zhu XD, Tan YF, Xiao WQ, Lu J, Xiao YM, Chen JY, Zhang XD. Controllable release of salmon-calcitonin in injectable calcium phosphate cement modified by chitosan oligosaccharide and collagen polypeptide. *J. Mater. Sci. Mater. Med.* 2007;18:2225-2231.

[379] Kamegai A, Shimamura N, Naitou K, Nagahara K, Kanematsu N, Mori M. Bone formation under the influence of bone morphogenetic protein/self-setting apatite cement composite as delivery system. *Biomed. Mater. Eng.* 1994;4:291-307.

[380] Fei Z, Hu Y, Wu D, Wu H, Lu R, Bai J, Song H. Preparation and property of a novel bone graft composite consisting of rhBMP-2 loaded PLGA microspheres and calcium phosphate cement. *J. Mater. Sci. Mater. Med.* 2008;19:1109-1116.

[381] Bodde EWH, Boerman OC, Russel FGM, Mikos AG, Spauwen PHM, Jansen JA. The kinetic and biological activity of different loaded rhBMP-2 calcium phosphate cement implants in rats. *J. Biomed. Mater. Res. Part A* 2008;87A:780-791.

[382] Meraw SJ, Reeve CM, Lohse CM, Sioussat TM. Treatment of perimplant defects with combination growth factor cement. *.J. Periodont.* 2000;71:8-13.

[383] Sasaki T, Ishibashi Y, Katano H, Nagumo A, Toh S. *In vitro* elution of vancomycin from calcium phosphate cement. *J. Arthroplasty* 2005;20:1055–1059.

[384] Blom EJ, Klein-Nulend J, Wolke JGC, van Waas MAJ, Driessens FCM, Burger EH. Transforming growth factor-β1 incorporation in a calcium phosphate bone cement: Material properties and release characteristics. *J. Biomed. Mater. Res.* 2002;59:265–272.

[385] Blom EJ, Klein-Nulend J, Yin L, van Waas MAJ, Burger EH. Transforming growth factor-β1 incorporated in calcium phosphate cement stimulates osteotransductivity in rat calvarial bone defects. *Clin. Oral Implants Res.* 2001;12:609-616.

[386] Link DP, van den Dolder J, van den Beucken JJ, Wolke JG, Mikos AG, Jansen JA. Bone response and mechanical strength of rabbit femoral defects filled with injectable CaP cements containing TGF-β1 loaded gelatin microparticles. *Biomaterials* 2008;29:675-682.

[387] Ruhé PQ, Boerman OC, Russel FGM, Mikos AG, Spauwen PHM, Jansen JA. *In vivo* release of rhBMP-2 loaded porous calcium phosphate cement pretreated with albumin. *J. Mater. Sci. Mater. Med.* 2006;17:919–927.

[388] Kisanuki O, Yajima H, Umeda T, Takakura Y. Experimental study of calcium phosphate cement impregnated with dideoxy-kanamycin B. *J. Orthopaedic Sci.* 2007;12:281-288.

[389] Blattert TR, Delling G, Weckbach A. Evaluation of an injectable calcium phosphate cement as an autograft substitute for transpedicular lumbar interbody fusion: A controlled, prospective study in the sheep model. *Eur. Spine J.* 2003;12:216 –223.

[390] Sanchez-Sotelo J, Munuera L, Madero R. Treatment of fractures of the distal radius with a remodellable bone cement: A prospective, randomised study using Norian SRS. *J. Bone Joint Surg. Br.* 2000;82:856–863.

[391] Lobenhoffer P, Gerich T, Witte F, Tscherne H. Use of an injectable calcium phosphate bone cement in the treatment of tibial plateau fractures: A prospective study of twenty-six cases with twenty-month mean follow-up. *J. Orthop. Trauma* 2002;16:143–149.

[392] Cassidy C, Jupiter JB, Cohen M, Delli-Santi M, Fennell C, Leinberry C, Husband J, Ladd A, Seitz WR, Constanz B. Norian SRS cement compared with conventional fixation in distal radial fractures: A randomized study. *J. Bone Joint Surg. Am.* 2003;85:2127–2137.

[393] Schmidt R, Cakir B, Mattes T, Wegener M, Puhl W, Richter M. Cement leakage during vertebroplasty: an underestimated problem? *Eur. Spine J.* 2005;14:466–473.

[394] Vlad MD, Torres R, López J, Barracó M, Moreno JA, Fernández E. Does mixing affect the setting of injectable bone cement? An ultrasound study. *J. Mater. Sci. Mater. Med.* 2007;18:347–352.

[395] Krebs J, Aebli N, Goss BG, Sugiyama S, Bardyn T, Boecken I, Leamy PJ, Ferguson SJ. Cardiovascular changes after pulmonary embolism from injecting calcium phosphate cement. *J. Biomed. Mater. Res. Part B: Appl. Biomater.* 2007;82B:526–532.

[396] Takagi S, Chow LC, Hirayama S, Sugawara A. Premixed calcium phosphate cement pastes. *J. Biomed. Mater. Res. Part B: Appl. Biomater.* 2003;67B:689–696.

[397] Carey LE, Xu HHK, Simon CG Jr, Takagi S, Chow LC. Premixed rapid-setting calcium phosphate composites for bone repair. *Biomaterials* 2005;26:5002–5014.

[398] Xu HHK, Carey LE, Simon CG Jr, Takagi S, Chow LC. Premixed calcium phosphate cements: Synthesis, physical properties, and cell cytotoxicity. *Dental Mater.* 2007;23:433-441.

[399] Lemaitre J, Pittet C, Brendlen D. *Pasty or liquid multiple constituent compositions for injectable calcium phosphate cements*. International PCT application, WO 03/041753 A1, May 22, 2003.

[400] Chow LC. Calcium phosphate materials: reactor response. *Adv. Dent. Res*. 1988;2:181-184.

[401] Bohner M. Calcium phosphate emulsions: possible applications. In: Giannini S, Moroni A, editors. *Bioceramics 13*. Zurich: Trans Tech Publications Ltd., 2001. p. 65–68.

[402] Troczynski T. A concrete solution. *Nature Materials* 2004;3:13-14.

[403] Xu HHK, Burguera EF, Carey LE. Strong, macroporous and *in situ*-setting calcium phosphate cement-layered structures. *Biomaterials* 2007;28:3786-3796.

[404] Xu HHK, Takagi S, Quinn JB, Chow LC. Fast-setting calcium phosphate scaffolds with tailored macropore formation rates for bone regeneration. *J. Biomed. Mater. Res. Part A* 2004;68A:725–734.

[405] Tajima S, Kishi Y, Oda M, Maruta M, Matsuya S, Ishikawa K. Fabrication of biporous low-crystalline apatite based on mannitol dissolution from apatite cement. *Dent. Mater. J.* 2006;25:616-620.

[406] Weir MD, Xu HHK, Simon CG Jr. Strong calcium phosphate cement-chitosan-mesh construct containing cell-encapsulating hydrogel beads for bone tissue engineering. *J. Biomed. Mater. Res. Part A* 2006;77A:487–496.

[407] Xu JH, Tan WQ, Lin J. Repair of madibular bone defect by combining calcium phosphate cement with bone morphogenetic protein composite as a bone graft material. *Chinese J. Biomed. Engin.* 2007;26:153-156.

[408] Niikura T, Tsujimoto K, Yoshiya S, Tadokoro K, Kurosaka M, Shiba R. Vancomycin-impregnated calcium phosphate cement for methicillin-resistant *staphylococcus aureus* femoral osteomyelitis. *Orthopedics* 2007;30:320-321.

[409] Lode A, Wolf-Brandstetter C, Reinstorf A, Bernhardt A, König U. Pompe W, Gelinsky M. Calcium phosphate bone cements, functionalized with VEGF: release kinetics and biological activity. *J. Biomed. Mater. Res. Part A* 2007;81A:474–483.

[410] Yoshikawa M, Toda T. *In vivo* estimation of periapical bone reconstruction by chondroitin sulfate in calcium phosphate cement. *J. Europ. Ceram. Soc*. 2004;24:521–531.

[411] Simon CG Jr, Guthrie WF, Wang FW. Cell seeding into calcium phosphate cement. *J. Biomed. Mater. Res. Part A* 2004;68A:628–639.

[412] dos Santos LA, Carrodéguas RG, Rogero SO, Higa OZ, Boschi AO, de Arruda AC. Alpha-tricalcium phosphate cement: "*in vitro*" cytotoxicity. *Biomaterials* 2002;23:2035-2042.

[413] Baroud G, Steffen T. A new cannula to ease cement injection during vertebroplasty. *Eur. Spine J.* 2005;14:474–479.

[414] Anderson JM. The future of biomedical materials. *J. Mater. Sci. Mater. Med.* 2006;17:1025–1028.

In: Bioceramics: Properties, Preparations and Applications ISBN: 978-1-60741-056-0
Editors: W. Kossler, J. Fuchs, pp. 67-161

Chapter II

Calcium Orthophosphates as Biomaterials and Bioceramics

Sergey V. Dorozhkin*
Kudrinskaja sq. 1-155, 123242 Moscow, Russia

Abstract

The present overview is intended to point the readers' attention to the important subject of calcium orthophosphates. This type of materials is of the special significance for the human beings because they represent the inorganic part of major normal (bones, teeth and antlers) and pathological (*i.e.* those appearing due to various diseases) calcified tissues of mammals. For example, atherosclerosis results in blood vessel blockage caused by a solid composite of cholesterol with calcium orthophosphates. Dental caries and osteoporosis mean a partial decalcification of teeth and bones respectively that results in replacement of a less soluble and harder biological apatite by more soluble and softer calcium hydrogenorthophosphates. Therefore, the processes of both normal and pathological calcifications are just an *in vivo* crystallization of calcium orthophosphates. Similarly, dental caries and osteoporosis might be considered as *in vivo* dissolution of calcium orthophosphates. Conversely, due to a great chemical similarity with the biological calcified tissues, many calcium orthophosphates possess remarkable biocompatibility and bioactivity. Materials scientists extensively use this property to construct artificial bone grafts that are either entirely made of or only surface-coated by the biologically relevant calcium orthophosphates. For example, self-setting hydraulic cements made of calcium orthophosphates are helpful in bone repair, while titanium substitutes covered by a surface layer of calcium orthophosphates are used for hip joint endoprostheses and tooth substitutes. Porous scaffolds made of calcium orthophosphates are very promising tools for tissue engineering applications. In addition, calcium orthophosphates of a technical grade are very popular mineral fertilizers. There is a great significance of calcium orthophosphates for the humankind and, in this paper, an overview on the current knowledge on this subject is provided. To assist and guide the

* E-mail: sedorozhkin@yandex.ru

readers, a great number of references to the related publications detalizing various specific aspects of the matter has been collected.

Keywords: Calcium orthophosphates, Antlers, Biological apatite, Biomaterials, Bioceramics, Biomimetics, Biomineralization, Bone grafts, Bones, Calcified tissues, Fluorapatite, Hydroxyapatite, Materials chemistry, Pathological calcification, Teeth, Tissue engineering.

1. Introduction

Calcium orthophosphates are the chemical compounds of a special interest in many interdisciplinary fields of science, including geology, chemistry, biology and medicine. According to the references, the initial attempts to establish their chemical composition were performed by J. Berzelius in the middle of the 19th century [1]. Approximately 70 years afterward the idea on existence of different crystal phases of calcium orthophosphates was introduced [2]; mixtures of calcium orthophosphates had been called apatites[14] until then.

By definition, all calcium orthophosphates consist of three major chemical elements: calcium (oxidation state +2), phosphorus (oxidation state +5) and oxygen (reduction state –2), as a part of orthophosphate anions. These three chemical elements are present in abundance on the surface of our planet: oxygen is the most widespread chemical element of the earth's surface (47 mass %), calcium occupies the fifth place (3.3 – 3.4 mass %) and phosphorus (0.08 – 0.12 mass %) is among the first twenty of the chemical elements most widespread on our planet [3]. In addition, the chemical composition of many calcium orthophosphates includes hydrogen, as an acidic orthophosphate anion (for example, HPO_4^{2-} or $H_2PO_4^-$), hydroxide (for example, $Ca_{10}(PO_4)_6(OH)_2$) and/or incorporated water (for example, $CaHPO_4{\cdot}2H_2O$). Diverse combinations of CaO and P_2O_5 (both in the presence of water and without it) provide a large variety of calcium phosphates, which are distinguished by the type of the phosphate anion: ortho- (PO_4^{3-}), meta- (PO_3^-), pyro- ($P_2O_7^{4-}$) and poly- ($(PO_3)_n^{n-}$). In the case of multi-charged anions (orthophosphates and pyrophosphates), calcium phosphates are also differentiated by the number of hydrogen ions attached to the anion. Examples include mono- ($Ca(H_2PO_4)_2$), di- ($CaHPO_4$), tri- ($Ca_3(PO_4)_2$) and tetra- ($Ca_2P_2O_7$) calcium phosphates [4-6]. However, only calcium orthophosphates will be reviewed in this paper.

The atomic arrangement of calcium orthophosphates is built up around a network of orthophosphate (PO_4) groups, which gives stability to the entire structure. The vast majority of calcium orthophosphates are sparingly soluble in water; however, all of them are easily soluble in acids but insoluble in alkaline solutions. All chemically pure calcium orthophosphates are crystals of white color and moderate hardness. However, natural

[14] As a mineral species, apatite was first recognized by the father of German geology Abraham Gottlob Werner (1750 – 1817) in 1786 and named by him from the Greek απατώ (apato) – "to mislead" or "to deceive", because it had previously been mistaken for other minerals, such as beryl, tourmaline, chrysolite, amethyst, fluorite, *etc.*

minerals of calcium orthophosphates are always colored due to impurities, the most widespread of which are ions of iron and rare earth elements. Biologically formed calcium orthophosphates are the major component of all mammalian calcified tissues [7], while natural calcium orthophosphates are the major raw material to produce phosphorus-containing fertilizers [8-11].

2. Geological and Biological Occurrence of Calcium Orthophosphates

Calcium orthophosphates are abundant in both nature and living organisms. Geologically, natural calcium orthophosphates are found in different regions mostly as deposits of apatites (mainly as natural fluorapatite (FA), chemical formula $Ca_{10}(PO_4)_6F_2$) or phosphorites [9,12]. The chemical composition of the latter cannot be described so easily. As phosphorites belong to sedimentary deposits, their general appearance and the chemical composition vary a lot. It is a common practice to consider francolite (or carbonate-hydroxyfluorapatite regarded as its synonym) as the basic phosphorite mineral [12-16]. A cryptocrystalline (almost amorphous) variety of francolite (partly of a biological origin) is called collophane (synonyms: collophanit, collophanita, collophanite, grodnolite, kollophan) [17]. It occurs in natural phosphorites predominantly as fossil bones and phosphatized microbial pseudomorphs: phosphatic crusts of chasmolithic biofilms (or microstromatolites) and globular clusters with intra-particular porosities [18]. Natural phosphorites (therefore, francolite and collophane as well) occur in various forms, such as nodules, crystals, or masses. Occasionally, other types of natural calcium orthophosphates are found as minerals, for example clinohydroxylapatite [19] and staffelite (synonyms: staffelit, staffelita) belonging to carbonate-rich fluorapatites (chemical formula: $Ca_5[(F,O)|(PO_4,CO_3)_3]$) [20]. The world deposits of natural calcium orthophosphates are estimated to exceed 150 billion tons; from which approximately 85 % belong to phosphorites and the remaining ~15 % belong to apatites [12].

Natural calcium orthophosphates occur in most geological environments usually as accessory minerals (< 5 %). Concentrations sufficient for economic use (> 15 %) are also available. The largest world deposits of natural apatites are located in Russia (the Khibiny and Kovdor massifs, Kola peninsula), Brazil and Zambia, while the largest world deposits of natural phosphorites are located in Morocco, Russia, Kazakhstan, USA (Florida, Tennessee), China and Australia, as well as in the oceans [8-12]. Most of natural calcium orthophosphates occur as small polycrystals. Larger crystals usually have the crystal structure of apatites (hexagonal system, space group $P6_3/m$). Giant crystals including "a solid but irregular mass of green crystalline apatite, 15 feet long and 9 feet wide" and a single euhedral crystal from the Aetna mine measuring 2.1 × 1.2 m with an estimated weight of 6 tons were found [13,14]. None of them is a pure compound; they always contain admixtures of other elements. For example, ions of calcium might be partially replaced by Sr, Ba, Mg, Mn, K, Na, Fe; ions of orthophosphate may be partly replaced by AsO_4^{3-}, CO_3^{2-} and VO_4^{3-} [21]; ions of hydroxide, chloride, bromide, carbonate and oxide may to a certain extent substitute fluoride in the crystal lattice of natural apatites [15]. In principle, the crystal structure of apatites can incorporate half the periodic chart in its atomic arrangement. These substitutions are usually in trace concentrations but large concentrations and even complete solid solutions exist for certain substituents (*e.g.*, F^- and OH^-). This might be related to the fact that the apatite structure type displays porous properties [22]. To make things even more complicated, some ions in the crystal structure may be missing, leaving the crystallographic defects, which leads to formation of non-stoichiometric compounds. Figure 1 shows examples of polycrystalline and single-crystalline samples of natural FA.

Manufacturing of elementary phosphorus (white and red), phosphoric acids, various phosphorus-containing chemicals and, especially, agricultural fertilizers (namely, superphosphate, ammonium orthophosphates) is the major industrial application of natural calcium orthophosphates. This consumes up to 85% of the world production of natural calcium orthophosphates. The total capacity of industrial plants in the world exceeds 25 million tons (as P_2O_5) of phosphate fertilizers per year with the annual increase of 2–3 % [9].

In biological systems, many organisms, ranging from isolated cells to invertebrates and vertebrates, synthesize calcium orthophosphates. Formation of calcium orthophosphates in primitive organisms is believed to enable the storage and regulation of essential elements such as calcium, orthophosphate and possibly magnesium. The morphology of precipitates in these organisms (small intracellular nodules of amorphous calcium phosphates often located in mitochondria) complies with the necessities for rapid mobilization and intracellular control of the concentration of these elements [23]. In vertebrates calcium orthophosphates occur as the principal inorganic constituent of normal (bones, teeth, fish enameloid, deer antlers and some species of shells) and pathological (dental and urinary calculus and stones, atherosclerotic lesions) calcifications [4,24-29]. Except for small portions of the inner ear, all hard tissue of the human body is formed of calcium orthophosphates.

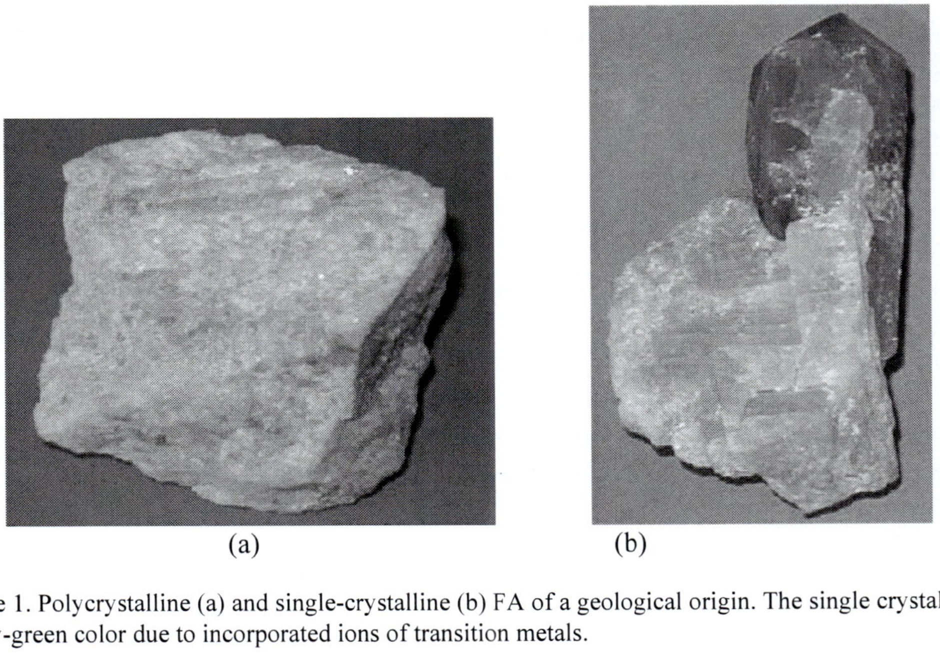

(a) (b)

Figure 1. Polycrystalline (a) and single-crystalline (b) FA of a geological origin. The single crystal has a grey-green color due to incorporated ions of transition metals.

Structurally, they occur mainly in the form of poorly crystallized non-stoichiometric Na-, Mg- and carbonate-containing hydroxyapatite (often called biological apatite[15] or dahllite[16]). The main constituents of human bones are calcium orthophosphates (~50-60 wt%), collagen[17] (~30-40 wt%) and water (up to 10 wt%) [28,33-35]. Detailed information on the chemical composition of the most important human normal calcified tissues is comprised in Table 1. One should note that the values mentioned in Table 1 are approximate; the main constituents can vary by a percent or more [36].

Table 1. Comparative composition and structural parameters of inorganic phases of adult human calcified tissues. Due to the considerable variation found in biological samples, typical values are given in these cases [4,35]

Composition, wt%	Enamel	Dentin	Cementum	Bone	HA
Calcium[a]	36.5	35.1	[c]	34.8	39.6
Phosphorus (as P)[a]	17.7	16.9	[c]	15.2	18.5
Ca/P (molar ratio)[a]	1.63	1.61	[c]	1.71	1.67
Sodium[a]	0.5	0.6	[c]	0.9	–
Magnesium[a]	0.44	1.23	[c]	0.72	–
Potassium[a]	0.08	0.05	[c]	0.03	–
Carbonate (as CO_3^{2-})[b]	3.5	5.6	[c]	7.4	–
Fluoride[a]	0.01	0.06	[c]	0.03	–
Chloride[a]	0.30	0.01	[c]	0.13	–
Pyrophosphate (as $P_2O_7^{4-}$)[b]	0.022	0.10	[c]	0.07	–
Total inorganic[b]	97	70	50	65	100
Total organic[b]	1.5	20	35	25	–
Water[b]	1.5	10	15	10	–
Crystallographic properties: Lattice parameters (± 0.003 Å)					
a-axis, Å	9.441	9.421	[c]	9.41	9.430
c-axis, Å	6.880	6.887	[c]	6.89	6.891
Crystallinity index, (HA=100)	70 – 75	33 – 37	[c]	33 – 37	100
Typical crystal sizes (nm) [242,283,285]	100 μm ×50×50	35×25×4	[c]	50×25×4	200 – 600
Ignition products (800 °C)	β-TCP + HA	β-TCP+ HA	β-TCP+ HA	HA + CaO	HA
Elastic modulus (GPa)	80	15	[c]	0.34 – 13.8	10
Tensile strength (MPa)	10	100	[c]	150	100

[a] Ashed samples.
[b] Unashed samples.
[c] Numerical values were not found in the literature but they should be similar to those for dentin.

[15] Occasionally "biological apatite" is called "bioapatite" [30-32].

[16] There are reports that dahllite belongs to the francolite group. Natural dahllite might be a rock forming mineral. For example, it is found in some phosphorite concretions of Podolia. In addition, it is found in both massive and accretionary crustal phosphorites [16].

[17] Collagens are fibrous, insoluble proteins found in the connective tissues, including skin, bone, ligaments and cartilage.

3. The Members of Calcium Orthophosphate Family

In the ternary system $Ca(OH)_2 - H_3PO_4 - H_2O$ [37,38] there are eleven[18] known non-ion-substituted calcium orthophosphates with the Ca/P molar ratio within 0.5 and 2.0 (Table 2). The most important parameters are the molar Ca/P ratio, basicity/acidity and solubility. These parameters strongly correlate with the solution pH. The lower the Ca/P molar ratio is, the more acidic and water-soluble the calcium orthophosphate is [4-6]. Due to the tripotic equilibrium that exists within orthophosphate-containing solutions, variations in pH alter the relative concentrations of the 4 polymorphs of orthophosphoric acid (Figure 2) and thus both the chemical composition and the amount of the calcium orthophosphates that forms by direct precipitation [43]. The solubility isotherms of different calcium orthophosphates are available in literature [44]. A brief description of all calcium orthophosphates is given below. Table 3 comprises their crystallographic data [45].

MCPM (monocalcium phosphate monohydrate, $Ca(H_2PO_4)_2{\cdot}H_2O$; the chemically correct name is calcium dihydrogen phosphate monohydrate) is both the most acidic and water-soluble compound. It precipitates from highly acidic solutions that are normally used in industry of phosphorus-containing fertilizer production ("triple superphosphate") [9]. At temperatures above 100 °C, it releases a molecule of water and transforms into MCPA. Due to high acidity and solubility, MCPM is never found in biological calcifications. Moreover, pure MCPM is not biocompartible[19] with bone [46]. However, in medicine MCPM is used as a component of several self-hardening calcium orthophosphate cements [47-49].

In addition, MCPM is used as a nutrient, acidulant and mineral supplement for dry baking powders, food, feed and some beverages [50]. Coupled with $NaHCO_3$, MCPM is used as a leavening agent for both dry baking powders and bakery dough. MCPM might be added to salt-curing preserves, pickled and marinated foods.

---

[18] In literature occasionally one might find notes on the 12th calcium orthophosphate, namely oxyapatite (Ca10(PO4)6O). A mixture of oxyapatite and HA might be prepared by dehydration of HA at temperatures exceeding ~900°C (e.g., during plasma-spray of HA) only in the absence of water vapor [5,6,39,40]. It also might be crystallized in glass-ceramics [41]. It has the hexagonal space group symmetry $P\bar{6}$ (174) of cesanite type [42], while the space group symmetry for partially dehydrated HA was found to change from hexagonal P63/m to triclinic $P\bar{1}$ when more than ca. 35% of the structurally bound water had been removed [40]. Oxyapatite is very reactive and transforms to HA in contact with water vapor [39]. Oxyapatite is still very poorly known; however, the following data on the solubility constant (Ks ~ 10-69 at 25°C) are available [5].

[19] Biocompatibility is the ability of a material to perform with an appropriate host response in a specific application [51].

Table 2. Properties of the biologically relevant calcium orthophosphates. The solubility is given as the logarithm of the ion product of the given formulae (excluding hydrate water) with concentrations in mol/l [44,266]

Ca/P Molar ratio	Compound	Formula	Solubility at 25 °C, –log(K_s)	Solubility at 37 °C, –log(K_s)	pH stability range in aqueous solutions at 25°C
0.5	Monocalcium phosphate monohydrate (MCPM)	$Ca(H_2PO_4)_2 \cdot H_2O$	1.14	data not found	0.0–2.0
0.5	Monocalcium phosphate anhydrous (MCPA)	$Ca(H_2PO_4)_2$	1.14	data not found	[c]
1.0	Dicalcium phosphate dihydrate (DCPD), mineral brushite	$CaHPO_4 \cdot 2H_2O$	6.59	6.63	2.0–6.0
1.0	Dicalcium phosphate anhydrous (DCPA), mineral monetite	$CaHPO_4$	6.90	7.02	[c]
1.33	Octacalcium phosphate (OCP)	$Ca_8(HPO_4)_2(PO_4)_4 \cdot 5H_2O$	96.6	95.9	5.5–7.0
1.5	α-Tricalcium phosphate (α-TCP)	α-$Ca_3(PO_4)_2$	25.5	25.5	[a]
1.5	β-Tricalcium phosphate (β-TCP)	β-$Ca_3(PO_4)_2$	28.9	29.5	[a]
1.2–2.2	Amorphous calcium phosphate (ACP)	$Ca_xH_y(PO_4)_z \cdot nH_2O$, n = 3–4.5; 15–20% H_2O	[b]	[b]	~5–12 [d]
1.5–1.67	Calcium-deficient hydroxyapatite (CDHA)	$Ca_{10-x}(HPO_4)_x(PO_4)_{6-x}(OH)_{2-x}$ ($0<x<1$)	~85.1	~85.1	6.5–9.5
1.67	Hydroxyapatite (HA or OHAp)	$Ca_{10}(PO_4)_6(OH)_2$	116.8	117.2	9.5–12
1.67	Fluorapatite (FA or FAp)	$Ca_{10}(PO_4)_6F_2$	120.0	119.2	7–12
2.0	Tetracalcium phosphate (TTCP or TetCP), mineral hilgenstockite	$Ca_4(PO_4)_2O$	38–44	37–42	[a]

[a] These compounds cannot be precipitated from aqueous solutions.

[b] Cannot be measured precisely. However, the following values were found: 25.7±0.1 (pH=7.40), 29.9±0.1 (pH=6.00), 32.7±0.1 (pH=5.28) [95]. The comparative extent of dissolution in acidic buffer is: ACP >> α-TCP >> β-TCP > CDHA >> HA > FA [35].

[c] Stable at temperatures above 100°C.

[d] Always metastable.

Table 3. Crystallographic data of calcium orthophosphates [5,42,160]

Compound	Space group	Unit cell parameters	Z[a]	Density, g cm^{-3}
MCPM	triclinic $P\bar{1}$	a=5.6261(5), b=11.889(2), c=6.4731(8) Å, α=98.633(6)°, β=118.262(6)°, γ=83.344(6)°	2	2.23
MCPA	triclinic $P\bar{1}$	a=7.5577(5), b=8.2531(6), c=5.5504(3) Å, α=109.87(1)°, β=93.68(1)°, γ=109.15(1)°	2	2.58
DCPD	monoclinic *I*a	a=5.812(2), b=15.180(3), c=6.239(2) Å, β=116.42(3)°	4	2.32
DCPA	triclinic $P\bar{1}$	a=6.910(1), b=6.627(2), c=6.998(2) Å, α=96.34(2)°, β=103.82(2)°, γ=88.33(2)°	4	2.89
OCP	triclinic $P\bar{1}$	a=19.692(4), b=9.523(2), c=6.835(2) Å, α=90.15(2)°, β=92.54(2)°, γ=108.65(1)°	1	2.61
α-TCP	monoclinic $P2_1$/a	a=12.887(2), b=27.280(4), c=15.219(2) Å, β=126.20(1)°	24	2.86
β-TCP	rhombohedral *R*3cH	a=b=10.4183(5), c=37.3464(23) Å, γ=120°	21[b]	3.08
HA	monoclinic $P2_1$/b or hexagonal $P6_3$/m	a=9.84214(8), b=2a, c=6.8814(7) Å, γ=120° (monoclinic) a=b=9.4302(5), c=6.8911(2) Å, γ=120° (hexagonal)	4 2	3.16
FA	hexagonal $P6_3$/m	a=b=9.367, c=6.884 Å, γ=120°	2	3.20
TTCP	monoclinic $P2_1$	a=7.023(1), b=11.986(4), c=9.473(2) Å, β=90.90(1)°	4	3.05

[a] Number of formula units per unit cell.

[b] Per the hexagonal unit cell.

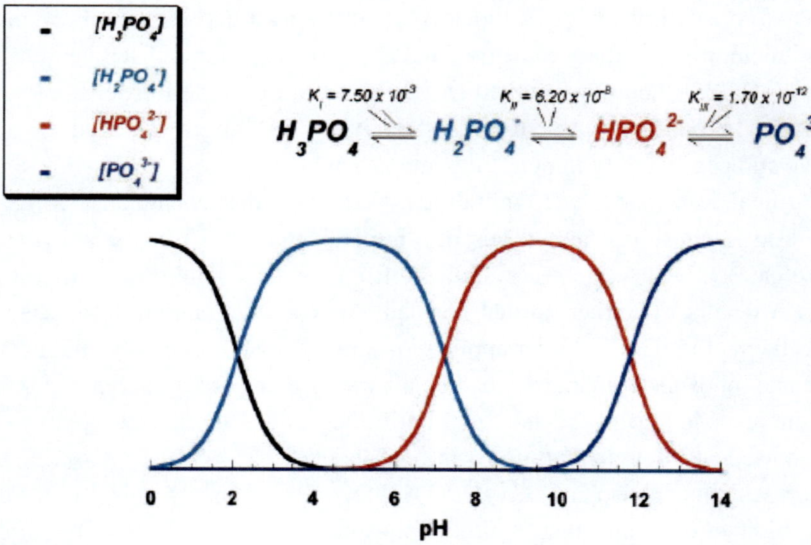

Figure 2. pH variation of ionic concentrations in tripotic equilibrium for phosphoric acid solutions. Reprinted from Ref. [43] with permission.

According to the European classification of food additives MCPM is marked as E341 additive. Occasionally, MCPM is added to tooth pastes. In addition, MCPM might be added to ceramics and glasses, while agriculture is the main consumer of a technical grade MCPM, where it is used as a fertilizer [9,50].

MCPA (monocalcium phosphate anhydrous, $Ca(H_2PO_4)_2$; the chemically correct name is calcium dihydrogen phosphate anhydrous) is the anhydrous form of MCPM. It crystallizes under the same conditions as MCPM but at temperatures above 100 °C (*e.g.*, from highly concentrated mother liquors during fertilizer production). Like MCPM, MCPA never appears in calcified tissues and is not biocompartible due to its acidity. There is no current application of MCPA in medicine. Due to the similarity with MCPM, in many cases MCPA might be used instead of MCPM [9,50]; however, highly hydroscopic properties of MCPA reduces its commercial application.

DCPD (dicalcium phosphate dihydrate, $CaHPO_4 \cdot 2H_2O$; the chemically correct name is calcium hydrogen phosphate dihydrate; the mineral brushite[20]) can be easily crystallized from aqueous solutions. It transforms into DCPA at temperatures above 80 °C. DCPD is of biological importance because it is often found in pathological calcifications (dental calculi, crystalluria, chondrocalcinosis [4,24,25] and urinary stones [26]) and some carious lesions. It has been proposed as an intermediate in both bone mineralization and dissolution of enamel in acids (dental erosion) [4,24-26]. In medicine, DCPD is used in calcium phosphate cements [48,52-56] and as an intermediate for tooth remineralization. DCPD is added to toothpaste both for caries protection (in this case, it is coupled with F-containing compounds such as NaF and/or Na_2PO_3F) and as a gentle polishing agent [57-61]. Other applications are: a flame retardant [62], a slow release fertilizer, glass production, as well as calcium supplement in

---

[20] To honor Prof. George Jarvis Brush (1831–1912), an American mineralogist, Yale University, New Haven, Connecticut, USA.

food, feed and cereals [50]. In food industry, it serves as a texturizer, bakery improver and water retention additive. In diary industry, DCPD is used as a mineral supplement. If added to food products, DCPD should be marked as E341 according to the European classification of food additives. In addition, plate-like crystals of DCPD might be used as a non-toxic, anticorrosive and passivating pigment for some ground coat paints.

DCPA (dicalcium phosphate anhydrous, $CaHPO_4$; the chemically correct name is calcium hydrogen phosphate anhydrous; the mineral monetite[21]) is the anhydrous form of DCPD. Like DCPD, DCPA can be crystallized from aqueous solutions but at 100 °C. Unlike DCPD, DCPA occurs in neither normal nor pathological calcifications. It is used in calcium phosphate cements [55,63-67]. Other applications include using as a polishing agent, a source of calcium and phosphate in nutritional supplements (*e.g.,* in prepared breakfast cereals, enriched flour and noodle products), a tabletting aid and a toothpaste component [50]. In addition, it is used as a dough conditioner in food industry.

OCP (octacalcium phosphate, $Ca_8(HPO_4)_2(PO_4)_4{\cdot}5H_2O$; the chemically correct name is octacalcium bis(hydrogenphosphate) tetrakis(phosphate) pentahydrate [45]) is often found as an unstable transient intermediate during the precipitation of the thermodynamically more stable calcium orthophosphates (*e.g.*, CDHA) in aqueous solutions. Its preparation technique might be found elsewhere [68-71]. Structurally OCP consists of apatitic layers (with atomic arrangements of calcium and orthophosphate ions similar to those of HA) separated by hydrated layers (with atomic arrangements of calcium and orthophosphate ions similar to those of DCPD) [4-6,72]. OCP is of a great biological importance because it is one of the stable components of human dental and urinary calculi [73-75]. OCP was first proposed by W. E. Brown [76] to participate as the initial phase in enamel mineral formation and bone formation through subsequent precipitation and stepwise hydrolysis of OCP was proposed [77]. It plays an important role in *in vivo* formation of apatitic biominerals. A "central OCP inclusion" (also known as "central dark line") is seen by transmission electron microscopy in many biological apatites and in some synthetically precipitated HA [78-81]. Although OCP has not been observed in vascular calcifications, it has been strongly suggested as a precursor phase to biological apatite found in natural and prosthetic heart valves [82,83]. In surgery, OCP is used for implantation into bone defects [84-87]. For the comprehensive information on OCP, the readers are referred to a monograph [75].

β-TCP (β-tricalcium phosphate, β-$Ca_3(PO_4)_2$; the chemically correct name is calcium phosphate tribasic beta) cannot be precipitated from aqueous solutions. It is a high temperature phase of calcium orthophosphates, which only can be prepared by thermal decomposition, *e.g.* of CDHA, at temperatures above 800 °C. Apart from the chemical preparation routes, ion-substituted β-TCP can be prepared by calcining of bones: such type of β-TCP is occasionally called "bone ash".

At temperatures above ~ 1125 °C, it transforms into the high-temperature phase α-TCP. Being the stable phase at room temperature, β-TCP is less soluble in water than α-TCP (Table 2). Pure β-TCP never occurs in biological calcifications. Only the Mg-substituted form called whitlockite[22] (β-TCMP – β-tricalcium magnesium phosphate, β-$(Ca,Mg)_3(PO_4)_2$) is found in

---

[21] For Moneta (now Monito) Island, which contains a notable occurrence.

[22] In 1941, to honor Mr. Herbert Percy Whitlock (1868–1948), an American mineralogist, the curator of the American Museum of Natural History, New York City, New York, USA, the term whitlockite was coined as a

dental calculi and urinary stones [4,24-26,91], dentinal caries, salivary stones, arthritic cartilage, as well as in some soft-tissue deposits [4,24-26]. In biomedicine, β-TCP is used in calcium phosphate bone cements [92-95]. In combination with HA, β-TCP forms a biphasic calcium phosphate (BCP)[23] [98-107]. Both β-TCP [108] and BCP [98-107] are widely used as a bone substitution bioceramics. Pure β-TCP is added to some brands of toothpaste as a gentle polishing agent. Multivitamin complexes with calcium orthophosphate are widely available in the market and β-TCP is used as the calcium phosphate there. In addition, it serves as a texturizer, bakery improver and anti-clumping agent for dry powdered food (flour, milk powder, dried cream, cocoa powder). In addition, β-TCP is added as a dietary or mineral supplement to food and feed, where it is marked as E341 according to the European classification of food additives. Occasionally, it might be used as inert filler in pelleted drugs. Other applications comprise porcelains, pottery, enamel, using as a component for mordants and ackey, as well as a polymer stabilizer [50]. β-TCP of a technical grade (as either calcined natural phosphorites or bone dust) is used as a slow release fertilizer for acidic soils [9].

α-TCP (α-tricalcium phosphate, α-$Ca_3(PO_4)_2$; the chemically correct name is calcium phosphate tribasic alpha) is usually prepared from β-TCP at heating above ~ 1125 °C and it might be considered as a high temperature phase of β-TCP. However, at the turn of the millennium, the previously forgotten data that the presence of silicates stabilized α-TCP at lower temperatures of 800 – 1000 °C [109] has been rediscovered again. Such type of α-TCP is called "silicon stabilized α-TCP" [110-115].

Although α-TCP and β-TCP have exactly the same chemical composition, they differ by the crystal structure (Table 3) and solubility (Table 2). In addition, β-TCP is more stable than the α-phase [116]. Therefore, of them, α-TCP is more reactive in aqueous systems, has a higher specific energy and it can be hydrolyzed to a mixture of other calcium phosphates. It never occurs in biological calcifications but in medicine chemically pure α-TCP is occasionally used in calcium phosphate cements [48,53-56,65-67,117]. Pure α-TCP has received not much interest in the biomedical field. The disadvantage for using α-TCP is its quick resorption rate, which limits its application in this area. However, the silicon stabilized α-TCP (more precisely as a biphasic composite with HA) has been commercialized as a starting material to produce bioresorbable porous ceramic scaffolds to be used as artificial bone grafts [108,110-114]. Theoretical insights into bone grafting properties of the silicon-stabilized α-TCP might be found in Ref. [118]. Surface and adsorption properties of α-TCP are available in Ref. [119]. α-TCP of a technical grade might be used as a fertilizer [50].

ACP (amorphous calcium phosphate, $Ca_xH_y(PO_4)_z{\cdot}nH_2O$, n = 3–4.5; 15–20% H_2O) is often encountered as a transient phase during the formation of calcium orthophosphates in aqueous systems. Usually, ACP is the first phase precipitated from a supersaturated solution

---

synonym for β-TCP identified by its X-ray diffraction pattern in phosphate rocks [88]. Therefore, strictly speaking, β-TCMP should be called as a "magnesium whitlokite". An iron-containing whitlockite with chemical formula $Ca_9(Mg,Fe^{2+})(PO_4)_6(PO_3,OH)$ exists in nature: is a relatively rare natural mineral but is found in granitic pegmatite and has also been found in meteorites. It can form small, but distinct and well-formed crystals [89,90].

[23] The term biphasic calcium phosphate (BCP) was first used by Nery *et. al.* [96] to describe the bioceramic, that consisted of a mixture of HA and β-TCP, based on the X-ray diffraction analysis which showed that the 'tricalcium phosphate" preparation material used in their early publication [97] was in fact a mixture of 20% HA and 80% β-TCP.

prepared by rapid mixing of solutions containing ions of calcium and orthophosphate [5,120-125]. ACP is thought to be formed at the beginning of the precipitation due to a lower surface energy than that of OCP and HA [121]. The amorphization level of ACP increases with the concentration increasing of Ca- and PO_4-containing solutions, as well as at a high solution pH and a low crystallization temperature. A continuous gentle agitation of as precipitated ACP in the mother solution, especially at elevated temperatures, results in a slow recrystallization and formation of better crystalline compounds, such as CDHA [4,5]. The chemical composition of ACP strongly depends on the solution pH and the concentrations of mixing solutions. For example, ACP with Ca/P ratios in the range of 1.18 (precipitated at solution pH=6.6) to 1.53 (precipitated at solution pH=11.7) [5,126] and even to 2.5 [4,24,25] have been described. The presence of ions of pyrophosphate, carbonate and/or magnesium in solution during the crystallization promotes formation of ACP and slows down its further transformation into more crystalline calcium orthophosphates, while the presence of fluoride has the opposite effect [4-6,35,127].

As all amorphous compounds are characterized by a lack of the long-range order, it is problematic to discuss the crystal structure of ACP (it is X-ray amorphous). Concerning the short-range order in ACP, it is uncertain either, because it depends on the preparation conditions, storage, admixtures, *etc.* Infra red spectra of ACP show broad featureless phosphate absorption bands. Electron microscopy of ACP usually shows featureless nearly spherical particles with diameters in the range of 20 to 200 nm. However, there is a questionable opinion that ACP has an apatitic structure but with a crystal size so small, that it is X-ray amorphous. This is supported by X-ray absorption spectroscopic data (EXAFS) on biogenic and synthetic samples [128-131]. On the other hand, it was proposed that the basic structural unit of ACP is a 9.5 Å diameter, roughly spherical cluster of ions with the composition $Ca_9(PO_4)_6$ [5,126]. These clusters were found experimentally as first nuclei during the crystallization of HA and a model was developed to describe the crystallization of HA as a step-wise assembly of these units [132] (see HA below). Biologically, ACP (often containing ions of Na, Mg, carbonate and pyrophosphate) is found in soft-tissue pathological calcifications (*e.g.*, heart valve calcifications of uremic patients) [4,24-26]. In medicine, pure ACP is used in calcium phosphate cements [53-55] and as a filling material in dentistry. Bioactive composites of ACP with polymers have properties suitable for use in dentistry [133-136] and surgery [137-140]. Due to a reasonable solubility and physiological pH of aqueous solutions, ACP appeared to be consumable by some microorganisms and for this reason it might be added as a mineral supplement to culture media. Non-biomedical applications of ACP comprise its using as a component for mordants and ackey. In food industry, ACP is used for syrup clearing. Occasionally, it might be used as inert filler in pelleted drugs. In addition, ACP is used in glass and pottery production and as a raw material for production of some organic phosphates. A good review on ACP is available in literature [141].

CDHA (calcium-deficient hydroxyapatite, $Ca_{10-x}(HPO_4)_x(PO_4)_{6-x}(OH)_{2-x}$ ($0<x<1$)) can be easily prepared by simultaneous addition of calcium- and orthophosphate-containing solutions into boiling water followed by boiling the suspension for several hours. During this time, initially precipitated ACP is restructured and transformed into CDHA[24]. Therefore, there are many similarities in the structure, properties and application between the precipitated in alkaline solutions (pH > 8) ACP and CDHA. CDHA crystals are poorly crystalline and of submicron dimensions. It has a very large specific surface area, typically 25-100 m^2/g. On heating above 700 °C, dry CDHA with Ca/P = 1.5 will convert to β-TCP and that with 1.5 < Ca/P < 1.67 will convert into a mixture of HA and β-TCP (the above-mentioned BCP) [98-106]. A reasonable solid-state mechanism of a high-temperature transformation of CDHA into BCP has been proposed [145,146].

The variability in Ca/P molar ratio of CDHA has been explained through different models: surface adsorption, lattice substitution and intercrystalline mixtures of HA and OCP [147]. Due to a lack of stoichiometry, CDHA usually contains other ions [23]. The extent depends on the counter-ions of the chemicals used for preparation (*e.g.*, Na^+, Cl^-). Direct determinations of the CDHA structures are still missing and the unit cell parameters remain uncertain. However, the long-range order exists and the following lattice parameters have been reported for formate (HCO_2^-) containing CDHA with Ca/P = 1.596 (ionic): *a*=9.4729(20) and *c*=6.8855(9) Å. Ca^{2+} ions were lost exclusively from Ca2 sites, while the PO_4 tetrahedron volume and P–O bonds were 4.4% and 1.4% smaller, respectively, than those in HA [148].

As a first approximation, CDHA may be considered as HA with some ions missing [149]. According to the chemical formula of CDHA (Table 2), there are vacancies of Ca^{2+} (mainly on Ca2 sites [148,150,151]) and OH^- ions in crystal structure of this compound. However, nothing is known about the vacancies of orthophosphate ions: in CDHA, a portion of PO_4^{3-} ions is either protonated (as HPO_4^{2-}) or substituted by other ions (*e.g.*, CO_3^{2-}) [152]. Theoretical investigations of the defect formation mechanism relevant to nonstoichiometry in CDHA are available elsewhere [153].

Unsubstituted CDHA (*i.e.* containing ions of Ca^{2+}, PO_4^{3-}, HPO_4^{2-} and OH^- only) does not exist in biological systems. The ion substituted CDHA: Na^+, K^+, Mg^{2+}, Sr^{2+} for Ca^{2+}; CO_3^{2-} for PO_4^{3-} or HPO_4^{2-}; F^-, Cl^-, CO_3^{2-} for OH^-, plus some water forms biological apatite – the main inorganic part of animal and human normal and pathological calcifications [4,23,24]. Therefore, CDHA is a very promising compound for industrial manufacturing of artificial bone substitutes. Non-biomedical applications of CDHA are similar to those of ACP. Very recently, CDHA was found to possess a catalytic activity to produce biogasoline [154].

HA (or OHAp) (hydroxyapatite[25], $Ca_5(PO_4)_3(OH)$, but is usually written as $Ca_{10}(PO_4)_6(OH)_2$ to denote that the crystal unit cell comprises two molecules) is the second most stable and least soluble calcium orthophosphate after FA. Chemically pure HA crystallizes in the monoclinic space group $P2_1/b$ [155]. However, at temperatures above 250 °C, there is a monoclinic to hexagonal phase transition in HA (space group $P6_3/m$) [5,45,126,156,157]. The detailed description of the HA structure was first reported in 1964 [158] and its interpretation in terms of aggregation of $Ca_9(PO_4)_6$ clusters, the so-called Posner's clusters, has been widely used since publication of the article by Posner and Betts

---

[24] In some research papers, CDHA is defined as "precipitated HA" [142-144].

[25] It is worth noting that the chemically correct name would be *hydroxylapatite* (perhaps, *hydroxidapatite* would be even better because it relates to calcium hydroxide) while by the medical and material communities it is usually called as *hydroxyapatite*.

[159]. Some impurities, like partial substitution of hydroxide by fluoride or chloride, stabilize the hexagonal structure of HA at ambient temperature. For this reason, the very rare single crystals of natural HA always exhibit a hexagonal space group. The crystal structure of HA is well described elsewhere [160], the detailed analysis of the electronic structure, bonding, charge transfer and optical properties are also available [161,162], while the readers interested in Posner's clusters are referred to other papers [163-166]. A shell model has been developed to study the lattice dynamics of HA [167].

Several techniques might be utilized for HA preparation; they can be divided into solid-state reactions and wet methods [168], which include precipitation, hydrothermal and hydrolysis of other calcium orthophosphates. HA can be prepared in aqueous solutions by mixing exactly stoichiometric quantities of Ca- and PO_4-containing solutions at pH > 9, followed by boiling for several days in CO_2-free atmosphere (the ageing or maturation stage), filtration, drying and, usually, sintering at about 1000 °C [169]. As the first precipitates are rich in non-apatitic environments (see ACP and CDHA), the ageing stage appears to be very important: the Ca/P molar ratio of 1.67 was found to attain in as little as 5 hours after the completion of the reaction at 90°C [170]. The surface of freshly precipitated HA is composed of a structured hydrated layer containing easily exchangeable mobile ionic species [171]. Usually unsintered HA is poorly crystalline and often non-stoichiometric, resembling the aforementioned CDHA. However, highly crystalline HA can be prepared from an aqueous solution [172]. Microcrystalline samples of HA can also be prepared by solid-state reaction of other calcium phosphates (e.g. MCPM, DCPA, DCPD, OCP) with CaO, $Ca(OH)_2$, or $CaCO_3$ at temperatures above 1200 °C in an atmosphere of equal volumes of water and nitrogen. HA can be prepared by hydrothermal synthesis [5,126,173]. A water-free synthesis can be performed in ethanol from $Ca(OEt)_2$ (Et=ethyl) and H_3PO_4 [174,175]. In addition, HA might be prepared by mechanochemical synthesis of a dry mixture of CaO and DCPD [176] or from coral skeletal carbonate by hydrothermal exchange [177,178]. Relatively large single crystals of HA might be prepared from those of chlorapatite [179] or by recently developed controlled homogeneous precipitation method [180]. Lower sized particles of HA might be prepared by a pyrosol technique, where an aerosol, containing calcium and orthophosphate ions in the adequate ratio, is transported to a furnace where the pyrolisis takes place [181]. Synthesis of nanosized HA has also been described [182,183], while the chronological development of nanosized HA synthesis might be found in another paper [184]. Two-dimensional nanocrystalline HA might be also synthesized [185]. Space-grown and terrestrial HA crystals were found to differ in size: the former appeared to be at least 1-1.5 orders of magnitude bigger in length [186,187]. Transparent HA ceramics might be prepared as well [188-191]. The detailed information on HA synthesis is available elsewhere [192-197]. In addition, there are good reviews on HA solubility, crystal growth and intermediate phases of HA crystallization [198], as well as on HA dissolution [199]. The electronic and crystallographic structures of apatites might be found in another paper [161].

Pure HA never occurs in biological systems. However, due to the chemical similarities to bone and teeth mineral (Table 1), HA is widely used as a coating on orthopedic (*e.g.*, hip joint prosthesis) and dental implants [200-206]. HA particles might be implanted as well [207]. A calcium phosphate cement with HA has been developed [52]. Due to a great similarity to biological apatite, over a long time HA has been used in liquid chromatography of nucleic acids, proteins and other biological compounds [208-215] and for drug delivery purposes [216,217]. Also, HA is added to some brands of toothpaste as a gentle polishing agent instead of calcium carbonate. Besides, it might be used as an environmentally friendly filler for elastomers [218], a sorbent of poisonous chemical elements [219] and a carrier for the catalyst [220,221]. To conclude this topic, one should mention on other reviews devoted to HA and its biomedical application [222-227].

FA (or FAp) (fluorapatite, $Ca_5(PO_4)_3F$, but is usually written as $Ca_{10}(PO_4)_6F_2$ to denote that the crystal unit cell comprises two molecules) is the hardest (5 according to the Mohs' scale of mineral hardness), most stable and least soluble compound among all calcium orthophosphates (Table 2). Perhaps, such "extreme" properties of FA are related to the specific position of F^- ions in the center of Ca2 triangles of the crystal structure [45]. Due to its properties, FA is the only calcium orthophosphate that naturally forms large deposits suitable for the commercial use [8-11] (see also Figure 1). Preparation techniques of the chemically pure FA are similar to the aforementioned ones for HA but the synthesis must be performed in presence of the necessary amount of F^- ions (usually, NaF or NH_4F is added). Under some special crystallization conditions, FA might form unusual dumbbell-like fractal morphology that finally closed to spheres (Figure 3) [228-233]. A hierarchical structure for FA was proposed [234]. The crystal structure of FA is well described elsewhere [160], while the detailed analysis of the electronic structure, bonding, charge transfer and optical properties is also available [162]. In addition, there are reviews on FA solubility [198] and the dissolution mechanism [199].

FA easily forms solid solutions with HA with any desired F/OH molar ratio. Such compounds are called fluorhydroxyapatites (FHA) or hydroxyfluorapatites (HFA) and described with a chemical formula $Ca_{10}(PO_4)_6(OH)_{2-x}F_x$, where $0<x<2$. If the F/OH ratio is either uncertain or not important, the chemical formula of FHA and HFA is often written as $Ca_{10}(PO_4)_6(F,OH)_2$. The lattice parameters, crystal structure, solubility and other properties of FHA and HFA lay in between of those for the chemically pure FA and HA [235-239].

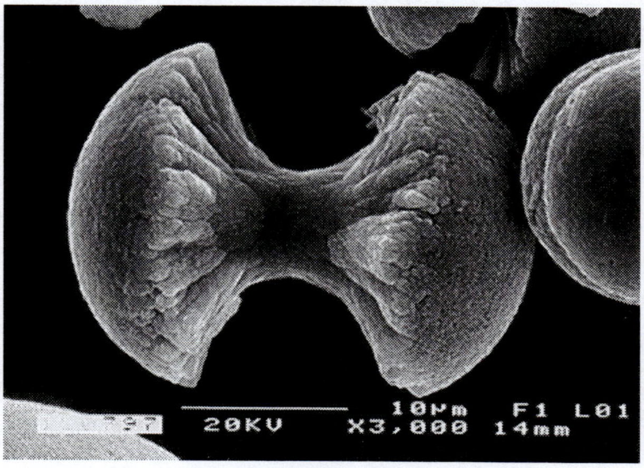

Figure 3. A biomimetically grown aggregate of FA that was crystallized in a gelatin matrix. Its shape can be explained and simulated by a fractal growth mechanism. Scale bar: 10 μm (taken from Ref. [229] with permission).

Similar to pure HA, pure FA never occurs in biological systems. Obviously, a lack of the necessary amount of toxic fluorides (the acute toxic dose of fluoride is ~5 mg/kg of body weight) in living organisms is the main reason of this fact (pure FA contains 3.7 % mass. F). Enameloid of shark teeth [35,240-245] and some exoskeletons of mollusks [246] seem to be the only exclusions because they contain substantial amounts of FA. Among all normal calcified tissues of humans, the highest concentration of fluorides is found in bones and the lowest – in dental enamel[26] (Table 1). However, even in bones, the total amount of fluorides is not enough to form FA; it is generally considered that the inorganic part of bones consists of ion-substituted CDHA. Due to the lowest solubility, good chemical stability and toxicity of high amounts of fluorides, chemically pure FA is rarely used as a bone substituting material [253]. However, due to the ability to form FHA and/or HFA, minor amounts of fluorides might be intentionally added to calcium orthophosphate biomaterials [254-260]. The effect of fluoride contents in FHA on both osteoblast behavior [261] and leukemia cells proliferation [262] has been described.

TTCP (or TetCP) (tetracalcium phosphate $Ca_4(PO_4)_2O$; the mineral hilgenstockite[27]) is the most basic calcium orthophosphate. However, its solubility in water is higher than that of HA (Table 2). TTCP cannot be precipitated from aqueous solutions. It can be prepared only by a solid-state reaction above 1300 °C, *e.g.*, by heating homogenized equimolar quantities of DCPA and $CaCO_3$ in dry air, or in a flow of dry nitrogen [5,126,265]. This reaction should be carried out in a dry atmosphere, in vacuum or with rapid cooling (to prevent uptake of water and formation of HA). TTCP is not very stable in aqueous solutions: it slowly hydrolyses to HA and calcium hydroxide [5,126]. Consequently, TTCP is never found in biological calcifications. In medicine, TTCP is widely used for preparation of various self-setting calcium phosphate cements [44,49,52,53,63,266]; however, to the best of my knowledge, there is no commercial bone-substituting product consisting solely of TTCP.

There is an opinion [45], that the aforementioned calcium orthophosphates might be classified into three major structural types: (i) the apatite type, $Ca_{10}(PO_4)_6X_2$, which includes HA, FA, CDHA, OCP and TTCP; (ii) the glaserite type, named after the mineral glaserite, $K_3Na(SO_4)_2$, which includes all polymorphs of TCP and, perhaps, ACP; (iii) the Ca-PO_4 sheet-containing compounds, which include DCPD, DCPA, MCPM and MCPA. However, a closer examination of the structures would reveal that all calcium orthophosphates, listed above, can be included as distorted glaserite type structures, but with varying degrees of distortion [45].

To conclude this part, one should briefly mention on carbonateapatite [267-271], chlorapatite [272,273] and various ion-substituted calcium orthophosphates [23]. Usually, they are of a non-stoichiometric nature and there are too many of them to be mentioned in one review; therefore, the readers are referred to books and monographs [4-

[26] The amount of fluorides on the very surface of dental enamel might be increased by using fluoride-containing toothpastes and mouthwashes [247-250]. Fluoride-containing toothpastes and mouthwashes are widely used in practice due to the well-known anti-cariogenic effect of fluorides that is related to the solubility decreasing [251,252].

[27] To honor a German metallurgist Gustav Hilgenstock (1844 - 1913), who first discovered it in Thomas slags nearly 120 years ago [263,264].

6,8,10,15,35,126,223,227]. In addition, there is a very good review, in which the structures of more than 75 chemically different apatites have been discussed [42].

It is interesting to note, that chemical elements not found in natural bones can be intentionally incorporated into calcium orthophosphate biomaterials to get special properties. For example, addition of Ag^{+} [274,275], Zn^{2+} and Cu^{2+} [275] has been used for imparting antimicrobial effect, while radioactive isotopes of ^{90}Y [276], ^{153}Sm [277,278,279] and ^{186}Re [277] have been incorporated into HA bioceramics and injected into knee joints to treat rheumatoid joint synovitis [276,277,279]. More to the point, apatites were found to be able to incorporate individual molecules, such as water, oxygen and carbon dioxide [23].

4. Biological Hard Tissues of Calcium Orthophosphates

Biological mineralization (biomineralization) is the process of *in vivo* formation of inorganic minerals [242,243]. As shown in Table 1 and discussed above, in the body of mammals the vast majority of both normal and pathological calcifications consist of ion-substituted calcium orthophosphates, mainly of apatitic structure [28]. At the element scale, bone apatite nanocrystals exhibit a variety of substitutions and vacancies that make the Ca/P molar ratio distinct from the stoichiometric HA ratio of 1.67. The impurities in biological apatite of bones and teeth introduce significant stresses into the crystal structure, which make it less stable and more reactive. Among all substituting ions, the presence of 4–8% of carbonates instead of orthophosphate anions (so called, B-type substitution [4-6,271]) and of 0.5–1.5 % of Mg is of the special importance because it leads to large lattice strain and significantly increases the solubility [280]. High concentrations of magnesium and carbonates in bone or dentin compared with enamel (Table 1) may explain a higher solubility and a lower crystallinity (smaller crystal size) of bone or dentin compared with enamel. In addition, the crystals of biological apatite are always very small which also increases its solubility when compared with that for the chemically pure HA and even CDHA [23]. Small dimensions and a low crystallinity are two distinct features of biological apatite, which, combined with their non-stoichiometric composition, inner crystalline disorder and presence of other ions in the crystal lattice, allow explaining their special behavior. For example, the small crystal size means that a large percentage of the atoms are on the surface of the crystal, providing a large specific surface area for sorption of ions, proteins and drugs [281]. The major properties of biological apatite are summarized in Figure 4.

The calcium orthophosphate nature of bones was first determined in 1926 [282]. Nowadays, according to Weiner and Wagner: "the term bone refers to a family of materials, all of which are built up of mineralized collagen fibrils" [283,284].

For mammals, this family of materials includes dentin – the material that constitutes the inner layers of teeth, cementum – the thin layer that binds the roots of teeth to the jaw, deer antlers and some other materials [283,285]. It is worth noting, that bones and teeth contain almost 99% of the total body calcium and about 85% of the total body phosphorus that amounts to a combined mass of approximately 2 kg in an average person [286,287]. In addition, it is important to recognize that calcium orthophosphates of bones are by no means inert; they play an important role in the metabolic functions of the body.

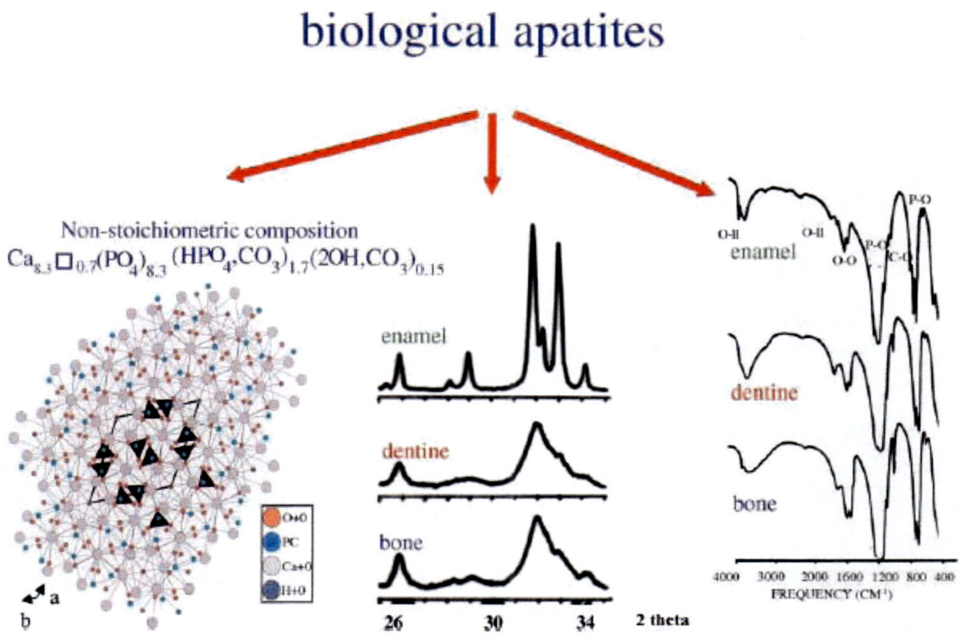

Figure 4. Crystal structure of biological apatite. Powder X-ray diffraction patterns and infrared spectra of enamel, dentine and bone. Reprinted from Ref. [281] with permission.

The recent data on the physico-chemical and crystallographic study of biological apatite have been reviewed elsewhere [288]. Besides, there is a comprehensive review on the application of surface science methods to study the properties of dental materials and related biomaterials [289].

4.1. Bone

Bone, also called osseous tissue (Latin: *os*), is a type of hard endoskeletal connective tissue found in many vertebrate animals. All bones of a single animal are, collectively, known as the skeleton. True bones are present in bony fish (osteichthyes) and all tetrapods. Bones support body structures, protect internal organs and in conjunction with muscles facilitate movement [290]. In addition, bones are also involved with cell formation, calcium metabolism and act for mineral storage. From the material point of view, bone is a complicated composite containing both inorganic (Table 1) and biological compounds (chiefly, collagen) [291-296]. The inorganic to biological ratio is approximately 75% to 25% by weight and 65% to 35% by volume. This ratio not only differs among animals, among bones in the same animal and over time in the same animal but also it exerts a major control on the material properties of bone, such as its toughness, ultimate strength and stiffness. In general, load-bearing ability of bones depends on not only architectural properties, such as cortical thickness and bone diameter, but also intrinsic, size-independent, material properties such as porosity, level of mineralization, crystal size and properties derived from the organic phase of bone [297]. A higher mineral to collagen ratio typically yields stronger, but more brittle, bones [298-300]. For example, bone from the leg of a cow has a relatively high concentration of calcium orthophosphates (for support), whereas bone from the antler of a deer has a relatively high concentration of collagen (for flexibility) [28]. It is interesting to note, that bone exhibits several physical properties such as piezoelectricity [301] and pyroelectricity [302].

Stability of the mineral composition of bones has a very long history: calcium orthophosphates were found in dinosaur fossils [303-306]. Therefore, organisms have had a great deal of time to exploit the feedback between composition and structure in apatite, on the one hand, and benefit from its biological functionality, on the other. Bones of modern animals is a relatively hard and lightweight porous composite material, formed mostly of biological apatite (*i.e.*, CDHA with ionic substitutions). It has relatively high compressive strength but poor tensile strength [307]. While bone is essentially brittle, it has a degree of significant plasticity contributed by its organic components. Usually bone is composed of a relatively dense outer layer (cortical or compact bone) covering an internal mesh-like structure (average porosity of 75–95%) of cancellous (other terms: spongy, trabecular) bone, the density of which is about 0.2 g/cm^3 but it may vary at different points (Figure 5). Cortical bone makes up a large portion of skeletal mass; but due to its high density (~ 1.80 g/cm^3) it has a low surface area. Cancellous bone has an open meshwork or honeycomb-like structure. It has a relatively high surface area but forms a smaller portion of the skeleton. Bone is a porous material with the pore sizes range from 1 to 100 μm in normal cortical bone and 200 to 400 μm in trabecular bone. 55 to 70% of the pores in trabecular bone are interconnected [4,24,25,33-35,242,283,292-296,308-311].

Bone can be either woven or lamellar. The fibers of woven bone are randomly aligned and as the result have a low strength. In contrast, lamellar bone has parallel fibers and is much stronger. Woven bone is put down rapidly during growth or repair but as growth continues, it is often replaced by lamellar bone. The replacement process is called "secondary bone formation" and described in details elsewhere [312 and references therein]. In addition, bones might be long, short, flat and irregular. The sizes and shapes of bones reflect their function. Namely, broad and flat bones, such as scapulae, anchor large muscle masses, flat skull bones protect the brain, ribs protect the lungs, pelvis protects other internal organs, short tubular bones in the digits of hands and feet provide specific grasping functions, hollow and thick-walled tubular bones, such as femur or radius, support weight and long bones enable locomotion [313,314]. Long bones are tubular in structure (*e.g.*, the tibia). The central shaft of a long bone is called the diaphysis and has a medullar cavity filled with bone marrow (Figure 5). Surrounding the medullar cavity is a thin layer of cancellous bone that also contains marrow. The extremities of the bone are called the epiphyses and are mostly cancellous bone covered by a relatively thin layer of compact bone. Short bones (*e.g.*, finger bones) have a similar structure to long bones, except that they have no medullar cavity. Flat bones (*e.g.*, the skull and ribs) consist of two layers of compact bone with a zone of cancellous bone sandwiched between them. Irregular bones (*e.g.*, vertebrae) do not conform to any of the previous forms. All bones contain living cells embedded in a mineralized organic matrix that makes up the main bone material [313,314]. The structure of bone is most easily understood by differentiating between 7 levels of organization because bone exhibits a strongly hierarchical structure (Figure 6) [223,242,283,291-296,301-306,308-311,315-317].

The mechanical properties of bone reconcile high stiffness and high elasticity in a manner that is not yet possible with synthetic materials. Cortical bone specimens have been found to have tensile strength in the range of 78.8–151.0 MPa in longitudinal direction and 51.0–56.0 MPa in transversal direction.

Bone's elasticity is also important for its function giving the ability to the skeleton to withstand impact. Estimates of modulus of elasticity of bone samples are of the order of 17.0–20.0 GPa in longitudinal direction and of 6.0–13.0 GPa in the transversal direction [318]. The elastic properties of bone were successfully modeled at the level of mineralized collagen fibrils via step-by-step homogenization from the staggered arrangement of collagen molecules up to an array of parallel mineralized fibrils [319]. Recent investigations revealed that bone deformation was not homogeneous but distributed between a tensile deformation of the fibrils and a shearing in the interfibrillar matrix between them [320,321].

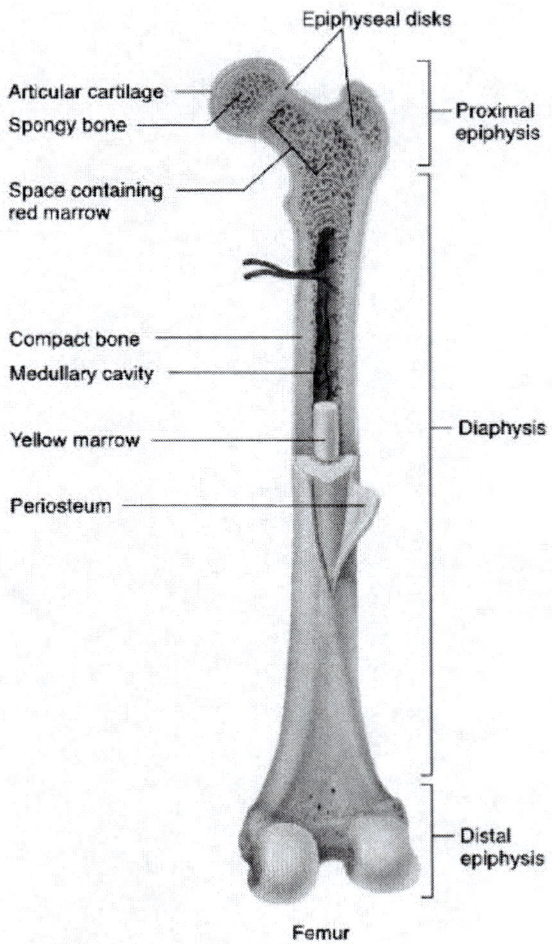

Figure 5. General structure of a mammalian bone. Other very good graphical sketches of the structure of a mammalian bone are available in Refs. [28,281].

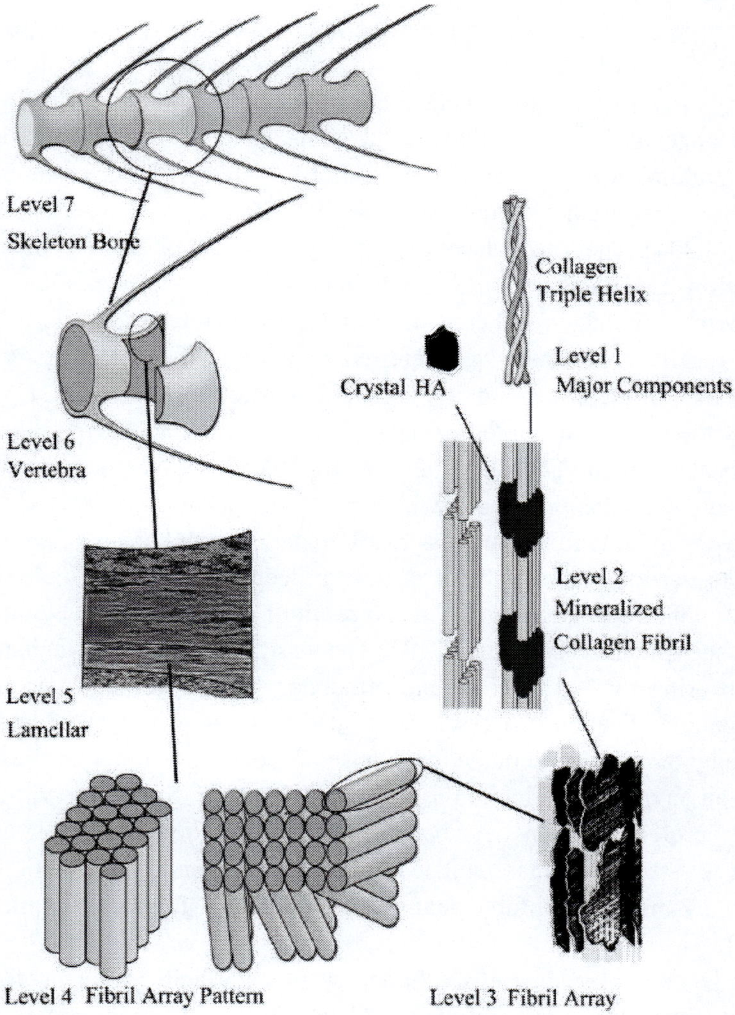

Figure 6. The seven hierarchical levels of organization of the zebrafish skeleton bone. Level 1: Isolated crystals and part of a collagen fibril with the triple helix structure. Level 2: Mineralized collagen fibrils. Level 3: The array of mineralized collagen fibrils with a cross-striation periodicity of nearly 60–70 nm. Level 4: Two fibril array patterns of organization as found in the zebrafish skeleton bone. Level 5: The lamellar structure in one vertebra. Level 6: A vertebra. Level 7: Skeleton bone. Reprinted from Ref. [332] with permission.

Nanoscopically, the constituting building blocks of bone are mineralized collagen fibrils of 80 to 100 nm thickness and a length of a few to tens of microns. These are composites of biological apatite and molecules of type I collagen [28,283,291,322]. Some evidences for direct physical bonding between the collagen fibers and apatite crystals in bone were found [323]. Eppell *et al.* used atomic force microscopy to measure the crystallites of mature cow bone [324]. They are always platelet-like (elongated along the crystallographic *c*-axis) and very thin [27,325-327], with remarkably uniform thicknesses (determined in transmission electron microscopy) of 2–4 nm (just a few unit cells thick – see Table 1)[28].

[28] Due to the nanoscopic dimensions, biological apatite is occasionally called "nano-apatite" [283].

The nanocrystals of biological apatite exist in bones not as discrete aggregates but rather as a continuous phase, which is indirectly evidenced by a very good strength of bones. This results in a very large surface area facing extracellular fluids, which is critically important for the rapid exchange of ions with these fluids. The nanocrystals of biological apatite are inserted in a parallel way into the collagen fibrils, while the latter are formed by self-assembly[29] of collagen triple helices [283,291,329-332] using the self-organization mechanism [333,334]. The lowest level of hierarchical organization of bone has successfully been simulated by HA precipitation on peptide-amphiphile nanofibers [334]. Unfortunately, the interface between collagen and crystals of biological apatite is still poorly understood; for the available details, the readers are referred to a review devoted to the structure and mechanical quality of the collagen/mineral nano-composite of bones [322]. There is still no clear idea why the crystals of biological apatite are platelet-shaped even though dahllite has hexagonal crystal symmetry [242,283,292-296,301-306,308-311]. One possible reason is that they grow via an OCP transition phase, which crystals are plate-shaped [283].

The processes of bone formation (ossification) and growth are very complicated ones and it is difficult to describe them without making a deep invasion into biology. Briefly, it is considered that bones appear and grow as the result of calcification (or biomineralization) of connective tissues, mainly cartilage [312]. The ossified tissue is invaginated with blood vessels, which bring ions of calcium and orthophosphate to be deposited in the ossifying tissue. The biomineralization process is controlled to some extent by cells and the organic matrices made by those cells facilitate the deposition of crystals. Initially, the mineral crystals are formed in an environment rich in the so-called SIBLING (Small Integrin-Binding LIgand N-linked Glycoprotein) proteins. As bone crystals grow, there is greater association with proteins, such as osteocalcin, that regulate remodeling. Thus, *in vivo* formation of hard tissues always occurs by mineral reinforcement of the previously formed network of soft tissues [312-314,332].

Cartilage is composed of cells (chondrocytes and their precursor forms known as chondroblasts), fibers (collagen and elastic fibers) and extracellular matrix (proteoglycans, which are a special class of heavily glycosylated glycoproteins) [335-337]. The initial stage involves the synthesis and extracellular assembly of the collagen matrix framework of fibrils. At the second stage, the chondrocytes calcify the matrix before undergoing the programmed cell death (apoptosis). At this point, blood vessels penetrate this calcified matrix, bringing in osteoblasts, which use the calcified cartilage matrix as a template to build bone, thus completing ossification [335-337].

During ossification, the crystals of biological apatite grow with a specific crystalline orientation – the *c*-axes of the crystals are roughly parallel to the long axes of the collagen fibrils within which they are deposited [283,285-289,292-294,312]. Probably, this process occurs via epitaxial growth mechanism [338]. The same is true for dentin and enamel [339,340] (see below), as well as for more primitive living organisms. For example, in the shell of the fossil mollusk *Lingula unguis* that consists of biological apatite, the crystal *c*-axes are oriented parallel to the β-chitin fibrils [246,341-343]. Therefore, the orientation of

[29] Self-assembling is the autonomous organization of components into patterns or structures without human intervention. It is considered that self-assembling processes are common throughout nature and technology [328].

biological apatite crystals parallel to the long axes of the organic framework could be a general feature of calcium orthophosphate biomineralization. However, the degree of biological apatite orientation appears to be a useful parameter to evaluate *in vivo* stress distribution, nano-scale microstructure and the related mechanical function, the regenerative process of the regenerated bone and to diagnose bone diseases such as osteoarthritis [344,345]. It is interesting to note, that contrary to what might be expected in accordance with possible processes of dissolution, formation and remineralization of hard tissues, no changes in phase composition of mineral part, crystal sizes (length, width and thickness) and arrangement of crystals on collagen fibers were detected in abnormal (osteoporotic) human bones compared to the normal ones [346].

Unlike other mineralized tissues, bone continuously undergoes a remodeling process, as it is resorbed by specialized cells called osteoclasts and formed by another type of cells called osteoblasts (so called "bone lining cells") in a delicate equilibrium [312,347,348]. The purpose of remodeling is the release of calcium and the repair of micro-damaged bones from everyday stress. Osteoblasts contain alkaline phosphatase – this is a weak base. It acts as a local pH increaser, which results in precipitation of biological apatite. In addition, there is one more type of the cells called osteocytes that originate from osteoblasts, which have migrated into, become trapped and surrounded by bone matrix, which they themselves produce [292-295,312-314].

If osteoblasts can be described as bone forming cells, the osteoclasts can be described as bone destroying cells because osteoclasts mature and migrate to discrete bone surfaces [347,348]. Upon arrival, active enzymes, such as acid phosphatase, are secreted against the mineral substrate that causes dissolution. This process, called bone resorption, allows stored calcium to be released into systemic circulation and is an important process in regulating calcium balance [347,348]. The iteration of remodeling events at the cellular level is influential on shaping and sculpting the skeleton both during growth and afterwards. That is why mature bone consists of a very complex mesh of bone patches, each of which has both a slightly different structure and a different age [242,283,285-289,292-294,312]. The interested readers are suggested to read a review on the interaction between biomaterials and osteoclasts [349].

Still there is no general agreement on the chemical mechanism of bone formation. It is clear that the inorganic part of bone consists of biological apatite, *i.e.* CDHA with ionic substitutions but without the detectable amounts of hydroxide [350-355]. However, various *in vitro* experiments on precipitation of CDHA and HA revealed that none of these compounds is directly precipitated from supersaturated aqueous solutions containing calcium and orthophosphate ions: some intermediate phases (precursors) are always involved [4,24,25,78-83,120-124]. Depending on the both solution pH and crystallization conditions, three calcium orthophosphates (DCPD, ACP and OCP) are discussed as possible precursors of CDHA precipitation *in vitro*. For this reason, the same calcium orthophosphates are suggested as the precursors of biological apatite formation *in vivo*.

The transient nature of the precursor phase of bone, if it exists at all, makes it very difficult to detect, especially *in vivo* [356]. However, in 1966 W. Brown proposed that OCP was the initial precipitate that then acted as a template upon which biological apatite nucleates [77]. This idea was extended in his further investigations [357-360]. The principal support for this concept derived from the following: (i) the close structural similarity of OCP and HA [361]; (ii) formation of interlayered single crystals of OCP and HA (pseudomorphs of OCP); (iii) the easier precipitation of OCP compared with HA; (iv) the apparent plate- or lath-like habit of biological apatites that does not conform to hexagonal symmetry, but looks like a pseudomorph of triclinic OCP; (v) the presence of HPO_4^{2-} in bone mineral, particularly in newly formed bones [288]. Some evidences supporting this idea were found using high-resolution transmission electron microscopy: computer-simulated lattice images of the "central dark line" in mineralized tissues revealed that it consisted of OCP [78-80]. Additional evidences of OCP to HA transformation, including a mechanistic model for central dark line formation, were obtained very recently [362].

Simultaneously with Brown, the research group led by A. Posner proposed that ACP was the initially precipitated phase of bone and dentin mineral formation *in vivo*, thus explaining the non-stoichiometric Ca/P ratio in bones and teeth [363-365]. This conclusion was drawn from the following facts: (i) when calcium orthophosphates are prepared by rapid precipitation from aqueous solutions containing ions of calcium and orthophosphate at pH > 8.5, the initial solid phase is amorphous; (ii) mature bone mineral is composed of a mixture of ion-substituted ACP and poorly crystallized ion-substituted CDHA; (iii) early bone mineral has a lower crystallinity than mature bone and the observed improvement in crystallinity with the age of the bone mineral is a result of a progressive reduction in the ACP content [288,363-371]. However, there are thermodynamic data proving that the transition of freshly precipitated ACP into CDHA involves intermediate formation of OCP [372,373]. Recently the discovery of a stable amorphous calcium carbonate in sea urchin spines [374] reawakened the suggestion that a transient amorphous phase might also exist in bone [312,375,376]. The modern points of view on the bone formation mechanisms have been summarized in a recent excellent review [312], where the interested readers are referred.

The maturation mechanism of bone minerals is not well established, mainly because of the difficulty involved in the nanostructural analyses of bone minerals [312,377]. Only indirect evidences for the *in vivo* bone mineral maturation are available. For example, X-ray diffraction patterns of bones from animals of different age show that the reflections become sharper with age increasing [32,378]. This effect is more pronounced in the crystallographic *a*-axis [(310) reflections] as compared to the *c*-axis [(002) reflections] [379,380]. In addition, other changes like an increase of Ca^{2+} content and a decrease of HPO_4^{2-} occur in bone mineral with age [381-384]. Both the crystal sizes and carbonate content were found to increase during aging in rats and cows [382,383]. From a chemical point of view, these changes indicate to a slow transformation of poorly crystallized non-apatitic calcium orthophosphates into a better-crystallized ion-substituted CDHA [237]. While there are still many gaps in our knowledge, the researchers seem to be comfortable in stating that in all but the youngest bone and dentin, the only phase present is a highly disordered, highly substituted biological apatite.

Occasionally, a debate relates to the question on whether bone formation is an active or a passive biomineralization process. Briefly, an "active process" means the assembly of calcium orthophosphate nanocrystals into bones due to an activity of the suitable cells (*e.g.*, osteoblasts), *i.e.* within a matrix vesicle. Such structures have been discovered by transmission electron microscopy for bone and teeth formation [385,386]. A "passive process" does not require involvement of cells and means mineralization from supersaturated solutions with respect to the precipitation of biological apatite. In the latter case, thermodynamically, biomineralization might occur at any suitable nucleus. The collagen fibrils have a specific structure with a 67 nm periodicity and 35–40 nm gaps or holes between the ends of the collagen molecules where bone mineral is incorporated in the mineralized fibril [242,283,284,313,314]. Such a nucleation within these holes would lead to discrete crystals with a size related to the nucleating cavity in the collagen fibril. It was proposed that a temporary absence of the specific inhibitors might regulate the process of bone formation [387-389].

To conclude the bone subject, let us briefly mention on the practical application of bones. Cut and polished bones from a variety of animals are sometimes used as a starting material for jewelry and other crafts. Ground cattle bone is occasionally used as a fertilizer. In the Stone Age, bone was used to manufacture art, weapons, needles, catchers, amulets, pendants, headdresses, *etc*.

4.2. Teeth

Teeth (singular: tooth) are dense structures found in the jaws of many vertebrates. They have various structures to allow them to fulfill their different purposes. The primary function of teeth is to tear, smell and chew food, while for carnivores it is also a weapon. Therefore, teeth have to withstand a range of physical and chemical processes, including compressive forces (up to ~ 700 N), abrasion and chemical attack due to acidic foods or products of bacterial metabolism [289]. The roots of teeth are covered by gums. From the surface teeth are covered by enamel of up to ~ 2 mm thick at the cutting edges of the teeth, which helps to prevent cavities on the teeth. The biggest teeth of some gigantic animals (elephants, hippopotamuses, walruses, mammoths, narwhals, *etc.*) are known as tusks or ivory.

Similar to the various types of bones, there are various types of teeth. The shape of the teeth is related to the animal's food, as well as its evolutionary descent. For example, plants are hard to digest, so herbivores have many molars for chewing. Carnivores need canines to kill and tear and since meat is easy to digest, they can swallow without the need for molars to chew the food well. Thus, the following types of teeth are known: molars (used for grinding up food), carnassials (used for slicing food), premolars (small molars), canines (used for tearing apart food) and incisors (used for cutting food). While humans only have two sets of teeth, some animals have many more: for example, sharks grow a new set of teeth every two weeks. Some other animals grow just one set during the life, while teeth of rodents grow and wear away continually through the animal gnawing, maintaining constant length [390,391].

Similar to bones, the inorganic part of teeth also consist of biological apatite [392]. The stability of the mineral composition of teeth also has a very long history: namely, calcium orthophosphates were found in fossil fish teeth [393]. Recent investigations of biological apatite from fossil human and animal teeth revealed its similarity to the modem biological apatite [394].

The structure of teeth appears to be even more complicated than that of bone (Figure 7). Unlike bone, teeth consist of at least two different materials: enamel that is a hard outer layer consisting of calcium orthophosphates and dentin, which is a bone-like inner layer, the bulk of the tooth.

In addition, there is a thin layer around the tooth roots called cementum – it covers the anatomic root of the tooth. Cementum is a bone-like material similar to dentin, which connects the teeth to the jaw. Finally, there is the core called pulp (commonly called "the nerve") – it is a remnant of the embryologic organ for tooth development and contains nerves and blood vessels necessary for tooth function (Figure 7) [313,314,390,391]. Both dentin and cementum are mineralized connective tissues with an organic matrix of collagenous proteins, while the inorganic component of them consists of biological apatite. As shown in Table 1, dentin, cementum and bone are quite similar and for general purposes of material scientists they can be regarded as being essentially the same material[30] [5,126,242,283,285-289,292-296,301,302,304-306,308-311,322,326,327,329,381,382]. Thus, most statements made in the previous chapter for bone are also valid for dentin and cementum; however, unlike bones, both dentin and cementum lack vascularization.

Dental enamel is the outermost layer of teeth. It is white and translucent and its true color might be observed at the cutting edges of the teeth only. Enamel is highly mineralized and acellular, so it is not a living tissue. Nevertheless, it is sufficiently porous for diffusion and chemical reactions to occur within its structure, particularly acidic dissolution (dental caries) and remineralization from saliva (possible healing of caries lesions). Enamel is the hardest substance in the body [307] and forms a solid, tough and wear-resistant surface for malaxation. In the mature state, it contains up to 98 % of inorganic phase (Table 1). The crystals of biological apatite of enamel are much larger as evidenced by higher crystallinity (reflecting greater crystal size and perfection) demonstrated in their X-ray diffraction patterns, than those of bone and dentin. Besides, enamel apatite has fewer ionic substitutions than bone or dentin mineral and more closely approximates the stoichiometric HA [313]. The organic phase of enamel does not contain collagen. Instead, enamel has two unique classes of proteins called amelogenins and enamelins. While the role of these proteins is not fully understood yet, it is believed that both classes of proteins aid in the enamel development by serving as a framework support [390,391,395]. The large amount of minerals in enamel accounts not only for its strength but also for its brittleness. Dentin, which is less mineralized and less brittle, compensates for enamel and is necessary as a support [390,391].

Shark enameloid is an intermediate form bridging enamel and dentin. It has enamel-like crystals of fluoridated biological apatite associated with collagen fibrils [23,240-245]. Due to the presence of fluorides, biological apatite of shark enameloid shows both higher crystal sizes and a more regular hexagonal symmetry if compared to non-fluoridated biological apatite of bones and teeth [35]. Similar correlation between the presence of fluorides and crystal dimensions was found for enamel [396].

Like that for bones, 7 levels of structural hierarchy have been also discovered in human enamel; moreover, the analysis of the enamel and bone hierarchical structure suggests similarities of the scale distribution at each level [397].

---

[30] Strictly speaking, there are some differences. For example, the hardness of live dentin is less than that of enamel but is greater than that of bone or cementum. When pulp of the tooth dies or is removed by a dentist, the properties of dentin change: it becomes brittle, liable to fracture and looses a reparative capability.

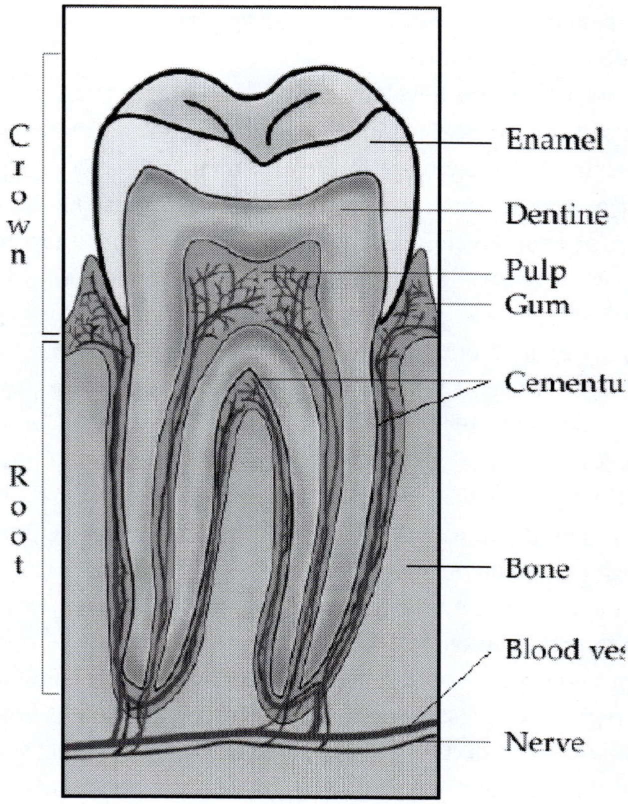

Figure 7. A schematic picture of a tooth.

The basic unit of enamel is called an enamel rod (formerly called an enamel prism), which is a tightly packed mass of biological apatite in an organized pattern. Each rod traverses uninterrupted through the thickness of enamel. They number 5 to 12 million rods per crown. The rods increase in diameter (4 up to 8 microns) as they flare outward from the dentin-enamel junction (DEJ). Needle-like enamel rods might be tens of microns long (up to 100 μm) but sometimes only 50 nm wide and 30 nm thick (Figure 8) [390,391,398-405]. They are quite different from the much smaller crystals of dentin and bone (Table 1), but all of them consist of biological apatite [230,406,407]. In cross section, an enamel rod is best compared to a keyhole, with the top, or head, oriented toward the crown of the tooth and the bottom, or tail, oriented toward the root of the tooth. Enamel is a selectively permeable membrane, allowing water and certain ions to pass via osmosis [390,391].

The arrangement of the crystals of biological apatite within each enamel rod is highly complex. Enamel crystals in the head of the enamel rod are oriented parallel to the long axis of the rod. When found in the tail of the enamel rod, the crystals' orientation diverges slightly from the long axis [390,391]. The arrangement of the enamel rods is understood more clearly than their internal structure. Enamel rods are found in rows along the tooth (Figure 8) and, within each row, the long axis of the enamel rod is generally perpendicular to the underlying dentin [390,391,398-402].

Recent AFM study indicated that CDHA crystals in enamel exhibited regular subdomains or subunits with distinct chemical properties related to topographical features and gave rise to patterned behavior in terms of the crystal surface itself and the manner in which it responded to low pH [408].

The *in vivo* formation and development of teeth appears to be even more complicated when compared with the afore-described process of bone formation. It is a very complex biological process, by which teeth are formed from embryonic cells, grow and erupt into the mouth. For human teeth enamel, dentin and cementum must all be developed during the appropriate stages of fetal development. Primary (baby) teeth start to form between the sixth and eighth weeks *in utero*, while the permanent teeth begin to form in the twentieth week *in utero* [390,391]. Recent data confirmed the necessity of calcium orthophosphates in the diet of pregnant and nursing mother to prevent early childhood dental caries [409].

As teeth consist of at least two materials with different properties (enamel and dentin), the tooth bud (sometimes called "the tooth germ" – that is an aggregation of cells that eventually forms a tooth) is organized into three parts: the enamel organ, the dental papilla and the dental follicle. The enamel organ is composed of at least four other groups of cells (for the biological details see Refs. [390,391]). Altogether, these groups of cells give rise to ameloblasts, which secret enamel matrix proteins.

The protein gel adjacent to ameloblasts is supersaturated with calcium orthophosphates, which leads to the precipitation of biological apatite. Similarly, the dental papilla contains cells that develop into odontoblasts, which are dentin-forming cells. The dental follicle gives rise to three important entities: cementoblasts, osteoblasts and fibroblasts. Cementoblasts form the cementum of a tooth. Osteoblasts give rise to the alveolar bone around the roots of teeth (see bone formation above). Fibroblasts develop the periodontal ligaments that connect teeth to the alveolar bone through cementum [313,314,390,391].

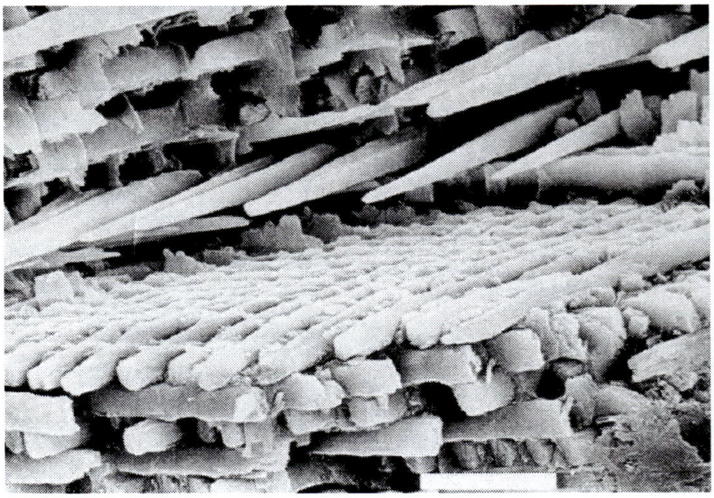

Figure 8. Scanning electron micrograph of the forming enamel of a continuously growing rat incisor showing ordered rods of calcium orthophosphates. Scale bar: 10 μm (taken from Ref. [242] with permission).

The first detectable crystals in enamel formation are flat thin ribbons [400-402], that were reported to be OCP [308,410-412], β-$(Ca,Mg)_3(PO_4)_2$ [411] or DCPD [350,353]. The crystallization process of enamel is different from that for bone or dentin: amelogenin being hydrophobic self-assembles into nanospheres that guide the growth of the ribbon-like dental enamel crystals. During maturation of enamel, the mineral content increases from initially ~45 wt. % up to ~98-99 wt. % [350,390,391]. The enamel crystal rods widen and thicken by additional growth [350,353,413] with a simultaneous increase of the Ca/P molar ratio [413] and a decrease in carbonate content [414-416], finally resulting in the most highly mineralized and hardest substance produced by vertebrates. It is interesting to note that in the radular teeth of chitons, ACP was found to be the first-formed calcium orthophosphate mineral, which over a period of weeks was transformed to dahllite [417].

The crystal faces expressed in enamel are always (100) face and at the ends presumably (001) [418,419], which are the ones usually found in HA. The centers of enamel crystals contain a linear structure known as the "central dark line" (this line was also observed in bone and dentin), which consists of OCP [78-81]. As described above for bones, X-ray diffraction shows that the crystals of younger dentin are less crystalline than those of more mature dentin [381]. Therefore, maturation of dentin also means a slow transformation of biological calcium orthophosphates from ion-substituted ACP to a better-crystallized ion-substituted CDHA.

The development of individual enamel and dentin crystals was studied by high-resolution transmission electron microscopy [420-422]. Both processes appear to be roughly comparable and were described in a four-step process. The first two steps include the initial nucleation and formation of nanometer-sized particles of biological apatite. They are followed by ribbon-like crystal formation, which until recently was considered as the first step of biological crystal formation [420-422]. These complicated processes, starting with the heterogeneous nucleation of inorganic calcium orthophosphates on an organic extracellular matrix, are controlled in both tissues by the organic matrix and are under cellular control [423]. To complicate the process even further, regular and discrete domains of various charges or charge densities on the surface of CDHA crystals derived from the maturation stage of enamel development were recently discovered by a combination of atomic and chemical force microscopy [424]. Binding of organic molecules (e.g., amelogenin [424]) at physiological solution pH appears to occur on the charged surface domains of CDHA.

The dentin-enamel junction (DEJ)[31] is the interface between the dentin and enamel. It is the remnant of the onset of enamel formation because enamel grows outwards from this junction [391,425,426]. The major steps of enamel crystal growth at the junction have been described above but the mechanism of the junction formation is still debatable. Some authors claim that the enamel crystals grow epitaxially on the pre-existing dentin crystals because of a high continuity between enamel and dentin crystals [427-429]. Others have shown that enamel crystals are formed at a given distance from the dentin surface [410-412,430] and could either reach dentin crystals by a subsequent growth [431] or remain distant [430,432].

Enamel is formed only during amelogenesis in the jaw. At some point before the tooth erupts into the mouth the ameloblasts are broken down. Consequently, enamel, unlike bones, has no way to regenerate itself using the process of "active mineralization" (see aforementioned debate on bone formation) because there is no biological process that repairs degraded or damaged enamel [390,391].

---

[31] In addition, there is a cementum-enamel junction (CEJ), which is quite similar to DEJ.

In addition, certain bacteria in the mouth feed on the remains of foods, especially sugars. They produce lactic acid, which dissolves the biological apatite of the enamel in a process known as enamel demineralization that takes place below the critical pH of about 5.5. Similar process called enamel erosion occurs when a person consumes acid (citric, lactic, phosphoric, *etc.*) containing soft drinks [398,433-436]. Evidences exist that there is a preferential loss of carbonates and Mg during the acid dissolution of mineral in dental caries. Luckily, saliva gradually neutralizes the acids that cause the pH of the tooth surface to rise above the critical pH. This might cause partial enamel remineralization, the return of the dissolved calcium orthophosphates to the enamel. Until recently, it was generally agreed, that if there was sufficient time between the intake of foods (generally, two to three hours) and the damage was very limited, the teeth could repair themselves by the "passive mineralization" process [437]. Data on increased remineralization of tooth enamel by milk containing added casein phosphopeptide-ACP nanocomplexes [438] are in support of this hypothesis.

Recently, by using atomic force microscopy nano-indentation technique it was discovered that the previously demineralized samples of enamel further exposed to remineralizing solutions did show a crystalline layer of calcium orthophosphates formed on the enamel surface. Unfortunately, the re-precipitated deposits of calcium orthophosphates always consisted of loosely packed crystals and did not protect the underlying enamel from a subsequent acid attack. Furthermore, these surface deposits have been completely removed by either a toothbrush or a short exposure to an erosive acidic solution [398,439-441].

In this context, it should be emphasized that the term remineralization, which is often misused in the literature, should imply the process of mineral growth that goes hand in hand with a strengthening effect of the weakened enamel surface. Since no strengthening of an exposure to remineralizing solutions was observed, it might be considered that no "passive mineralization" was found (in spite of the real evidence of the re-precipitated surface deposits of calcium orthophosphates) [398,440,441].

Thus, the enamel self-repairing ability by the passive remineralization appears to be doubtful, while the active remineralization is impossible. However, investigations in this field keep going [442,443].

A content of fluoride added to either toothpaste or mouthwash lowers the solubility of calcium orthophosphates (by formation of FHA on the surface) and therefore improves the acid-resistance of dental enamel [230,247-252,444]. Furthermore, fluorides also reduce the production of acids by bacteria in the mouth by reducing their ability to metabolize sugars.

To conclude the teeth subject, let us briefly mention on the practical application of teeth. Due to relatively small dimensions of normal teeth, only tusks and ivory of giant animals are used. For example, both the Greek and Roman civilizations used large quantities of ivory to make high value works of art, precious religious objects and decorative boxes for costly objects. Ivory was often used to form the whites of the eyes of statues. Prior to the introduction of plastics, it was used for billiard balls, piano keys, buttons and ornamental items. The examples of modern carved ivory objects are small statuary, netsukes, jewelry, flatware handles and furniture inlays.

4.3. Antlers

Deer antlers (Figure 9) are unique biological structures since their growth rate is without parallel in vertebrates and because they are the only bony appendages in mammals capable of complete regeneration. This allows for basic research in bone biology without the interference of surgical procedures and their adverse effects in animals where samples are obtained. In addition, antlers also allow for the gathering of a large amount of samples from different populations to assess nutritional and ecological effects on bone composition and structure [445-448]. They are costly sexual secondary characters of male deer and constitute 1 to 5% of the body weight [449]. Antlers are not true horns; they are a simple extension of bone, so they have a matrix of biological apatite similar to that of mammalian bones. Antlers are large and complex horn-like appendages of deer consisting of bony outgrowths from the head with no covering of keratin as is found in true horns.

Similar to bones, antlers contain pores and can withstand applied stresses of over 300 MPa [450-452], which is even higher than that of bones (Table 1). Therefore, antlers are occasionally considered an almost unbreakable bone [300]. Each antler grows from an attachment point on the skull called a pedicle. While an antler is growing, it is covered with highly vascular skin called velvet, which supplies oxygen and nutrients to the growing bone.

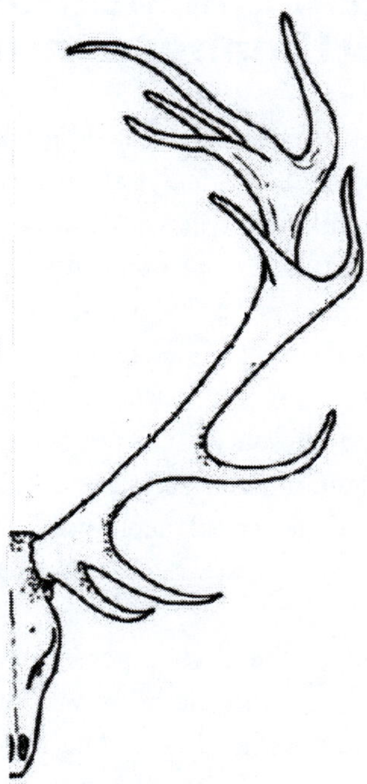

Figure 9. A schematic picture of a deer antler.

Once the antler has achieved its proper size, the velvet starts to dry out, cracks and breaks off, while the antler's bone dies. Fully developed antlers consist of dead bone only [453-462].

It was found that food processing cannot supply the mineral needs required for antler growth and thus, male deer must temporary resorb calcium orthophosphate minerals from their own skeleton for antler growth [453-465]. Detailed studies revealed that daily food intake provided between 25 and 40% of calcium needed for antler mineralization, which resulted in a temporary skeleton demineralization [464,465].

Antlers are a good model to study bone biology because they are accessible, shed after mating season and cast every year [466]. However, people seldom come across the antlers in the woods. Rabbits and rodents such as mice and chipmunks eat antlers (and bones of wild animals after they die) for calcium. Rodents and rabbits also gnaw bones and antlers to sharpen their incisors. Due to an extremely high growth rate, which can achieve 2-4 cm per day [453], combined with a very fast biomineralization, these unique appendages might be a well-suited animal model for studying the disturbances of bone formation induced by additives (*e.g.*, by excess of fluoride) [455]. Antler size and external characteristics were found to be influenced by nutrition, climatic variability and other factors. Thus, since antlers are periodically replaced, the analysis of naturally cast antlers offers the opportunity for a continuous, noninvasive monitoring of the environmental pollution by these additives [455]. Recently, the first attempt to evaluate a potential use of deer antlers as a bone regeneration biomaterial has been performed [467].

5. Pathological Calcification of Calcium Orthophosphates

In the body of mammals, osteoblasts and odontoblasts fix ions of calcium and orthophosphate and then precipitate biological apatite onto an organic matrix. This is the process of physiological biomineralization that is restricted to the specific sites in skeletal tissues, including growth plate cartilage, bones and teeth [35,242]. Normally, mammals are supposed to die with calcium orthophosphates located in bones and teeth (and antlers for male deer) only and nowhere else, because under the normal conditions soft tissues are not mineralized. Unfortunately, owing to ageing, various diseases and under certain pathological conditions blood vessels and some internal organs are calcified as well. This process is called pathological calcification or ectopic mineralization and leads to a morbidity and a mortality [35,242]. In general, any type of abnormal accumulation of calcium orthophosphates in wrong places is accounted for by a disruption of systemic defense mechanism against calcification [468].

To the best of my knowledge, the first paper on a negative influence of unwanted depositions of calcium orthophosphates in the body was published in 1946 [469]; however, apatite in urinary calculi was found earlier [470]. The unwanted depositions always lead to various diseases, for instance: soft tissue calcification (in damaged joints, blood vessels, dysfunctional areas in the brain, diseased organs, scleroderma, prostate stones) [471-476], kidney and urinary stones [4,477,478], dental pulp stones and dental calculus [73,74,479], salivary stones, gall stones, pineal gland calcification, atherosclerotic arteries and veins [26,480-483], coronary calcification [484], cardiac skeleton, damaged cardiac valves [485], calcification on artificial heart valves [486-490], carpal tunnel [491], cataracts, malacoplakia, calcified menisci [492,493], dermatomyositis [494,495] and others [35]. In addition, there is a metastatic calcification of nonosseous viable tissue occurring throughout the body, but it primarily affects the interstitial tissue of the blood vessels, kidney, lungs and gastric mucosa [496]. A metastatic calcification is defined as a deposition of calcium orthophosphates in previously normal tissue due to an abnormal biochemistry with disturbances in the calcium or phosphorus metabolism [497]. Common causes of the metastatic calcification include hyperparathyroidism, chronic renal disease, massive bone destruction in widespread bone metastases and increased intestinal calcium absorption. One author has mentioned on "apatite diseases" which are characterized by the appearance of needle-like crystals comparable to those of bone apatite in the fibrous connective tissue [498]. All these cases are examples of a calcinosis, which might be described as a formation of calcium orthophosphate deposits in any soft tissue. In dentistry, a calculus or a tartar refers to a hardened plaque on the teeth, formed by the presence of saliva, debris and minerals. Its rough surface provides an ideal medium for bacterial growth, threatening the health of the gums and absorbing unaesthetic stains far more easily than natural teeth [4].

Contrary to the mineral phases of the normal calcifications (bone, dentine, enamel, cementum, antlers), which consist of only one type of calcium orthophosphate (namely, biological apatite), the mineral phases of abnormal and/or pathological calcifications are found to occur as single or mixed phases of other types of calcium orthophosphates (ACP, DCPD, OCP, β-$(Ca,Mg)_3(PO_4)_2$) and/or other phosphatic and non-phosphatic compounds (*e.g.*, magnesium orthophosphates, calcium pyrophosphates, calcium oxalates, *etc.*) in addition to or in place of biological apatite (Table 4) [4,6,25,35,99,499-503]. In some cases, the chemical composition of an unwanted inorganic phase might depend on the age of the pathological calcification and its location. For example, DCPD is more frequently found in young (3 months or younger) calculus, biological apatite is present in all ages of calculus, while β-$(Ca,Mg)_3(PO_4)_2$ occurs more frequently in sub-gingival calculus. In mature calculus, the relative abundance of OCP, β-$(Ca,Mg)_3(PO_4)_2$ and biological apatite also differ between the inner and outer layers [25].

It is interesting to note that the mineral phases of animal calculus (*e.g.*, from dog) was found to consist of calcium carbonate and biological apatite, while human calculi do not contain calcium carbonate [25,504]. Recent findings suggest that the mechanisms and factors regulating physiological biomineralization may be identical or similar to those regulating ectopic mineralization: both are initiated by matrix vesicles, *i.e.*, membrane-enclosed particles released from the plasma membrane of mineralization-competent cells [505-507].

Table 4. Occurrence of calcium phosphates in biological systems (human) [25]

Calcium phosphate	Occurrence
biological apatite	enamel, dentin, bone, dental calculi, stones, urinary stones, soft-tissue deposits
OCP	dental and urinary calculi
DCPD	dental calculi, crystalluria, chrondrocalcinosis, in some carious lesions
β-$(Ca,Mg)_3(PO_4)_2$	dental calculi, salivary stones, arthritic cartilage, soft-tissue deposits
$Ca_2P_2O_7\cdot 2H_2O$	pseudo-gout deposits in synovium fluids
ACP	heart calcifications in uremic patients

In addition, other regulators (activators and inhibitors) of physiological mineralization have been identified and characterized. Besides, some evidences indicate that the same factors also contribute to the regulation of ectopic mineralization [505-512].What's more, the biological fluids (*e.g.*, serum, saliva, synovial fluids) are normally supersaturated with respect to biological apatite precipitation [4,25,242]; therefore, in principle, calcification is thermodynamically feasible in any part of the body. However, normally it is not the case. Therefore, in the healthy body, the appropriate inhibitory mechanisms must be at work to prevent a superfluous calcification of soft tissues. These inhibition mechanisms are a hot research topic in molecular medicine but this subject is beyond the scope of current review. The interested readers are forwarded, for example, to a very interesting review on molecular recognition at the protein-HA interface [513]. More to the point, molecular, endocrine and genetic mechanisms of arterial calcification have been reviewed in another paper [514].

To conclude this part, it is worth reminding that calcium orthophosphates of biological origin are sparingly soluble in aqueous solutions. Removing them from the places of unwanted deposition would be an equivalent of demineralizing bone; that is a challenge. Therefore, the majority of therapeutic approaches are directed at preventing the progression of pathological calcifications. Among them, a chelation therapy might be of some interest to chemists and materials researchers because it deals with chemical processes [515,516]. Very recently, the general principles of demineralization and decalcification (*i.e.*, removing the mineral Ca-containing compounds (phosphates and carbonates) from the organic matrix) have been extensively reviewed [517,518], where the interested readers are referred.

6. Calcium Orthophosphates as Biomaterials and Bioceramics

A number of definitions have been developed for the term "biomaterials". The consensus developed by experts in this field is the following: biomaterials are defined as synthetic or natural materials to be used to replace parts of a living system or to function in intimate contact with living tissue [51]. In general, they are intended to interface with biological systems to evaluate, treat, augment or replace any tissue, organ or function of the body and are now used in a number of different applications throughout the body [519,520]. *Biomaterials* are different from *biological materials* because the former are the materials that are accepted by living tissues and, therefore, might be used for tissue replacements, while the latter are the materials being produced by biological systems (wood, cotton, bones, *etc.*). In addition, there are *biomimetic materials*, which are not made by living organisms but have the composition, structure and properties similar to those of biological materials. Bioceramics might be defined as biomaterials of the ceramic origin. In general, it can have structural functions as joint or tissue replacements, be used as coatings to improve the biocompatibility of metal implants and function as resorbable lattices, which provide temporary structures and a framework that is dissolved and/or replaced as the body rebuilds tissue. Some types of bioceramics even feature a drug-delivery capability [521].

The performance of living tissues is the result of millions years of evolution, while the performance of acceptable artificial substitutions those humankind has designed to repair damaged hard tissues are only a few decades old. Archaeological findings exhibited in museums showed that materials used to replace missing human teeth have included ox teeth, shells, coral, ivory (elephant tusk), wood, human teeth from corpses and metals (gold or silver). For instance, the Etruscans learned to substitute missing teeth with bridges made from artificial teeth carved from the bones of oxen, while in the 17th century a piece of dog skull was successfully transplanted into the damaged skull of a Dutch duke. The Chinese recorded the first use of dental amalgam to repair decayed teeth in the year 659 AD, while pre-Columbian civilizations used gold sheets to heal cranial cavities following trepanation [522]. Unfortunately, many other implantations failed because of infection or a lack of knowledge about toxicity of the selected materials. In this frame, the use of calcium orthophosphates as biomaterials and bioceramics is based upon their similarity with the mineral phase of bone and teeth [242,243,283,284]. However, according to available literature, the first attempt to use calcium orthophosphates (it was TCP) as an artificial material to repair surgically created defects in rabbits was performed in 1920 [523]. In general, calcium orthophosphate-based biomaterials can be prepared from various sources [524,525]. Unfortunately, up to now, all attempts to synthesize bone replacement materials for clinical applications featuring the physiological tolerance, biocompatibility and a long term stability have had only a relative success; it comes to show a superiority and a complexity of the natural structures [281].

Generally, living organisms might treat artificial implants as bioinert, biotolerant, bioactive or bioresorbable materials [51,519,520]. Bioinert (*e.g.*, zirconia, alumina, carbon and titanium) and biotolerant (*e.g.*, polymethyl methacrylate (PMMA), titanium and Co–Cr alloy) materials will evoke a physiological response to form a fibrous capsule, thus, isolating the material from the body. Calcium orthophosphates (both non-substituted and ion-substituted) fall into the categories of bioactive and bioresorbable materials. A bioactive material will dissolve slightly but promote the formation of a layer of biological apatite before interfacing directly with the tissue at the atomic level, that result in the formation of a direct chemical bond with bone. Such an implant will provide a good stabilization for materials that are subject to mechanical loading. A bioresorbable material will dissolve and allow a newly formed tissue to grow into any surface irregularities but may not necessarily interface directly with the material [223,526-530]. Bioceramics made of dense HA would be a good example of a bioactive material, while porous scaffolds made of BCP (*i.e.,* β-TCP + HA [98-107], α-TCP + HA [110-113]) or bone grafts made of CDHA [531], TCP [532] and/or ACP [139,533] appear to be the examples of bioresorbable materials. Unfortunately, any calcium orthophosphate bioceramics possesses poor mechanical properties that do not allow them to be used in load-bearing areas [534]. Due to this reason, the medical application of calcium orthophosphates is currently focused on the production of non-load-bearing implants, such as pieces for middle ear surgery, filling of bone defects in oral or orthopedic surgery, as well as coating of dental implants and metallic prosthesis [281]. The mechanical properties of calcium orthophosphate biomaterials and bioceramics were reviewed elsewhere [200,535]. In addition, there is a good review on the recent developments in processing and surface modification of HA [536].

In spite of serious mechanical limitations, biomaterials and bioceramics of calcium orthophosphates are available in various physical forms: particles, blocks (dense or porous), injectable compositions, self-setting cements, coatings on metal implants, composites with polymers, *etc.* [537]. A porous surface provides mechanical fixation in addition to providing sites on the surface that allow chemical bonding between biomaterials and bone. For example, porous HA bioceramics can be colonized by bone tissues [538-540]. Therefore, macroporosity (pore size > 100 μm) in solid biomaterials is intentionally introduced by addition of various porogens, which consist of crystals or particles of either volatile or soluble substances (*e.g.*, naphthalene, sucrose, $NaHCO_3$, gelatin, PMMA microbeads) [99,223,541-545]. Sintering particles, preferably spheres of equal size, is another way to generate porous three-dimensional (3D) bioceramics of calcium orthophosphates. A wetting solution such as polyvinyl alcohol is usually used to aid compaction, which is achieved by cold isostatic pressing the particles into cylinders at approximately 200 MPa [546]. As hardly any effect of macropore sizes (150, 260, 510 and 1220 μm) was observed on the *in vivo* response [547], there is no need to create bioceramics with very big pores; however, the pores must be interconnected. Microporosity (pore size < 10 μm) results from the sintering process, while dimensions of the pores depend on temperature and sintering time. Creation of the desired porosity in bioceramics is a rather complicated engineering task and the interested readers are referred to the special literature [99,139,543,548-557].

The sintering stage appears to be of a great importance to produce bioceramics with the required properties. Several processes occur during sintering of calcium orthophosphates. Firstly, moisture, carbonates and all volatile chemicals remaining from the synthesis stage, such as ammonia, nitrates and any organic compounds, are removed as gaseous products. Secondly, the removal of these gases facilitates the production of dense materials during sintering. Thirdly, these chemical changes are accompanied by a concurrent increase in crystal size and a decrease in the specific surface area. Fourthly, there is the chemical decomposition of all acidic orthophosphates and their transformation into other phosphates (*e.g.*, $2HPO_4^{2-} \rightarrow P_2O_7^{4-} + H_2O$). Besides, sintering causes toughening of the ceramics [558]. Further details on the sintering process of calcium orthophosphates are available elsewhere [4,5,169,200,223,530].

Studies showed that increasing the specific surface area and pore volume of biomaterials for tissue repair might greatly accelerate the kinetic process of biological apatite deposition and therefore enhance the bone-forming bioactivity[32]. More importantly, the precise control over porosity, pore size and internal pore architecture of biomaterials on different length scales is essential for understanding of the structure-bioactivity relationship and the rational design of better bone-forming biomaterials [559,560].

Calcium orthophosphates in a number of forms and compositions are currently either in use or under consideration in many areas of dentistry and orthopedics, with even more in development. For example, bulk material, available in dense and porous forms, is used for alveolar ridge augmentation, immediate tooth replacement and maxillofacial reconstruction [4,24,561]. Further applications include orbital implants (Bio-Eye®) [562,563], increment of the hearing ossicles, spine fusion and repair of bone defects [564,565]. In order to permit growth of new bone into bone defects, a suitable bioresorbable material should fill the defects. Otherwise, ingrowth of fibrous tissue might prevent bone formation within the

[32] Bioactivity is defined as the property of the material to develop a direct, adherent and strong bonding with bone [205,206].

defects. Today, a large number of different calcium orthophosphate bioceramics for the treatment of bone defects is available on the market. As an example, the readers are referred to a thorough physicochemical characterization of 14 calcium phosphate-based bone substitution materials in comparison to natural bone [566]. Commercial and trade names of several very important types of calcium orthophosphate bioceramics might be found in literature [566,567].

Chemically, calcium orthophosphate bioceramics is based on HA, β-TCP, α-TCP and/or BCP (*i.e.*, a composite of HA with α- or β-TCP) [4,24,98-108,111-114,116,118,119,561,568]. The BCP concept is determined by the optimum balance of a more stable phase of HA and a more soluble TCP. General requirements for the ideal bone grafts are as follows: pores of some 100 μm size, a biodegradation rate comparable to the formation of bone tissue (*i.e.*, between a few months and about two years) and the sufficient mechanical stability. When compared to α- and β-TCP, HA is a more stable phase under the physiological conditions, as it has a lower solubility and a slower resorption kinetics [4,24,561]. As implants made of calcined HA are present in bone defects for many years after implantation, bioceramics made of β-TCP, α-TCP, CDHA or BCP [35,100,102,103,110-114,116,118,119,569] is more preferable for medical purposes. According to both observed and measured bone formation parameters, calcium orthophosphates were ranked in order of increasing magnitude as follows: low sintering temperature BCP (rough and smooth) ≈ medium sintering temperature BCP ≈ TCP > calcined low sintering temperature HA > non-calcined low sintering temperature HA > high sintering temperature BCP (rough and smooth) > high sintering temperature HA (calcined and non-calcined) [569]. Figure 10 shows some examples of the commercially available calcium orthophosphate bioceramics to be used as bone grafts. The need of biomaterials for minimal invasive surgery has induced the development of a concept of self-setting bone cements made from calcium orthophosphates to be applied as injectable and/or mouldable bone substitutes [44,47-49,52-56,63-67,92-95,117,266,541,542,555,569-573].

This type of biomaterials might be defined as a low temperature bioceramics. Two major types of cements are possible. The first one is a dry mixture of two different calcium orthophosphates (a basic one and an acidic one), in which, after being wetted, the setting reaction occurs according to an acid-base reaction. The second type of calcium orthophosphate cements is when the initial and final calcium orthophosphates have the same Ca/P molar ratio.

Typical examples are ACP with Ca/P molar ratio within 1.50-1.67 and α-TCP: they form CDHA upon contact with an aqueous solution [569,570]. Upon mixing with water, initial calcium orthophosphate(s) are dissolved and precipitated into less soluble calcium orthophosphates, which causes the cement setting.

During the precipitation reaction, new crystals grow and become entangled, thus providing a mechanical rigidity to the cement. Setting of these cements occurs mostly within the initial 6 hours, yielding a ~ 80% conversion to the final products and a compressive strength of 40-60 MPa. The rate of hardening is strongly influenced by a powder to liquid ratio and addition of other chemicals [63,117,569-571,573]. Despite a large number of formulations, all calcium orthophosphate cements can only form two different end products: CDHA and DCPD [569,570].

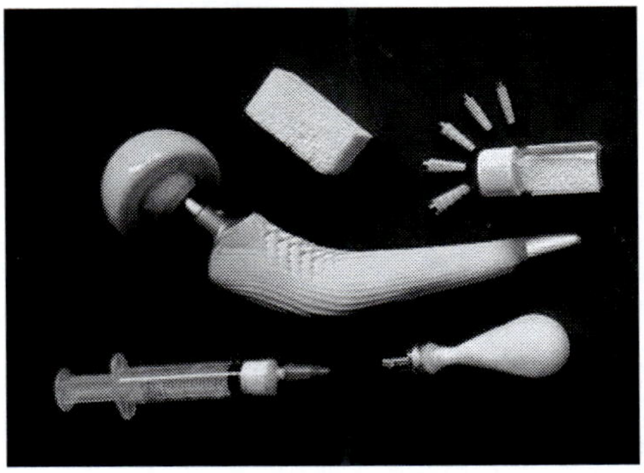

Figure 10. Examples of calcium orthophosphate-based bone substitution materials.

The first animal study on a calcium orthophosphate cement was performed in 1991: the cement consisting of TTCP and DCPA was investigated histologically by implanting disks made of this cement within the heads of nine cats [574,575]. All calcium orthophosphate cements are biocompartible, bioactive and bioresorbable. The structure and composition of the hardened cements is close to that of bone mineral; therefore, the material of these cements can easily be used by bone remodeling cells for reconstruction of damaged parts of bones [117,569,570]. The biomechanical evaluation of calcium orthophosphate cements for use in vertebroplasty might be found elsewhere [576]. Unfortunately, the cements possess a low mechanical strength; this property might be improved by reinforcement with polymers [577]. A good adaptation to the defect geometry is the major advantage of bone cements, when compared to implantation of bulk ceramics and scaffolds [44,117,200,266,569,570,573].

Injectable bone substitutes (IBS) made of calcium orthophosphates and an aqueous solution of a hydrophilic biodegradable polymer are another type of biomaterials for minimal invasive surgery [103,578-584]. They look as pastes of high viscosity but possessing enough fluidity to be injected into bone defects by a standard syringe with a needle. These materials are perfectly biocompatible and potentially resorbable and, thanks to their initial plasticity, they can fit bone defects very easily, without necessity to elaborate shaping of implantation site. During bioresorption of IBS, bone cells are able to invade the spaces released by disappearance of the biodegradable polymer. Creation of the required level of viscosity to prevent IBS from segregation and phase separation during the shelf life is the major task of the polymer in IBS, while calcium orthophosphates is the building material for bone healing. In terms of application, IBS more or less similar to the aforementioned hydraulic bone cements but, unlike the cements, IBS do not possess the self-setting abilities since no chemical reactions occur between the components [585]. Besides, there are paste-like formulations consisting of a suspension of pure HA in water prepared by a wet chemical reaction [586-588]. Further details on IBS are available elsewhere [103,578-584]. Recently, injectable and macroporous calcium orthophosphate cement scaffolds, combining the advantages of IBS and bone cements, have been developed [589]. The future development of both IBS and calcium orthophosphate bone cements might be seen in introduction of living cells into their composition [590,591]. Calcium orthophosphate coatings on metals are often applied in medicine [222]. Metallic implants are encountered in endoprostheses (total hip joint replacements) and artificial teeth sockets. The requirement for a sufficient mechanical stability necessitates the use of a metallic body for such devices. As metals usually do not undergo bone bonding, *i.e.* do not form a mechanically stable link between the implant and bone tissue, ways have been sought to improve the mechanical contact at the interface [592,593]. The major way is to coat the metal with calcium orthophosphate ceramics that generally exhibit bone-bonding ability between the metal and bone [594,595]. The list of most important coating techniques is comprised in Table 5, while the main advantages and drawbacks of each coating technique, as well as the important properties of the deposed calcium orthophosphates, are discussed in details elsewhere [202,222,223,596-601]. Clinical results for HA-coated metallic implants revealed that they had much longer life times after implantation than uncoated devices. Namely, HA coating as a system of fixation of hip implants was found to work well in the short to medium term (8 years [602], 15 years [603], 17 years [604] and 19 years [605]). Similar data for HA-coated dental implants are also available [606,607]. The longer-term clinical results are awaited with a great interest. The biomedical aspects of osteoconductive[33] coatings for total joint arthroplasty have been reviewed elsewhere [608].

The perfect biomaterial for medical applications would not only be biocompatible but also have physical properties similar to those of the tissue being replaced or repaired. Researchers therefore have sought ways of combining calcium orthophosphate bioceramics with other materials to tailor properties such as strength and elasticity to meet system requirements. This has led to a large variety of bone substituting composites and hybrid biomaterials made of calcium orthophosphate bioceramics and (bio)organic compounds (usually, polymers, preferably, biodegradable ones).

This approach appeared due to the poor mechanical properties (namely: a low elasticity, a high brittleness, a low tensile strength, a low fracture toughness and a poor impact resistance) of bone substitutes made of calcium orthophosphates only [200,205,206].

In addition, it is worth reminding that all biologically formed calcified tissues (bones, teeth, antlers, shells, *etc.*) appear to be very complicated composites of (bio)organic and inorganic phases [4,24,25,35,192,242,283,284]. In such composites, the mineral component provides the strength whereas the (bio)organic component contributes to the ductility. This combination of strength and ductility leads to an energy absorption prior to failure [310].

A list of the suitable calcium orthophosphates (except of MCPM and MCPA – both are too acidic and, therefore, are not biocompatible) is mentioned in Table 2, while there is an even greater choice of biocompatible polymers those can be divided into two major groups: synthetic polymers (*e.g.*, polyesters, PMMA, poly-ε-caprolactone) and polymers of biological origin (*e.g.*, collagen, gelatin, chitosan, alginate, modified starch, cellulose esters).

Various ways have been already realized to bring these two components together into biocomposites, like simple mechanical mixing or co-precipitation. Usually, powder forms of calcium orthophosphates are used to produce biocomposites. It is also possible to introduce porosity into such biocomposites that is advantageous for most applications as bone substitution material. Such biocomposites might possess the unique properties; for example, there is a recent report on shape memory properties of poly(D,L-lactide)/HA biocomposites [609].

---

[33] Osteoconductivity is the ability to provide a scaffold or template for the formation of new bone on its surface by attachment, migration, proliferation, and differentiation of bone-forming cells [537].

Table 5. Different techniques to deposit bioresorbable coatings of calcium orthophosphates on metal implants [202,596]

Technique	Thickness	Advantages	Disadvantages
Thermal spraying	30–200 μm	High deposition rates; low cost	Line of sight technique; high temperatures induce decomposition; rapid cooling produces amorphous coatings
Sputter coating	0.5–3 μm	Uniform coating thickness on flat substrates; dense coating	Line of sight technique; expensive; time consuming; produces amorphous coatings
Pulsed laser deposition	0.05–5 μm	Coating by crystalline and amorphous phases; dense and porous coating	Line of sight technique
Dynamic mixing method	0.05–1.3 μm	High adhesive strength	Line of sight technique; expensive; produces amorphous coatings
Dip coating	0.05–0.5 mm	Inexpensive; coatings applied quickly; can coat complex substrates	Requires high sintering temperatures; thermal expansion mismatch
Sol-gel technique	< 1 μm	Can coat complex shapes; low processing temperatures; relatively cheap as coatings are very thin	Some processes require controlled atmosphere processing; expensive raw materials
Electrophoretic deposition	0.1–2.0 mm	Uniform coating thickness; rapid deposition rates; can coat complex substrates	Difficult to produce crack-free coatings; requires high sintering temperatures
Biomimetic coating	< 30 μm	Low processing temperatures; can form bonelike apatite; can coat complex shapes; can incorporate bone growth stimulating factors	Time consuming; requires replenishment and a pH constancy of simulated body fluid
Hot isostatic pressing	0.2–2.0 μm	Produces dense coatings	Cannot coat complex substrates; high temperature required; thermal expansion mismatch; elastic property differences; expensive; removal/interaction of encapsulation material
Electrochemica l deposition	0.05–0.5 mm	Uniform coating thickness; rapid deposition rates; can coat complex substrates; moderate temperature, low cost	The coating/substrate bonding is not strong enough

The topic of the composite biomaterials made of calcium orthophosphates and organic/biological compounds was first introduced in 1981 by Prof. William Bonfield, who realized the application potential of calcium orthophosphates as fillers in polymer-bioceramics biocomposites and the move was envisaged towards an improved mechanical performance of HA bioceramics [610]. Biocomposites of polymers and calcium orthophosphate bioceramics can confer favorable mechanical properties, including strength due to the ceramic phase, toughness and plasticity due to the polymer phase, as well as a graded mechanical stiffness. Another advantage of such biomaterials is that they are sufficiently soft and ductile to be shaped by a surgeon in the operating theatre. Although current technologies cannot yet reproduce the multistage biosynthesis, the hierarchical structure and the mechanical properties of bones, the synthesis of various types of calcium orthophosphate-based biocomposites and hybrid biomaterials is a strong and very promising research area and the readers are referred to other papers and reviews [223,310,311,611-622].

To conclude the subject, the bioactivity mechanism of calcium orthophosphate biomaterials and bioceramics should be described. Strange enough but careful seeking in the literature resulted in only two publications [202,623], where the bioactivity mechanism of calcium orthophosphates had been briefly described. For example, the chemical changes occurring after exposure of a synthetic HA ceramic to both *in vivo* (implantation in human) and *in vitro* (cell culture) conditions were studied. A small amount of HA was phagocytized but the major remaining part behaved as a secondary nucleator as evidenced by the appearance of a newly formed mineral [623]. Therefore, one should better rely on the bioactivity mechanism of other biomaterials, particularly of bioactive glasses – the concept introduced by Prof. Larry Hench [205,206].

The mechanism of bonding of bioactive glasses to living tissue involves a sequence of 11 successive reaction steps. The initial 5 steps occurred on the surface of biomaterials are "chemistry" only, while the remaining 6 steps belong to "biology" because the latter include colonization by osteoblasts, followed by proliferation and differentiation of the cells to form a new bone that had a mechanically strong bond to the implant surface (Figure 11). Therefore, in the case of bioactive glasses the border between "dead" and "alive" is located between stages 5 and 6.

According to L. Hench, all bioactive materials "form a bone-like apatite layer on their surfaces in the living body and bond to bone through this apatite layer. The formation of bone-like apatite on artificial material is induced by functional groups, such as Si–OH (in the case of biological glasses), Ti–OH, Zr–OH, Nb–OH, Ta–OH, –COOH and $-H_2PO_4$ (in the case of other materials). These groups have specific structures revealing negatively charge and induce apatite formation via formations of an amorphous calcium compound, *e.g.*, calcium silicate, calcium titanate and ACP" [205,206].

For want of anything better, the bioactivity mechanism of calcium orthophosphates should also be described by Figure 11 with omitting of several initial stages, as it was actually made for HA in Ref. [202], where 3 initial chemical stages of the Hench's mechanism were replaced by partial dissolution of HA.

7. Biomimetic Crystallization of Calcium Orthophosphates

In general, biomimetics[34] (also known as bionics, biognosis and/or biomimicry) might be defined as application of the methods and systems found in nature to the study, design and construction of new engineering systems, materials, chemical compounds and modern technology. The concept is very old (*e.g.*, the Chinese wanted to make artificial silk ~ 3000 years ago; Daedalus' wings was one of the early design failure) but the implementation is gathering momentum only recently. In spite of the tremendous achievements of modern science and technology, the nature's ability to assemble inorganic compounds into hard tissues (shells, spicules, teeth, bones, antlers, skeletons, *etc.*) is still not achievable by the synthetic procedures. This is not surprising – designs found in nature are the result of millions of years of evolution and competition for survival. The models that failed are fossils; those that survived are the success [624]. In the frames of this review, biomimetics is considered as mimicking natural manufacturing methods to generate artificial calcified tissues (grafts, implants, prostheses) those might be used as temporary or permanent replacements of the missing, lost, injured or damaged bones and teeth.

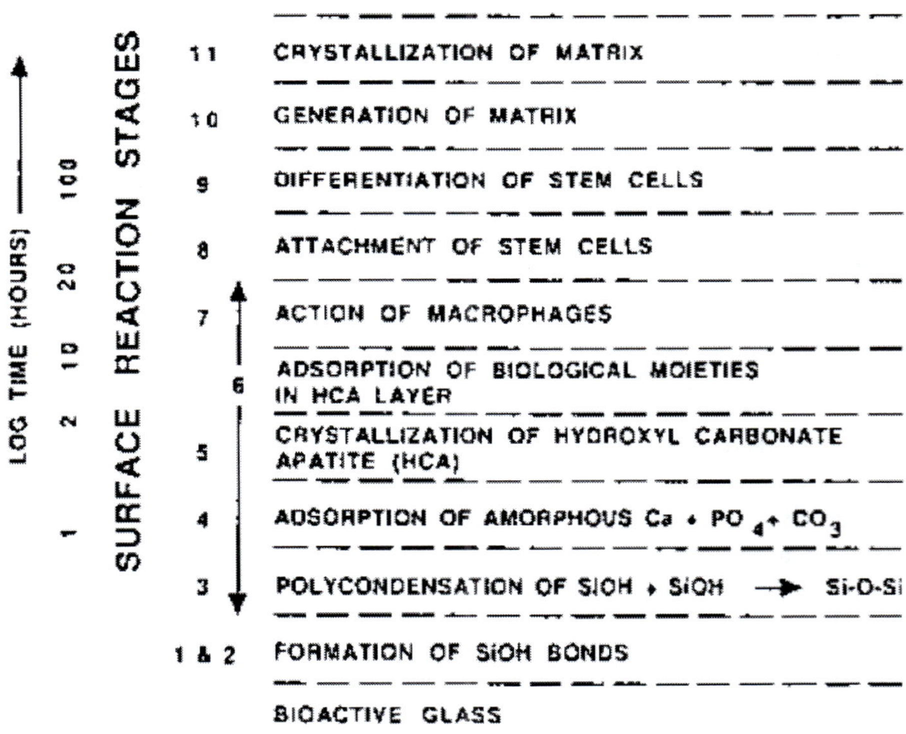

Figure 11. The sequence of interfacial reactions involved in forming a bond between tissue and bioactive glasses. The border between "dead" and "alive" occurs approximately at stage 6. Reprinted from Ref. [206] with permission.

[34] The term "biomimetics" ("the mimicry of life") was coined by an American inventor, engineer and biophysicist Otto Herbert Schmitt (1913 – 1998) in the 1950-s.

As this is mainly the subject of crystallization of calcium orthophosphates, the matter of choosing the correct experimental conditions and well-mimicking solutions is of the primary importance. The easiest way to perform the crystallization would be mixing of aqueous solutions containing the ions of calcium and orthophosphate [4-6]. Unfortunately, such type of crystallization provides precipitates with the properties (chemical composition, Ca/P ratio, crystallinity level, particle size distribution, *etc.*) far different from those of biological apatite. This can be explained by the following paramount differences between the *in vivo* and *in vitro* crystallization conditions [625]:

(i) *In vitro* crystallization normally occurs at permanently depleting concentrations of calcium and orthophosphate, while the concentrations of all ions and molecules are kept strictly constant during biological mineralization (the same is valid for the solution pH);
(ii) Chemical crystallization is a fast process (time scale of minutes to days), while the biological process is a slow one (time scale of weeks to years);
(iii) Many inorganic, bioorganic, biological and polymeric compounds are present in biological liquids (blood plasma, serum, saliva). Each of these compounds might act as an inhibitor, promoter, nucleator or even as a template for the growth of biological apatite [281]. In addition, each of them somehow influences the crystallization kinetics and might be either incorporated into the solid structure or co-precipitated with calcium orthophosphates.
(iv) Chemical crystallization is, by all means, a "passive" process, while the biological mineralization is strongly influenced by cells and occurs by the self-organization mechanisms [333,334]. Still there are no good ways to overcome this difference.

The first and the second differences might be overcome by using the appropriate crystallization techniques. The details are available elsewhere [625] but, briefly, the first problem might be overcome by either a continuous flow of a supersaturated solution [626, 627] or using a constant-composition (CC) technique [83,628,629]. The second difference might be surpassed by a restrained diffusion of calcium and orthophosphate ions from the opposite directions in, for example, a double-diffusion (DD) crystallization device or in viscous gels [228-230,232,233,630]. The CC and DD techniques have been combined into a single constant-composition double-diffusion (CCDD) device, which currently seems to be the most advanced experimental tool to perform biomimetic crystallization [625,631-635]. However, in no case the CCDD device should be considered as the final construction; it still has much room for further improvement, *e.g.* by upgrading the design of the crystallization chamber [636]. Other constructions, *e.g.* to study calcification of biological heart valve prostheses [637], are also possible. In addition, one should keep in mind that the potential of the standard CC technique has not reached its limit yet: for example, recently a good mimicking of the self-organized microstructure of tooth enamel has been achieved [638].

The third major difference between the *in vivo* and *in vitro* crystallization conditions might be overcome by using the appropriate crystallization solutions [625]. The best way would be to perform experiments using natural liquids (blood serum, saliva, lymph, *etc.*), but this is not easy due to variability of the chemical and biochemical composition of natural liquids and problems with their storage. As stated before, using supersaturated aqueous solutions containing only the ions of calcium and orthophosphate appears to be unable to mimic the crystallization of biological apatite; therefore, more advanced solutions have been elaborated. To the best of my knowledge, Hanks' balanced salt solution (HBSS) [639] was the first successful simulating medium, containing the ions of calcium and orthophosphate together with other inorganic ions and glucose. HBSS is commercially available and still used in biomimetic experiments [640-642]; its chemical composition might be taken, *e.g.*, from Refs. [643,644]. Other physiological solutions include α-modified Eagle's medium (α-MEM), which contains numerous bioorganic (*e.g.*, alanine, aspartic acid, glycine, biotin, vitamin C, folic acid, riboflavin) and inorganic (*e.g.*, $CaCl_2$, KCl, NaCl, NaH_2PO_4) compounds [645-647], phosphate buffered saline (PBS) that contains only inorganic components (*e.g.*, $CaCl_2$, $MgCl_2$, KCl, KH_2PO_4, NaCl, NaH_2PO_4) [648,649], as well as an artificial saliva containing both bioorganic (*e.g.*, xantan gum or sodium carboxymethylcellulose, sorbitol, *etc.*) and inorganic (*e.g.*, $CaCl_2$, $MgCl_2$, KCl, KH_2PO_4, NaCl, KH_2PO_4) compounds [650,651]. All these simulating solutions are commercially available.

However, the most popular biomimetic solution is a protein-free acellular simulated body fluid (SBF). It was introduced by Kokubo *et al.* [652] and occasionally named as Kokubo's SBF. It is a metastable aqueous solution with pH ~ 7.40, supersaturated with respect to the precipitation of HA, containing only inorganic ions in concentrations nearly equal to those in human blood plasma. However, the standard SBF, firstly, contains the tris/HCl buffer, and, secondly, the concentration of hydrogencarbonate (4.2 mM) is only a fraction of that in blood plasma (27 mM) [652]. The problem of a low concentration of hydrogencarbonate ions has been overcome by first introducing a "synthetic body fluid" [653-655] and later a revised SBF (rSBF) [656,657]. Due to the chemical similarity with human blood plasma, rSBF currently seems to be the best simulating solution. However, it contains Hepes buffer, loses CO_2 in open vessels and does not contain any organic and/or biological molecules [656,657]. Other types of SBF are also available; the interested readers are referred to a recent leading opinion co-authored by the SBF inventor [658], where the entire history and the preparation technique of SBF are well described. The application of SBF for the surface mineralization of various materials *in vitro* has been reviewed in Ref. [659], while the theoretical analysis of calcium orthophosphate precipitation (the driving force and the nucleation rate based on the classical crystallization theory) in SBF is also available [660].

Further attempts to improve the biomimetic properties of SBF and rSBF have been performed. Efforts were made to replace artificial buffers (tris/HCl, Hepes) with simultaneous increasing the concentration of hydrogencarbonates for SBF [661,662] or avoiding losses of CO_2 from open vessels for rSBF [625,631-635] by means of permanent bubbling of gaseous CO_2 through the solutions. Addition of the most important organic and biological compounds like glucose [633] and albumin [631] is another direction to improve biomimetic properties of SBFs; further improvements of biomimetic solutions are to be made in future. Occasionally, condensed solutions of SBF (*e.g.*, 1.5-fold, 2-fold [663,664], 5-fold [665,666] and even 10-fold [667]) are used to accelerate the precipitation; however, whenever possible this should be avoided because the application of condensed solutions of SBF leads to changes in the chemical composition of the precipitates; namely, the concentration of carbonates increases, while the concentration of orthophosphates decreases [668].

It is very difficult to mimic exactly the calcification process that occurs in bones and teeth. A step further would be to perform the precipitation from the simulating solutions on templates of biomineralization proteins for the control of crystal organization and properties. For example, there are successful attempts to crystallize calcium orthophosphates on collagen in order to obtain bone-like composites [311,669-674]. Although the ultrastructure of bone has not been realized yet, such collagen/calcium orthophosphate composites are currently under investigation for clinical use. Other popular biomimetic matrixes to perform calcium orthophosphate crystallization comprise gelatin [228-230,232,233,675-677], chitosan [675,678,679], organic polyelectrolytes [680-683], titanium and its alloys [684-690], polymers [691], cellulose [692], self-assembled monolayers [693] and many other materials.

8. Calcium Orthophosphates in Tissue Engineering

All present day orthopedic implants lack three of the most critical characteristics of living tissues: (i) the ability to self-repair; (ii) the ability to maintain a blood supply; (iii) the ability to modify their structure and properties in response to environmental factors such as mechanical load [554]. Needless to mention, that bones not only possess all aforementioned properties but, in addition, they are self-generating, hierarchical, multifunctional, nonlinear, composite and biodegradable; therefore, good artificial bone substitutes must possess similar properties [281].

The last two decades have seen a surge in creative ideas and technologies developed to tackle the problem of repairing or replacing diseased and damaged tissues, leading to the emergence of a new field in healthcare technology now referred to as *tissue engineering*. Tissue engineering is an interdisciplinary field that exploits a combination of living cells, engineering materials and suitable biochemical factors in a variety of ways to improve, replace, restore, maintain or enhance living tissues and whole organs [694]. This field of science[36] started more than a decade ago [696] and nowadays is at full research potential due to the following key advantages: (i) the solutions it provides are long-term, much safer than other options and cost-effective as well; (ii) the need for a donor tissue is minimal, which eliminates the immuno-suppression problems; (iii) the presence of residual foreign material is eliminated as well. As 2 of 3 major components (namely, living cells and biochemical factors) of tissue engineering appear to be far beyond the scope of this review, here the topic of tissue engineering is narrowed down to the engineering materials only.

[36] In 2003, the NSF published a report titled: "*The emergence of tissue engineering as a research field*", which provides a thorough description of the history of this field [695].

Cells are generally implanted or seeded into an artificial structure, usually referred to as a scaffold, capable of supporting 3D tissue formation. The scaffolds are temporary matrices for bone growth and provide a specific environment and architecture for tissue development. They serve at least one of the following purposes: (i) allow cell attachment and migration; (ii) deliver and retain cells and biochemical factors; (iii) enable diffusion of vital cell nutrients and expressed products; (iv) exert certain mechanical and biological influences to modify the behavior of the cell phase [697]. To achieve the goal of tissue reconstruction, the scaffolds must meet some specific requirements. A reasonable surface roughness is necessary to facilitate cell seeding and fixation [698-700]. A high porosity and an adequate pore size are very important to provide diffusion throughout the whole structure of both cells and nutrients [699-705]. Biodegradability is very essential since scaffolds need to be resorbed by the surrounding tissues without the necessity of a surgical removal. The resorption rate has to coincide as much as possible with the rate of tissue formation [706]: this means that while cells are fabricating their own natural matrix structure around themselves, the scaffold is able to provide a structural integrity within the body and eventually it will break down leaving the newly formed tissue that will take over the mechanical load. Injectability is also an important factor for the clinical use [569,570,578-583].

In the case of bone grafts, the aim of tissue engineering is to provide an artificially prepared porous scaffold made of calcium orthophosphates that provides the physical and chemical cues to guide cell seeding, differentiation and assembly into 3D tissues of a newly formed bone [707-710]. More to the point, bone-forming functions of cells can be dependent on grain morphology of the scaffolds. For example, osteoblast functions were found to be increased on nanofiber structures if compared to nanospherical ones because nanofibers more closely approximated the shape of biological apatite in bones [711]. To meet these needs, much attention is devoted to further modification of calcium orthophosphates [712]. From the chemical point of view, the modifications include synthesis of novel ion-substituted calcium orthophosphates [713-718], while from the material point of view the major research topics include nanocrystalline structures [224,719-728], organic-inorganic composites and hybrid biomaterials [223,611-619,728-730], fibers and whiskers [731-738], micro- and nanospheres [729,739-742], porous 3D scaffolds made of ACP [139], HA [743-746] and BCP [747], structures with graded porosity [748] and hierarchically organized ones [749]. The influence of the porosity of HA ceramics on *in vitro* and *in vivo* bone formation studied by cultured rat bone marrow stromal cells has been studied [750]. The feasible production of ceramic scaffolds with tailored structure and properties opens up a spectacular future for calcium orthophosphates.

There are three principal therapeutic strategies for treating diseased or injured tissues in patients: (i) implantation of freshly isolated or cultured cells; (ii) implantation of tissues assembled *in vitro* from cells and scaffolds; (iii) *in situ* tissue regeneration. For cellular implantation, individual cells or small cellular aggregates from the patient or a donor are either injected into the damaged tissue directly or are combined with a degradable scaffold *in vitro* and then implanted. For tissue implantation, a complete 3D tissue is grown *in vitro* using patient or donor cells and a bioresorbable scaffold and then is implanted into the patients to replace diseased or damaged tissues. For *in situ* regeneration, a scaffold implanted directly into the injured tissue stimulates the body's own cells to promote local tissue repair

[694,751]. In any case, simply trapping cells at a particular point on a surface is not enough: the cells must be encouraged to differentiate, which is impossible without the presence of suitable biochemical factors [752]. All previously mentioned clearly indicates that for the purposes of tissue engineering, calcium orthophosphates play only an auxiliary role; namely, they act as a suitable material to manufacture an appropriate 3D template, substrate or scaffold to be colonized by living cells before the successive implantation. However, the scaffolds themselves might be prepared from not only pure calcium orthophosphates but also organic-inorganic composites [753-756]. The *in vitro* evaluation of potential calcium orthophosphate scaffolds for tissue engineering has been described elsewhere [757], while the data on mechanical properties and porosity of calcium orthophosphates for use in tissue engineering are also available [758,759]. The effect of a HA-based biomaterial on gene expression in osteoblast-like cells was reported [760], while the influence of adsorbed serum proteins, RGD and proteoglycan-binding peptides on the adhesion of mesenchymal stem cells to HA be also studied [761]. To conclude, the excellent biocompatibility of calcium orthophosphates and their high affinity for proteins and cells makes them very functional for hard tissue regeneration [178,762-764].

Conclusions and Outlook

By the end of the XX-th century, it became clear that calcium orthophosphate biomaterials and bioceramics by themselves could not give a complete response to the clinical needs for artificial implants. Biomaterials with more demanding properties were required. Namely, in 1998, Prof. Larry Hench published a forecast for the future of biomaterials development [765], where he noted that available that time bioactive materials (calcium orthophosphates, bioactive glasses and glass ceramics) had already improved prostheses lifetime but, unfortunately, any type of prosthesis had mechanical limitations. As the solution, he proposed that biomaterial researchers would need to focus on tissue regeneration instead of tissue replacement. A working hypothesis was announced: "Long-term survivability of prosthesis will be increased by the use of biomaterials that enhance the regeneration of natural tissues" [765]. One path to follow is the regeneration of bone using calcium orthophosphate scaffolds that mimic the structure of biological apatite, bond to bone and in some cases activate the genes within bone cells to stimulate new bone growth [554,694,751]. Thus, 10 years ago Prof. Hench predicted a rapid development of tissue engineering field, where calcium orthophosphates play an auxiliary role. The history has shown that tissue engineering, indeed, is a very rapidly developed field of science and research [766].

However, what can be said about calcium orthophosphates themselves? The major questions on chemistry, crystallization, ion-substitution, crystallography, thermodynamics and phase relationships for the chemically pure calcium orthophosphates have been answered in the XX-th century. Some topics for DCPD and CDHA have been additionally investigated in the field of calcium orthophosphate cements [570]. Conversely, calcium orthophosphates of biological origin, including the control of their morphology and interaction of calcium orthophosphate bioceramics with various bio- and organic compounds are not well investigated yet. The same is valid for nanocrystalline samples of calcium orthophosphates. Small amounts of bone-like apatite might be easily prepared by crystallization from SBF and rSBF but what can be said about larger quantities? A standard way of the concentration increasing causes chemical changes in the precipitates [668]. After a necessary technology is developed, one will have to think on scaffold preparation from this material, keeping in mind that any thermal treatment would destroy this material. Perhaps, spark plasma sintering approach based on the use of pulsed current and enabling very fast heating and cooling rates might be a first hint to overcome this problem [767]. Furthermore, the existence of oxyapatite remains to be questionable, as well as the bioactivity mechanism of calcium orthophosphates requires improving.

To date, although calcium orthophosphate biomaterials and bioceramics have been extensively studied for over 50 years, their ability to trigger bone formation is still incomparable with other biomaterials. Naturally, the biomaterials' field is shifting towards biologically active systems in order to improve their performance and to expand their use. Due to this case, tissue engineering is the strongest subject of current research, which, in the case of calcium orthophosphates, means fabrication of proper substrates and scaffolds for cells, hormones and biochemical factors to be used in tissue engineering. Presumably, the synthesis of various types of calcium orthophosphate-based hybrid biomaterials occupies the second important place. For example, even composites of HA with carbon nanotubes already exist [768-770]! The third important place is occupied by investigations devoted to the synthesis and characterization of various nanoparticles and nanocrystals of calcium orthophosphates, as well as by synthesis of calcium orthophosphates with controlled particle geometry. In general, the geometry of crystal phases can be varied by controlling the precipitation conditions, such as temperature, solution pH, concentration of the reagents, hydrodynamics, presence of various admixtures, inhibitors or promoters, ultrasonication, *etc.* All these approaches might be useful in preparation of calcium orthophosphate fibers, whiskers, hollow microspheres, *etc.* In addition, a great attention is paid to manufacturing of calcium orthophosphate cements [570] and multiphase[37] mixtures mimicking as closely as possible the mineral component of biological apatite. The study of nanostructured and nanocrystalline materials made of calcium orthophosphates, similar to the complex hierarchical structures of hard tissues (bone and teeth), is also a very attractive field [281]. A work along the ecological ways of synthesis of calcium orthophosphates might be of a great importance as well [772]. A deeper study of the fascinating growth rate of deer antlers might provide new and unexpected approaches to the bone-healing concept, as well as this will be important for further development of both biomimetics and biomineralization fields. Unfortunately, no currently available bone substitutes can substitute the bones' mechanical function, illustrating yet unmet medical need that would entirely substitute and regenerate a damaged tissue or organ. In a close future, the foreseeable application of calcium orthophosphates will be as a component of the third generation biomaterials [751,765], where calcium orthophosphates will support cells and/or other biologically active substances

---

[37] For multiphase compositions of various calcium orthophosphates, the problem of accurate phase quantification often arises. The problem is usually solved by the Rietveld refinement and the readers are referred to a recent paper on this subject [771].

(peptides, growth factors, hormones, drugs, *etc.*) to guide regeneration of hard tissues [178,521,712,773-778].

To finalize this review, one should note that, in spite of a rather long history of calcium orthophosphate research, there are still many gaps in our knowledge to be investigated in future.

References

[1] J. Berzelius, Ueber basische phosphorsaure kalkerde. *Ann. Chem. Pharmac.* 1845, 53, 286–288.

[2] H. Hausen, Die Apatite, deren chemische zusammensetzung, und ihrer Verhältnis zu physikalischen und morphologischen Eigenschaften. *Acta Acad. Abo. Ser. B: Mater. Phys. Mater. Natur. Teknik.* 1929, 5, 62–65.

[3] D. R. Lide, *The CRC handbook of chemistry and physics.* 86th Ed., CRC Press, Boca Raton, Florida, 2005, 2544 pp.

[4] R. Z. LeGeros, *Calcium phosphates in oral biology and medicine.* Karger, Basel, 1991, 201 pp.

[5] J. C. Elliot, Structure and chemistry of the apatites and other calcium orthophosphates. *Studies in inorganic chemistry.* Vol. 18. Elsevier, Amsterdam, 1994, 389 pp.

[6] Z. Amjad (Ed.), *Calcium phosphates in biological and industrial systems.* Kluwer Academic Publishers, Boston, MA, 1997, 529 pp.

[7] S. V. Dorozhkin, M. Epple, Biological and medical significance of calcium phosphates. *Angew. Chem. Int. Ed. Engl.* 2002, 41, 3130-3146.

[8] D. McConnell, in: *Apatite: its crystal chemistry, mineralogy, utilization, and biologic occurrences.* Springer, New York, 1973, pp. 111-115.

[9] P. Becker, Phosphates and phosphoric acid: raw materials technology and economics of the wet process. in: *Fertilizer science and technology series,* 2nd edition, Marcel Dekker, New York, 1989, 760 pp.

[10] D. K. Smith, Calcium phosphate apatites in nature. in: *Hydroxyapatite and related materials.* (Eds.: P. W. Brown, B. Constantz), CRC Press Inc., Boca Raton, Florida, 1994, pp. 29-44.

[11] A. I. Angelov, B. V. Levin, Yu. D. *Chernenko, Phosphate ore. A reference book.* (in Russian), Nedra busyness centre, Moscow, 2000, 120 pp.

[12] P. J. Cook, J. H. Shergold (Eds.), *Phosphate deposits of the world.* Cambridge University Press, 2005, 404 pp.

[13] D. D. Hogarth, The discovery of apatite on the Lievre River, *Quebec. Mineral. Rec.* 1974, 5, 178-182.

[14] J. van Velthuizen, Giant fluorapatite crystals: a question of locality. *Mineral. Rec.* 1992, 23, 459-463.

[15] Y. Pan, M. E. Fleet, Compositions of the apatite-group minerals: substitution mechanisms and controlling factors. in: Phosphates: geochemical, geobiological and materials importance. *Series: Reviews in Mineralogy and Geochemistry.* Vol. 48, J. M.

Hughes, M. Kohn, J. Rakovan (Eds.). *Mineralogical Society of America*, Washington, D.C. 2002, pp. 13-49.

[16] Yu. N. Zanin, The classification of calcium phosphates of phosphorites. *Lithology and Mineral Resources* 2004, 39, 281–282.

[17] http://www.mindat.org/min-10072.html (accessed in September 2008).

[18] B. Hubert, J. J. Álvaro, J. Y. Chen, Microbially mediated phosphatization in the Neoproterozoic Doushantuo Lagerstätte, South China. *Bull. Soc. Géol.* Fr. 2005, 176, 355-361.

[19] A. R. Chakhmouradian, L. Medici, Clinohydroxylapatite: a new apatite-group mineral from northwestern Ontario (Canada), and new data on the extent of Na-S substitution in natural apatites. *Eur. J. Mineralogy* 2006, 18, 105-112.

[20] http://www.mindat.org/gallery.php?min=9293 (accessed in September 2008).

[21] N. A. Trueman, Substitutions for phosphate ions in apatite. *Nature* 1966, 210, 937–938.

[22] T. White, C. Ferraris, J. Kim, S. Madhavi, Apatite – an adaptive framework structure. In: *Micro- and mesoporous mineral phases. Series: Reviews in Mineralogy and Geochemistry*. Vol. 57, G. Ferraris, S. Merlino (Eds.). Mineralogical Society of America, Washington, D.C. 2005, pp. 307-401.

[23] C. Rey, C. Combes, C. Drouet, H. Sfihi, Chemical diversity of apatites. *Advances in Science and Technology* 2006, 49, 27-36.

[24] W. C. O'Neill, The fallacy of the calcium-phosphorus product. *Kidney International* 2007, 72, 792-796.

[25] R. Z. LeGeros, Formation and transformation of calcium phosphates: relevance to vascular calcification. *Z. Kardiol.* 2001, 90, Suppl. 3, III116-III125.

[26] A. Becker, M. Epple, K. M. Müller, I. Schmitz, A comparative study of clinically well-characterized human atherosclerotic plaques with histological, chemical, and ultrastructural methods. *J. Inorg. Biochem.* 2004, 98, 2032-2038.

[27] B. Wopenka, J. D. Pasteris, A mineralogical perspective on the apatite in bone. *Mater. Sci. Engin.* C 2005, 25, 131-143.

[28] J. D. Pasteris, B. Wopenka, E. Valsami-Jones, Bone and tooth mineralization: why apatite? *Elements* 2008, 4, 97-104.

[29] Y. Sun, E. N. Hanley, Jr. Calcium-containing crystals and osteoarthritis. *Curr. Opin. Orthopedics*. 2007, 18, 472-478.

[30] S. N. Danil'chenko, A. N. Kulik, A. N. Bugai, P. A. Pavlenko, T. G. Kalinichenko, N. V. Ul'yanchich, L. F. Sukhodub, Thermally activated diffusion of magnesium from bioapatite crystals. *J. Appl. Spectroscopy* 2005, 72, 899-905.

[31] B. H. Passey, T. F. Robinson, L. K. Ayliffe, T. E. Cerling, M. Sphonheimer, M. D. Dearing, B. L. Roeder, J. R. Ehleringer, Carbon isotopic fractionation between diet, breath and bioapatite in different mammals. *J. Arch. Sci.* 2005, 32, 1459-1470.

[32] C. Meneghini, M. C. Dalconi, S. Nuzzo, S. Mobilio, R. H. Wenk, Rietveld refinement on X-ray diffraction patterns of bioapatite in human fetal bones. *Biophys. J.* 2003, 84, 2021-2029.

[33] H. C. W. Skinner, *Biominerals. Mineralogical Magazine* 2005, 69, 621-641.

[34] G. Daculsi, Physicochemical and ultrastructural analysis of bone bioactive interface. *Biomater. Tissue Int.* 1992, 10, 296-304.

[35] G. Daculsi, J. M. Bouler, R. Z. LeGeros, Adaptive crystal formation in normal and pathological calcifications in synthetic calcium phosphate and related biomaterials. *Int. Rev. Cytology* 1997, 172, 129-191.

[36] F. C. M. Driessens, R. M. H. Verbeeck, *Biominerals*. CRC Press, Boca Raton, Florida, 1990, 440 pp.

[37] P. W. Brown, Phase relationships in the ternary system $CaO-P_2O_5-H_2O$ at 25°C. *J. Amer. Ceram. Soc.* 1992, 75, 17-22.

[38] R. I. Martin, P. W. Brown, Phase equilibria among acid calcium phosphates. *J. Amer. Ceram. Soc*. 1997, 80, 1263–1266.

[39] K. A. Gross, C.C. Berndt, R. Dinnebier, P. Stephens, Oxyapatite in hydroxyapatite coatings, *J. Mater. Sci. Mater. Med.* 1998, 33, 3985-3991.

[40] P. Alberius-Henning, E. Adolfsson, J. Grins, A. Fitch, Triclinic oxy-hydroxyapatite. *J. Mater. Sci.* 2001, 36, 663-668.

[41] C. van't Hoen, V. Rheinberger, W. Höland, E. Apel, Crystallization of oxyapatite in glass-ceramics. *J. Eur. Ceram. Soc*. 2007, 27, 1579-1584.

[42] T. J. White, Z. L. Dong, Structural derivation and crystal chemistry of apatites. *Acta Crystallogr.* B 2003, B59, 1-16.

[43] A. K. Lynn, W. Bonfield, A novel method for the simultaneous, titrant-free control of pH and calcium phosphate mass yield. *Acc. Chem. Res*. 2005, 38, 202-207.

[44] E. Fernandez, F. J. Gil, M. P. Ginebra, F. C. M. Driessens, J. A. Planell, S. M. Best, Calcium phosphate bone cements for clinical applications. Part I: solution chemistry. *J. Mater. Sci. Mater. Med.* 1999, 10, 169-176.

[45] M. Mathew, S. Takagi, Structures of biological minerals in dental. *Research. J. Res. Natl. Inst. Stand. Technol*. 2001, 106, 1035–1044.

[46] K. Köster, H. Heide, R. König, Resorbierbare Calciumphosphatkeramik im Tierexperiment unter Belastung. *Langenbecks Arch. Chir*. 1977, 343, 173–181.

[47] O. Bermúdez, M. G. Boltong, F. C. M. Driessens, J. A. Planell, Optimization of a calcium orthophosphate cement formulation occurring in the combination of monocalcium phosphate monohydrate with calcium oxide. *J. Mater. Sci. Mater. Med.* 1994, 5, 67-71.

[48] O. Bermúdez, M. G. Boltong, F. C. M. Driessens, J. A. Planell, Development of some calcium phosphate cements from combinations of α-TCP, MCPM and CaO. *J. Mater. Sci. Mater. Med.* 1994, 5, 160-163.

[49] F. C. M. Driessens, M. G. Boltong, O. Bermúdez, J. A. Planell, M. P. Ginebra, E. Fernández, Effective formulations for the preparation of calcium phosphate bone cements. *J. Mater. Sci. Mater. Med.* 1994, 5, 164-170.

[50] S. Budavari, M. J. O'Neil, A. Smith, P. E. Heckelman, J. F. Kinneary (Eds.), *The Merck Index: An encyclopedia of chemicals, drugs, and biologicals.* 12th Ed., Chapman and Hall, 1996, 1741 pp.

[51] D. F. Williams. *The Williams dictionary of biomaterials*. Liverpool University Press. Liverpool, 1999, 368 pp.

[52] C. Hamanishi, K. Kitamoto, K. Ohura, S. Tanaka, Y. Doi, Self-setting, bioactive, and biodegradable TTCP-DCPD apatite cement. *J. Biomed. Mater. Res*. 1996, 32, 383-389.

[53] K. Kurashina, H. Kurita, M. Hirano, A. Kotani, C. P. Klein, K. de Groot, *In vivo* study of calcium phosphate cements: implantation of an α-tricalcium phosphate/dicalcium phosphate dibasic/tetracalcium phosphate monoxide cement paste. *Biomaterials* 1997, 18, 539-543.

[54] F. C. M. Driessens, J. A. Planell, M. G. Boltong, I. Khairoun, M. P. Ginebra, Osteotransductive bone cements. *Proc. Inst. Mech. Eng.* [H] 1998, 212, 427-435.

[55] S. Takagi, L. C. Chow, K. Ishikawa, Formation of hydroxyapatite in new calcium phosphate cements. *Biomaterials* 1998, 19, 1593-1599.

[56] H. Yamamoto, S. Niwa, M. Hori, T. Hattori, K. Sawai, S. Aoki, M. Hirano, H. Takeuchi, Mechanical strength of calcium phosphate cement *in vivo* and *in vitro*. *Biomaterials* 1998, 19, 1587-1591.

[57] J. J. Crall, J. M. Bjerga, Effects of DCPD/APF application and prolonged exposure to fluoride on caries-like lesion formation *in vitro*. *J. Oral Pathol.* 1987, 16, 488-491.

[58] J. S. Wefel, J. D. Harless, The use of saturated DCPD in remineralization of artificial caries lesions *in vitro*. *J. Dent. Res.* 1987, 66, 1640-1643.

[59] P. M. Hoppenbrouwers, E. Groenendijk, N. R. Tewarie, F. C. M. Driessens, Improvement of the caries resistance of human dental roots by a two-step conversion of the root mineral into fluoridated hydroxylapatite. *J. Dent. Res.* 1988, 67, 1254-1256.

[60] A. Gaffar, J. Blake-Haskins, J. Mellberg, *In vivo* studies with a dicalcium phosphate/MFP system for caries prevention. *Int. Dent. J.* 1993, 43 (Suppl. 1), 81-88.

[61] R. J. Sullivan, A. Charig, J. Blake-Haskins, Y. P. Zhang, S. M. Miller, M. Strannick, A. Gaffar, H. C. Margolis, *In vivo* detection of calcium from dicalcium phosphate dihydrate dentifrices in demineralized human enamel and plaque. *Adv. Dent. Res.* 1997, 11, 380-387.

[62] S. M. Mostashari, H. Haddadi, Z. Hashempoor, Effect of deposited calcium hydrogen phosphate dihydrate on the flame retardancy imparted to cotton fabric. *Asian J. Chem.* 2006, 18, 2388-2390.

[63] Y. Fukase, E. D. Eanes, S. Takagi, L. C. Chow, W. E. Brown, Setting reactions and compressive strengths of calcium phosphate cements. *J. Dent. Res.* 1990, 69, 1852-1856.

[64] K. S. TenHuisen, P. W. Brown, The formation of hydroxyapatite-ionomer cements at 38 degrees C. *J. Dent. Res.* 1994, 73, 598-606.

[65] E. Fernandez, M. P. Ginebra, M. G. Boltong, F. C. M. Driessens, J. Ginebra, E. A. de Maeyer, R. M. H. Verbeeck, J. A. Planell, Kinetic study of the setting reaction of a calcium phosphate bone cement. *J. Biomed. Mater. Res.* 1996, 32, 367-374.

[66] E. Fernandez, F. J. Gil, S. M. Best, M. P. Ginebra, F. C. M. Driessens, J. A. Planell, The cement setting reaction in the $CaHPO_4$ – α-$Ca_3(PO_4)_2$ system: an X-ray diffraction study. *J. Biomed. Mater. Res.* 1998, 42, 403-406.

[67] E. Fernandez, F. J. Gil, M. P. Ginebra, F. C. M. Driessens, J. A. Planell, S. M. Best, Production and characterization of new calcium phosphate bone cements in the $CaHPO_4$ – α-$Ca_3(PO_4)_2$ system: pH, workability and setting times. *J. Mater. Sci. Mater. Med.* 1999, 10, 223-230.

[68] R. Z. LeGeros, Preparation of octacalcium phosphate (OCP): a direct fast method. Calcif. *Tissue Intern.* 1985, 37, 194-197.

[69] A. Bigi, E. Boanini, M. Borghi, G. Cojazzi, S. Panzavolta, N. Roveri, Synthesis and hydrolysis of octacalcium phosphate: effect of sodium polyacrylate. *J. Inorg. Biochem.* 1999, 75, 145-151.

[70] A. Nakahira, S. Aoki, K. Sakamoto, S. Yamaguchi, Synthesis and evaluation of various layered octacalcium phosphates by wet-chemical processing. *J. Mater. Sci. Mater. Med.* 2001, 12, 793-800.

[71] R. M. Shelton, Y. Liu, P. R. Cooper, U. Gbureck, M. J. German, J. E. Barralet, Bone marrow cell gene expression and tissue construct assembly using octacalcium phosphate microscaffolds. *Biomaterials* 2006, 27, 2874–2881.

[72] W. E. Brown, M. Mathew, M. S. Tung, Crystal chemistry of octacalcium phosphate. *Prog. Cryst. Growth Charact.* 1981, 4, 59-87.

[73] R. Z. LeGeros, Variations in the crystalline components of human dental calculus: I. crystallographic and spectroscopic methods of analysis. *J. Dent. Res.* 1974, 53, 45-50.

[74] H. Schroeder, Formation and inhibition of dental calculus. *J. Periodontol.* 1969, 40, 643-646.

[75] L. C. Chow, E. D. Eanes (Eds.), Octacalcium phosphate. *Monogr. Oral Sci.* vol. 18. Karger, Basel, 2001, 167 pp.

[76] W. E. Brown, Octacalcium phosphate and hydroxyapatite. *Nature* 1962, 196, 1048-1050.

[77] W. E. Brown, Crystal growth of bone mineral. *Clin. Orthop. Relat. Res.* 1966, 44, 205-220.

[78] D. G. A. Nelson, G. J. Wood, J. C. Barry, J. D. B. Featherstone, The structure of (100) defects in carbonated apatite crystallites: a high-resolution electron microscope study. *Ultramicroscopy* 1986, 19, 253-265.

[79] M. Iijima, D. G. A. Nelson, Y. Pan, A. T. Kreinbrink, M. Adachi, T. Goto, Y. Moriwaki, Fluoride analysis of apatite crystals with a central planar OCP inclusion: concerning the role of F^- ions on apatite/OCP/apatite structure formation. *Calcif. Tissue Int.* 1996, 59, 377-384.

[80] P. Bodier-Houllé, P. Steuer, J. C. Voegel, F. J. G. Cuisinier, First experimental evidence for human dentine crystal formation involving conversion of octacalcium phosphate to hydroxyapatite. *Acta Crystallogr. D: Biol. Crystallogr.* 1998, 54, 1377-1381.

[81] T. Aoba, H. Komatsu, Y. Shimazu, H. Yagishita, Y. Taya, Enamel mineralization and an initial crystalline phase. *Connect. Tissue Res.* 1998, 38, 129-137.

[82] B. B. Tomazic, W. E. Brown, F. J. Shoen, Physicochemical properties of calcific deposits isolated from porcine bioprosthetic heart valves removed from patients following 2-13 years function. *J. Biomed. Mater. Res.* 1994, 28, 35-47.

[83] G. H. Nancollas, W. Wu, Biomineralization mechanisms: a kinetics and interfacial energy approach. *J. Cryst. Growth* 2000, 211, 137-142.

[84] S. Kamakura, Y. Sasano, H. Homma, O. Suzuki, M. Kagayama, K. Motegi, Implantation of octacalcium phosphate (OCP) in rat skull defects enhances bone repair. *J. Dent. Res.* 1999, 78, 1682-1687.

[85] S. Kamakura, Y. Sasano, H. Homma, O. Suzuki, M. Kagayama, K. Motegi, Implantation of octacalcium phosphate nucleates isolated bone formation in rat skull defects. *Oral Dis*. 2001, 7, 259-265.

[86] F. Sargolzaei-Aval, A. Sobhani, M.R. Arab, S.A. Sarani, M.H. Heydari, The efficacy of implant of octacalcium phosphate in combination with bone matrix gelatin (BMG) on bone regeneration in skull defects in rat. *Iran J. Med. Sci*. 2004, 29, 124-129.

[87] O. Suzuki, S. Kamakura, T. Katagiri, M. Nakamura, B. Zhao, Y. Honda, R. Kamijo, Bone formation enhanced by implanted octacalcium phosphate involving conversion into Ca-deficient hydroxyapatite. *Biomaterials* 2006, 27, 2671-2681.

[88] A. T. Jensen, S. L. Rowles, Magnesium whitlockite, a major constituent of dental calculus. *Acta Odont. Scand*. 1957, 16, 121-139.

[89] C. Calvo, R. Gopal, The crystal structure of whitlockite from the Palermo Quarry. *Amer. Mineral*. 1975, 60, 120-133.

[90] http://rruff.geo.arizona.edu/doclib/hom/whitlockite.pdf (accessed in September 2008).

[91] T. Kodaka, K. Debari, S. Higashi, Magnesium-containing crystals in human dental calculus. *J. Electron Microsc*. (Tokyo) 1988, 37, 73-80.

[92] A. A. Mirtchi, J. Lemaître, E. Munting, Calcium phosphate cements: study of the β-tricalcium phosphate – dicalcium phosphate – calcite cements. *Biomaterials* 1990, 11, 83-88.

[93] A. A. Mirtchi, J. Lemaître, E. Munting, Calcium phosphate cements: effect of fluorides on the setting and hardening of β-tricalcium phosphate – dicalcium phosphate – calcite cements. *Biomaterials* 1991, 12, 505-510.

[94] J. Lemaître, E. Munting, A. A. Mirtchi, Setting, hardening and resorption of calcium phosphate ionic cements. *Rev. Stomatol. Chir. Maxillofac*. 1992, 93, 163-165.

[95] K. Ohura, M. Bohner, P. Hardouin, J. Lemaître, G. Pasquier, B. Flautre, Resorption of, and bone formation from, new β-tricalcium phosphate-monocalcium phosphate cements: an *in vivo* study. *J. Biomed. Mater. Res*. 1996, 30, 193-200.

[96] R. F. Ellinger, E. B. Nery, K. L. Lynch, Histological assessment of periodontal osseous defects following implantation of hydroxyapatite and biphasic calcium phosphate ceramics: a case report. *Int. J. Periodont. Restor. Dent*. 1986, 3, 22-33.

[97] E. B. Nery, K. L. Lynch, W. M. Hirthe, K. H. Mueller, Bioceramic implants in surgically produced infrabony defects. *J. Periodontol*. 1975, 46, 328-347.

[98] A. Lecomte, H. Gautier, J. M. Bouler, A. Gouyette, Y. Pegon, G. Daculsi, C. Merle, Biphasic calcium phosphate: a comparative study of interconnected porosity in two ceramics. *J. Biomed. Mater. Res. B Appl. Biomater*. 2008, 84B, 1-6.

[99] F. Tancret, J. M. Bouler, J. Chamousset, L. M. Minois, Modelling the mechanical properties of microporous and macroporous biphasic calcium phosphate bioceramics. *J. Eur. Ceram. Soc*. 2006, 26, 3647-3656.

[100] J. M. Bouler, M. Trecant, J. Delecrin, J. Royer, N. Passuti, G. Daculsi, Macroporous biphasic calcium phosphate ceramics: Influence of five synthesis parameters on compressive strength. *J. Biomed. Mater. Res*. 1996, 32, 603-609.

[101] J. Wang, W. Chen, Y. Li, S. Fan, J. Weng, X. Zhang, Biological evaluation of biphasic calcium phosphate ceramic vertebral laminae. *Biomaterials* 1998, 19, 1387-1392.

[102] G. Daculsi, Biphasic calcium phosphate concept applied to artificial bone, implant coating and injectable bone substitute. *Biomaterials* 1998, 19, 1473-1478.

[103] G. Daculsi, P. Weiss, J. M. Bouler, O. Gauthier, F. Millot, E. Aguado, Biphasic calcium phosphate/hydrosoluble polymer composites: a new concept for bone and dental substitution biomaterials. *Bone* 1999, 25, Suppl. 2, 59S-61S.

[104] R. Z. LeGeros, S. Lin, R. Rohanizadeh, D. Mijares, J. P. LeGeros, Biphasic calcium phosphate bioceramics: preparation, properties and applications. *J. Mater. Sci. Mater. Med.* 2003, 14, 201-209.

[105] G. Daculsi, O. Laboux, O. Malard, P. Weiss, Current state of the art of biphasic calcium phosphate bioceramics. *J. Mater. Sci. Mater. Med.* 2003, 14, 195-200.

[106] I. Alam, I. Asahina, K. Ohmamiuda, S. Enomoto, Comparative study of biphasic calcium phosphate ceramics impregnated with rhBMP-2 as bone substitutes. *J. Biomed. Mater. Res.* 2001, 54, 129-138.

[107] G. Daculsi, Biphasic calcium phosphate granules concept for injectable and mouldable bone substitute. *Advances in Science and Technology* 2006, 49, 9-13.

[108] D. S. Metsger, T. D. Driskell, J. R. Paulsrud, Tricalcium phosphate ceramic – a resorbable bone implant: review and current status. *J. Amer. Dent. Assoc.* 1982, 105, 1035-1038.

[109] R. W. Nurse, J. B. Welch, W. Gun, High-temperature phase equilibria in the system dicalcium silicate – tricalcium phosphate. *J. Chem. Soc.* 1959, 1077-1083.

[110] S. D. Langstaff, M. Sayer, T. J. N. Smith, S. M. Pugh, S. A. M. Hesp, W. T. Thompson, Resorbable bioceramics based on stabilized calcium phosphates. Part I: Rational design, sample preparation and material characterization. *Biomaterials* 1999, 20, 1727-1741.

[111] S. D. Langstaff, M. Sayer, T. J. N. Smith, S. M. Pugh, Resorbable bioceramics based on stabilized calcium phosphates. Part II: Evaluation of biological response. *Biomaterials* 2001, 22, 135-150.

[112] M. Sayer, A. D. Stratilatov, J.W. Reid, L. Calderin, M. J. Stott, X. Yin, M. MacKenzie, T. J. N. Smith, J. A. Hendry, S. D. Langstaff, Structure and composition of silicon-stabilized tricalcium phosphate. *Biomaterials* 2003, 24, 369–382.

[113] J. W. Reid, A. M. Pietak, M. Sayer, D. Dunfield, T. J. N. Smith, Phase formation and evolution in the silicon substituted tricalcium phosphate/apatite system. *Biomaterials* 2005, 26, 2887-2897.

[114] J. W. Reid, L. Tuck, M. Sayer, K. Fargo, J. A. Hendry, Synthesis and characterization of single-phase silicon substituted α-tricalcium phosphate. *Biomaterials*, 2006, 27, 2916-2925.

[115] R. Astala, L. Calderin, X. Yin, M. J. Stott, *Ab initio* simulation of Si-doped hydroxyapatite. *Chem. Mater*. 2006, 18, 413-422.

[116] X. Yin, M. J. Stott, A. Rubio, α- and β-tricalcium phosphate: a density functional study. *Phys. Rev*. B 2003, 68, 205205 (7 pages).

[117] B. R. Constantz, I. C. Ison, M. T. Fulmer, R. D. Poser, S. T. Smith, M. Vanwagoner, J. Ross, S. A. Goldstein, J. B. Jupiter, D. I. Rosenthal, Skeletal repair by *in situ* formation of the mineral phase of bone. *Science* 1995, 267, 1796-1799.

[118] X. Yin, M. J. Stott, Theoretical insights into bone grafting Si-stabilized α-tricalcium phosphate. *J. Chem. Phys*. 2005, 122, 024709 (9 pages).

[119] X. Yin, M. J. Stott, Surface and adsorption properties of α-tricalcium phosphate. *J. Chem. Phys.* 2006, 124, 124701 (9 pages).

[120] J. D. Termine, E. D. Eanes, Comparative chemistry of amorphous and apatitic calcium phosphate preparations. *Calcif. Tissue Res*. 1972, 10, 171-197.

[121] E. D. Eanes, J. D. Termine, M. U. Nylen, An electron microscopic study of the formation of amorphous calcium phosphate and its transformation to crystalline apatite. *Calcif. Tissue Res*. 1973, 12, 143-158.

[122] J. L. Meyer, E. D. Eanes, A thermodynamic analysis of the amorphous to crystalline calcium phosphate transformation. *Calcif. Tissue Res.* 1978, 28, 59-68.

[123] J. L. Meyer, E. D. Eanes, A thermodynamic analysis of the secondary transition in the spontaneous precipitation of calcium phosphate. *Calcif. Tissue Res*. 1978, 28, 209-216.

[124] R. E. Wuthier, G. S. Rice, J. E. Wallace, R. L. Weaver, R. Z. LeGeros, E. D. Eanes, *In vitro* precipitation of calcium phosphate under intracellular conditions: formation of brushite from an amorphous precursor in the absence of ATP. *Calcif. Tissue Int*. 1985, 37, 401-410.

[125] V. A. Sinyaev, E. S. Shustikova, L. V. Levchenko, A. A. Sedunov, Synthesis and dehydration of amorphous calcium phosphate. *Inorg. Materials* 2001, 37, 619-622.

[126] J. C. Elliot, Recent studies of apatites and other calcium orthophosphates. in: Les matériaux en phosphate de calcium. Aspects fondamentaux. / Calcium phosphate materials. *Fundamentals.* (Eds.: E. Brès, P. Hardouin), Sauramps Medical, Montpellier, 1998, pp. 25-66.

[127] D. Tadic, F. Peters, M. Epple, Continuous synthesis of amorphous carbonated apatites. *Biomaterials* 2002, 23, 2553-2559.

[128] J. E. Harries, D. W. L. Hukins, S. S. Hasnain, Analysis of the EXAFS spectrum of hydroxyapatite. *J. Phys. C: Solid State Phys*. 1986, 19, 6859-6872.

[129] J. E. Harries, D. W. L. Hukins, C. Holt, S. S. Hasnain, Conversion of amorphous calcium phosphate into hydroxyapatite investigated by EXAFS spectroscopy. *J. Cryst. Growth* 1987, 84, 563-570.

[130] M. G. Taylor, K. Simkiss, J. Simmons, L. N. Y. Wu, R. E. Wuthier, Structural studies of a phosphatidyl serine-amorphous calcium phosphate complex. *Cell. Mol. Life Sci.* 1998, 54, 192-202.

[131] F. Peters, K. Schwarz, M. Epple, The structure of bone studied with synchrotron X-ray diffraction, X-ray absorption spectroscopy and thermal analysis. *Thermochim. Acta* 2000, 361, 131-138.

[132] K. Onuma, A. Ito, Cluster growth model for hydroxyapatite. *Chem. Mater*. 1998, 10, 3346-3351.

[133] D. Skrtic, A. W. Hailer, S. Takagi, J. M. Antonucci, E. D. Eanes, Quantitative assessment of the efficacy of amorphous calcium phosphate/methacrylate composites in remineralizing caries-like lesions artificially produced in bovine enamel. *J. Dent. Res.* 1996, 75, 1679-1686.

[134] D. Skrtic, J. M. Antonucci, E. D. Eanes, Improved properties of amorphous calcium phosphate fillers in remineralizing resin composites. *Dent. Mater*. 1996, 12, 295-301.

[135] D. Skrtic, J. M. Antonucci, E. D. Eanes, Amorphous calcium phosphate-based bioactive polymeric composites for mineralized tissue regeneration. *J. Res. Natl. Inst. Stand. Technol.* 2003, 108, 167-182.

[136] D. Skrtic, J. M. Antonucci, E. D. Eanes, F. C. Eichmiller, G. E. Schumacher, Physicochemical evaluation of bioactive polymeric composites based on hybrid amorphous calcium phosphates. *J. Biomed. Mater. Res.* (Appl. Biomater.) 2000, 53, 381-391.

[137] C. Schiller, M. Siedler, F. Peters, M. Epple, Functionally graded materials of biodegradable polyesters and bone-like calcium phosphates for bone replacement. *Ceramic Trans.* 2001, 114, 97-108.

[138] W. Linhart, F. Peters, W. Lehmann, A. F. Schilling, K. Schwarz, M. Amling, J. M. Rueger, M. Epple, Biologically and chemically optimized composites of carbonated apatite and polyglycolide as bone substitution materials. *J. Biomed. Mater. Res.* 2001, 54, 162-171.

[139] D. Tadic, F. Beckmann, K. Schwarz, M. Epple, A novel method to produce hydroxylapatite objects with interconnecting porosity that avoids sintering. *Biomaterials* 2004, 25, 3335-3340.

[140] D. Tadic, M. Epple, Amorphous calcium phosphates as bone substitution materials. *Eur. J. Trauma* 2002, 28, 136-137.

[141] E. D. Eanes, Amorphous calcium phosphate. In: L. C. Chow, E. D. Eanes (Eds.), Octacalcium phosphate. *Monogr. Oral Sci.* vol. 18. Karger, Basel, 2001, pp. 130-147.

[142] J. C. Knowles, S. Callcut, G. Georgiou, Characterisation of the rheological properties and zeta potential of a range of hydroxyapatite powders. *Biomaterials* 2000, 21, 1387-1392.

[143] R. Kumar, K. H. Prakash, P. Cheang, K. A. Khor, Temperature driven morphological changes of chemically precipitated hydroxyapatite nanoparticles. *Langmuir* 2004, 20, 5196-5200.

[144] Y. M. Sung, J. C. Lee, J. W. Yang, Crystallization and sintering characteristics of chemically precipitated hydroxyapatite nanopowder. *J. Cryst. Growth* 2004, 262, 467-472.

[145] E. I. Dorozhkina, S. V. Dorozhkin, Mechanism of the solid-state transformation of a calcium-deficient hydroxyapatite (CDHA) into biphasic calcium phosphate (BCP) at elevated temperatures. *Chem. Mater.* 2002, 14, 4267–4272.

[146] S. V. Dorozhkin, Mechanism of solid-state conversion of non-stoichiometric hydroxyapatite to diphase calcium phosphate. *Russ. Chem. Bull.* (Int. Ed.) 2003, 52, 2369–2375.

[147] L. Rodríguez-Lorenzo, Studies on calcium deficient apatites structure by means of MAS-NMR spectroscopy. *J. Mater. Sci. Mater. Med.* 2005, 16, 393-398.

[148] R. M. Wilson, J. C. Elliott, S. E. P. Dowker, Formate incorporation in the structure of Ca-deficient apatite: Rietveld structure refinement. *J. Solid State Chem.* 2003, 174, 132-140.

[149] P. W. Brown, R. I. Martin, An analysis of hydroxyapatite surface layer formation. *J. Phys. Chem.* B 1999, 103, 1671-1675.

[150] A. Mortier, J. Lemaître, L. Rodrique, P. G. Rouxhet, Synthesis and thermal behavior of well-crystallized calcium-deficient phosphate apatite. *J. Solid State Chem.* 1989, 78, 215-219.

[151] J. Jeanjean, S. McGrellis, J. C. Rouchaud, M. Fedoroff, A. Rondeau, S. Perocheau, A. Dubis. A crystallographic study of the sorption of cadmium on calcium hydroxyapatites: incidence of cationic vacancies. *J. Solid State Chem.* 1996, 126, 195-201.

[152] T. I. Ivanova, O. V. Frank-Kamenetskaya, A. B. Kol'tsov, V. L. Ugolkov, Crystal structure of calcium-deficient carbonated hydroxyapatite thermal decomposition. *J. Solid State Chem.* 2001, 160, 340-349.

[153] K. Matsunaga, Theoretical investigation of the defect formation mechanism relevant to nonstoichiometry in hydroxyapatite. *Phys. Rev. B* 2008, 77, 104106 (14 pages).

[154] T. Tsuchida, T. Yoshioka, S. Sakuma, T. Takeguchi, W. Ueda, Synthesis of biogasoline from ethanol over hydroxyapatite catalyst. *Ind. Engin. Chem. Res.* 2008, 47, 1443-1452.

[155] J. C. Elliott, P. E. Mackie, R. A. Young, Monoclinic hydroxyapatite. *Science* 1973, 180, 1055–1057.

[156] N. Rangavittal, A. R. Landa-Cánovas, J. M. González-Calbet, M. Vallet-Regi, Structural study and stability of hydroxyapatite and β-tricalcium phosphate: two important bioceramics. *J. Biomed. Mater. Res.* 2000, 51, 660-668.

[157] J. Y. Kim, R. R. Fenton, B. A. Hunter, B. J. Kennedy, Powder diffraction studies of synthetic calcium and lead apatites. *Austr. J. Chem.* 2000, 53, 679-686.

[158] M. I. Kay, R. A. Young, A. S. Posner, Crystal structure of hydroxyapatite. *Nature* 1964, 204, 1050-1052.

[159] A. S. Posner, F. Betts, Synthetic amorphous calcium phosphate and its relation to bone mineral structure. *Acc. Chem. Res.* 1975, 8, 273-281.

[160] J. M. Hughes, J. Rakovan, The crystal structure of apatite, $Ca_5(PO_4)_3(F,OH,Cl)$. in: Phosphates: geochemical, geobiological and materials importance. *Series: Reviews in Mineralogy and Geochemistry*. Vol. 48, J. M. Hughes, M. Kohn, J. Rakovan (Eds.). Mineralogical Society of America, Washington, D.C. 2002, pp. 1-12.

[161] L. Calderin, M. J. Stott, A. Rubio, Electronic and crystallographic structure of apatites, *Phys. Rev.* B, 2003, 67, 134106 (6 pages).

[162] P. Rulis, L. Ouyang, W. Y. Ching, Electronic structure and bonding in calcium apatite crystals: hydroxyapatite, fluorapatite, chlorapatite and bromapatite. *Phys. Rev.* B 2004, 70, 155104 (8 pages).

[163] G. Treboux, P. Layrolle, N. Kanzaki, K. Onuma, A. Ito, Symmetry of Posner's cluster. *J. Amer. Chem. Soc.* 2000, 122, 8323-8324.

[164] G. Treboux, P. Layrolle, N. Kanzaki, K. Onuma, A. Ito, Existence of Posner's cluster in vacuum. *J. Phys. Chem.* A 2000, 104, 5111-5114.

[165] X. Yin, M. J. Stott, Biological calcium phosphates and Posner's cluster. *J. Chem. Phys.* 2003, 118, 3717-3723.

[166] N. Kanzaki, G. Treboux, K. Onuma, S. Tsutsumi, A. Ito, Calcium phosphate clusters. *Biomaterials* 2001, 22, 2921-2929.

[167] L. Calderin, D. Dunfield, M. J. Stott, Shell-model study of the lattice dynamics of hydroxyapatite. *Phys. Rev.* B 2005, 72, 224304 (12 pages).

[168] El Briak-Ben, H. Abdeslam, M. P. Ginebra, M. Vert, P. Boudeville, Wet or dry mechanochemical synthesis of calcium phosphates? Influence of the water content on DCPD-CaO reaction kinetics. *Acta Biomater.* 2008, 4, 378-386.

[169] R. Z. LeGeros, J. P. LeGeros, Dense hydroxyapatite. In: *An introduction to bioceramics*. (Eds.: L. L. Hench, J. Wilson), World Scientific, London, 1993, 139-180.

[170] L. M. Rodriguez-Lorenzo, M. Vallet-Regi, Controlled crystallization of calcium phosphate apatites. *Chem. Mater.* 2000, 12, 2460-2465.

[171] S. Cazalbou, C. Combes, D. Eichert, C. Rey, Adaptive physico-chemistry of bio-related calcium phosphates. *J. Mater. Chem.* 2004, 14, 2148–2153.

[172] M. Markovic, B. O. Fowler, M. S. Tung, Preparation and comprehensive characterization of a calcium hydroxyapatite reference material. *J. Res. Natl. Inst. Stand. Technol.* 2004, 109, 553-568.

[173] K. Ioku, G. Kawachi, S. Sasaki, H. Fujimori, S. Goto, Hydrothermal preparation of tailored hydroxyapatite. *J. Mater. Sci.* 2006, 41, 1341-1344.

[174] P. Layrolle, A. Lebugle, Characterization and reactivity of nanosized calcium phosphates prepared in anhydrous ethanol. *Chem. Mater.* 1994, 6, 1996-2004.

[175] P. Layrolle, A. Lebugle, Synthesis in pure ethanol and characterization of nanosized calcium phosphate fluoroapatite. *Chem. Mater.* 1996, 8, 134-144.

[176] B. Yeong, X. Junmin, J. Wang, Mechanochemical synthesis of hydroxyapatite from calcium oxide and brushite. *J. Amer. Ceram. Soc.* 2001, 84, 465–467.

[177] D. M. Roy, S. K. Linnehan, Hydroxyapatite formed from coral skeletal carbonate by hydrothermal exchange. *Nature* 1974, 247, 220-222.

[178] B. Ben-Nissan, Natural bioceramics: from coral to bone and beyond. *Curr. Opin. Solid State Mater.* Sci. 2003, 7, 283–288.

[179] J. C. Elliott, R. A. Young, Conversion of single crystals of chlorapatite into single crystals of hydroxyapatite. *Nature* 1967, 214, 904-906.

[180] Preparation of large-sized hydroxyapatite single crystals using homogeneous releasing controls. *J. Cryst. Growth* 2007, 308, 151-158.

[181] M. Vallet-Regi, M. T. Gutièrrez Rios, M. P. Alonso, M. I. de Frutos, S. Nicolopoulos, Hydroxyapatite particles synthesized by pyrolysis of an aerosol. *J. Solid State Chem.* 1994, 112, 58-64.

[182] M. L. Montero, A. Sáenz, J. G. Rodríguez, J. Arenas, V. M. Castaño, Electrochemical synthesis of nanosized hydroxyapatite. *J. Mater. Sci.* 2006, 41, 2141-2144.

[183] A. R. Kumar, S. Kalainathan, Growth and characterization of nano-crystalline hydroxyapatite at physiological conditions. *Crystal Res. Technology* 2008, 43, 640-644.

[184] S. J. Kalita, A. Bhardwaj, H. A. Bhatt, Nanocrystalline calcium phosphate ceramics in biomedical engineering. *Mater. Sci. Engin.* C 2007, 27, 441–449.

[185] I. V. Melikhov, V. F. Komarov, A. V. Severin, V. E. Bozhevolnov, V. N. Rudin, Two-dimensional crystalline hydroxyapatite. *Doklady Phys. Chem*, 2000, 373, 125-128.

[186] E. I. Suvorova, P. A. Buffat, Electron diffraction and HRTEM characterization of calcium phosphate precipitation from aqueous solutions under biomineralization conditions. *Eur. Cells Mater.* 2001, 1, 27-42.

[187] E. I. Suvorova, P. A. Buffat, Model of the mechanism of Ca loss by bones under microgravity and earth conditions. *J. Biomed. Mater. Res.* 2002, 63, 424-432.

[188] K. Uematsu, M. Takagi, T. Honda, N. Uchida, K. Saito, Transparent hydroxyapatite prepared by hot isostatic pressing of filter cake. *J. Amer. Ceram. Soc.* 1989, 72, 1476-1478.

[189] K. Takikawa, M. Akao, Fabrication of transparent hydroxyapatite and application to bone marrow derived cell/hydroxyapatite interaction observation *in vivo*. *J. Mater. Sci. Mater. Med.* 1996, 7, 439-445.

[190] Y. Watanabe, T. Ikoma, A. Monkawa, Y. Suetsugu, H. Yamada, J. Tanaka, Y. Moriyoshi, Fabrication of transparent hydroxyapatite sintered body with high crystal orientation by pulse electric current sintering. *J. Amer. Ceram. Soc.* 2005, 88, 243-245.

[191] N. Kotobuki, K. Ioku, D. Kawagoe, H. Fujimori, S. Goto, H. Ohgushi, Observation of osteogenic differentiation cascade of living mesenchymal stem cells on transparent hydroxyapatite ceramics. *Biomaterials* 2005, 26, 779-785.

[192] R. Z. LeGeros, J. P. LeGeros, G. Daculsi, R. Kijkowska, Calcium phosphate biomaterials: preparation, properties and biodegradation. In: *Encyclopedic Handbook of Biomaterials and Bioengineering*. Part A: Materials Vol. 2. Wise DL, Trantolo DJ, Altobelli DE, Yaszemski MJ, Gresser JD, Schwartz ER (Eds.). Marcel Dekker, New York. 1995, pp. 1429-1463.

[193] T. S. B. Narasaraju, D. E. Phebe, Some physico-chemical aspects of hydroxylapatite. *J. Mater. Sci.* 1996, 31, 1-21.

[194] V. P. Orlovskii, S. M. Barinov, Hydroxyapatite and hydroxyapatite-matrix materials: a survey. *Russ. J. Inorg. Chem.* 2001, 46, Suppl. 2, S129-S149.

[195] V. P. Orlovskii, V. S. Komlev, S. M. Barinov, Hydroxyapatite and hydroxyapatite-based ceramics. *Inorganic Materials* 2002, 38, 973-984.

[196] J. Peña, M. Vallet-Regi, Hydroxyapatite, tricalcium phosphate and biphasic materials prepared by a liquid mix technique. *J. Eur. Ceram. Soc.* 2003, 23, 1687–1696.

[197] S. Koutsopoulos, Synthesis and characterization of hydroxyapatite crystals: a review study on the analytical methods. *J. Biomed. Mater. Res.* 2002, 62, 600-612.

[198] J. Rakovan, Growth and surface properties of apatite. In: *Phosphates: geochemical, geobiological and materials importance. Series: Reviews in Mineralogy and Geochemistry.* Vol. 48, J. M. Hughes, M. Kohn, J. Rakovan (Eds.). Mineralogical Society of America, Washington, D.C. 2002, pp. 51-86.

[199] S. V. Dorozhkin, A review on the dissolution models of calcium apatites. *Prog. Cryst. Growth Charact.* 2002, 44, 45–61.

[200] W. Suchanek, M. Yoshimura, Processing and properties of hydroxyapatite-based biomaterials for use as hard tissue replacement implants. *J. Mater. Res.* 1998, 13, 94-117.

[201] G. Willmann, Coating of implants with hydroxyapatite – material connections between bone and metal. *Adv. Engin. Materials* 1999, 1, 95-105.

[202] L. Sun, C. C. Berndt, K. A. Gross, A. Kucuk, Review: material fundamentals and clinical performance of plasma sprayed hydroxyapatite coatings. *J. Biomed. Mater. Res.* (Appl. Biomater.) 2001, 58, 570–592.

[203] J. L. Ong, D. C. N. Chan, Hydroxyapatites and their use as coatings in dental implants: a review. *Crit. Rev. Biomed. Engin.* 1999, 28, 667-707.

[204] R. G. Geesink, Osteoconductive coatings for total joint arthroplasty. *Clin. Orthop. Rel. Res.* 2002, 395, 53-65.

[205] L. L. Hench, Bioceramics: from concept to clinic. *J. Amer. Ceram. Soc.* 1991, 74, 1487-1510.

[206] L. L. Hench, Bioceramics. *J. Amer. Ceram. Soc.* 1998, 81, 1705-1728.

[207] C. Mangano, A. Piattelli, V. Perrotti, G. Iezzi, Dense hydroxyapatite inserted into postextraction sockets: a histologic and histomorphometric 20-year case report. J. *Periodontology* 2008, 79, 929-933.

[208] W. Dickinson, Chromatography of insulin on calcium phosphate columns. *Nature,* 1956, 178, 994–995.

[209] G. Bernardi, Chromatography of nucleic acids on hydroxyapatite. *Nature* 1965, 206, 779-783.

[210] Z. Xia, X. Duan, R. M. Locklin, M. Quijano, R. L. Dobson, J. T. Triffitt, F. H. Ebetino, G. R. Russell, Evaluation of the relative mineral-binding affinities of clinically-relevant bisphosphonates by using hydroxyapatite-column chromatography and adsorption isotherms combined with mass spectrometric analysis. *Bone* 2008, vol. 42, Supp. 1, S90-S91.

[211] M. Brand, S. Rampalli, C. P. Chaturvedi, F. J. Dilworth, Analysis of epigenetic modifications of chromatin at specific gene loci by native chromatin immunoprecipitation of nucleosomes isolated using hydroxyapatite chromatography. *Nature Protocols*, 2008, 3, 398-409.

[212] T. Yoshitake, S. Kobayashi, T. Ogawa, T. Okuyama, Hydroxyapatite chromatography of guanidine denatured proteins: 1. Guanidine containing phosphate buffer system. *Chromatography*, 2006, 27, 19-26.

[213] G. P. Smith, T. R. Gingrich, Hydroxyapatite chromatography of phage-display virions. *Biotechniques,* 2005, 39, 879-884.

[214] A. Jungbauer, R. Hahn, K. Deinhofer, P. Luo, Performance and characterization of a nanophased porous hydroxyapatite for protein chromatography. *Biotechnol. Bioengin.* 2004, 87, 364-375.

[215] S. Doonan, Chromatography on hydroxyapatite. *Methods Mol. Biol.* 2004, 244, 191-194.

[216] T. Y. Liu, S. Y. Chen, D. M. Liu, S. C. Liou, On the study of BSA-loaded calcium-deficient hydroxyapatite nano-carriers for controlled drug delivery. *J. Controlled Release,* 2005, 107, 112-121.

[217] B. Palazzo, M. C. Sidoti, N. Roveri, A. Tampieri, M. Sandri, L. Bertolazzi, F. Galbusera, G. Dubini, P. Vena, R. Contro, Controlled drug delivery from porous hydroxyapatite grafts: an experimental and theoretical approach. *Mater. Sci. Engin. C* 2005, 25, 207-213.

[218] J. Pietrasik, K. Szustakiewicz, M. Zaborski, K. Haberko, Hydroxyapatite: environmentally friendly filler for elastomers. *Molecular Crystals and Liquid Crystals* 2008, 483, 172-178.

[219] A. Corami, S. Mignardi, V. Ferrini, Cadmium removal from single- and multi-metal (Cd plus Pb plus Zn plus Cu) solutions by sorption on hydroxyapatite. *J. Coll. Interface Sci.* 2008, 317, 402-408.

[220] N. Phonthammachai, Z. Ziyi, G. Jun, H. Y. Fan, T. J. White, Synthesis of high performance hydroxyapatite-gold catalysts for CO oxidation. *Gold Bulletin* 2008, 41, 42-50.

[221] W. Chen, Z. L. Huang, Y. Liu, Q. J. He, Preparation and characterization of a novel solid base catalyst hydroxyapatite loaded with strontium. *Catalysis Comm.* 2008, 9, 516-521.

[222] K. de Groot, J. G. C. Wolke, J. A. Jansen, Calcium phosphate coatings for medical implants. *Proc. Inst. Mech. Eng. Part H: J. Eng. Med.* 1998, 212, 137-147.

[223] K. A. Gross, C. C. Berndt, Biomedical application of apatites. In: *Phosphates: geochemical, geobiological and materials importance. Series: Reviews in Mineralogy and Geochemistry*. Vol. 48, J. M. Hughes, M. Kohn, J. Rakovan (Eds.). Mineralogical Society of America, Washington, D.C. 2002, pp. 631-672.

[224] M. P. Ferraz, F. J. Monteiro, C. M. Manuel, Hydroxyapatite nanoparticles: a review of preparation methodologies. *J. Appl. Biomater. Biomech.* 2004, 2, 74-80.

[225] E. Damien, P. A. Revell, Coralline hydroxyapatite bone graft substitute: a review of experimental studies and biomedical applications. *J. Appl. Biomater. Biomech.* 2004, 2, 65-73.

[226] H. Aoki, *Science and medical applications of hydroxyapatite*. Tokyo, JAAS, 1991, 245 pp.

[227] S. M. Barinov, V. S. Komlev, Calcium phosphate based bioceramics for bone tissue engineering. *Materials Science Foundations* (monograph series), v. 48. Trans Tech Publications, Inc., 2008, 170 pp.

[228] R. Kniep, S. Busch, Biomimetic growth and self-assembly of fluorapatite aggregates by diffusion into denatured collagen matrices. *Angew. Chem. Int. Ed. Engl.* 1996, 35, 2624-2626.

[229] S. Busch, H. Dolhaine, A. Duchesne, S. Heinz, O. Hochrein, F. Laeri, O. Podebrad, U. Vietze, T. Weiland, R. Kniep, Biomimetic morphogenesis of fluorapatite-gelatin composites: fractal growth, the question of intrinsic electric fields, core/shell assemblies, hollow spheres and reorganization of denatured collagen. *Eur. J. Inorg. Chem.* 1999, 1643-1653.

[230] S. Busch, U. Schwarz, R. Kniep, Morphogenesis and structure of human teeth in relation to biomimetically grown fluorapatite-gelatine composites. *Chem. Mater.* 2001, 13, 3260-3271.

[231] O. Prymak, V. Sokolova, T. Peitsch, M. Epple, The crystallization of fluoroapatite dumbbells from supersaturated aqueous solution. *Cryst. Growth Des.* 2006, 6, 498-506.

[232] H. Tlatlik, P. Simon, A. Kawska, D. Zahn, R. Kniep, Biomimetic fluorapatite-gelatine nanocomposites: pre-structuring of gelatine matrices by ion impregnation and its effect on form development. *Angew. Chem. Int. Ed. Engl.* 2006, 45, 1905-1910.

[233] P. Simon, D. Zahn, H. Lichte, R. Kniep, Intrinsic electric dipole fields and the induction of hierarchical form developments in fluorapatite-gelatine nanocomposites: a

general principle for morphogenesis of biominerals? *Angew. Chem. Int. Ed. Engl.* 2006, 45, 1911-1915.

[234] S. V. Dorozhkin, A hierarchical structure for apatite crystals. J. *Mater. Sci. Mater. Med.* 2007, 18, 363–366.

[235] S. M. Barinov, L. I. Shvorneva, D. Ferro, I. V. Fadeeva, S. V. Tumanov, Solid solution formation at the sintering of hydroxyapatite–fluorapatite ceramics. *Sci. Technol. Advanc. Mater.* 2004, 5, 537-541.

[236] I. Nikcevic, V. Jokanovic, M. Mitric, Z. Nedic, D. Makovec, D. Uskokovic, Mechanochemical synthesis of nanostructured fluorapatite/fluorhydroxyapatite and carbonated fluorapatite/fluorhydroxyapatite. *J. Solid State Chem.* 2004, 177, 2565-2574.

[237] K. Cheng, W. Weng, H. Qu, P. Du, G. Shen, G. Han, J. Yang, J. M. F. Ferreira, Sol-gel preparation and *in vitro* test of fluorapatite/hydroxyapatite films. *J. Biomed. Mater. Res.* B 2004, 69B, 33-37.

[238] L. M. Rodriguez-Lorenzo, J. N. Hart, K. A. Gross, Influence of fluorine in the synthesis of apatites. Synthesis of solid solutions of hydroxy-fluorapatite. *Biomaterials,* 2003, 24, 3777-3785.

[239] M. Wei, J. H. Evans, T. Bostrom, L. Grondahl, Synthesis and characterization of hydroxyapatite, fluoride-substituted hydroxyapatite and fluorapatite. *J. Mater. Sci. Mater. Med.,* 2003, 14, 311-320.

[240] G. Daculsi, L. M. Kerebel, Ultrastructural study and comparative analysis of fluoride content of enameloid in sea-water and fresh-water sharks. *Arch. Oral Biol.* 1980, 25, 145–151.

[241] G. Daculsi, L. M. Kerebel, B. Kerebel, Effects of fluoride on human enamel and selachian enameloid *in vitro*: a high-resolution TEM and electron diffraction study. *Calcif. Tissue Int.* 1981, 33, 9-13.

[242] H. A. Lowenstam, S. Weiner, *On biomineralization*, Oxford University Press, 1989, 324 pp.

[243] S. Weiner, P. M. Dove, An overview of biomineralization processes and the problem of the vital effect. In: *Biomineralization. Series: Reviews in Mineralogy and Geochemistry.* Vol. 54. P. M. Dove, J. J. de Yoreo, S. Weiner (Eds.). Mineralogical Society of America, Washington, D.C. 2003, pp. 1-29.

[244] S. Dahm, S. Risnes, A comparative infrared spectroscopic study of hydroxide and carbonate absorption bands in spectra of shark enameloid, shark dentin, and a geological apatite. *Calcif. Tissue Int.* 1999, 65, 459-465.

[245] A. Carr, A. Kemp, I. Tibbetts, R. Truss, J. Drennan, Microstructure of pharyngeal tooth enameloid in the parrotfish *Scarus rivulatus* (Pisces: *Scaridae*). *J. Microscopy* 2006, 221, 8-16.

[246] I. Leveque, M. Cusack, S. A. Davis, S. Mann, Promotion of fluorapatite crystallization by soluble-matrix proteins from *Lingula Anatina* shells. *Angew. Chem. Int. Ed. Engl.* 2004, 43, 885-888.

[247] C. S. R. Fonteles, D. T. Zero, M. E. Moss, J. Fu, Fluoride concentrations in enamel and dentin of primary teeth after pre- and postnatal fluoride exposure. *Caries Res.* 2005, 39, 505-508.

[248] A. Wiegand, C. Krieger, R. Attin, E. Hellwig, T. Attin, Fluoride uptake and resistance to further demineralisation of demineralised enamel after application of differently concentrated acidulated sodium fluoride gels. *Clinical Oral Investigations* 2005, 9, 52-57.

[249] D. Waszkiel, K. Opalko, R. Lagocka, D. Chlubek, Fluoride and magnesium content in superficial enamel layers of teeth with erosions. *Fluoride* 2004, 37, 271-277.

[250] A. P. G. F. Vieira, R. Hancock, M. Dumitriu, M. Schwartz, H. Limeback, M. D. Grynpas, How does fluoride affect dentin microhardness and mineralization? *J. Dental Res.* 2005, 84, 951-957.

[251] F. C. M. Driessens, Relation between apatite solubility and anti-cariogenic effect of fluoride. *Nature* 1973, 243, 420-421.

[252] E. C. Moreno, M. Kresak, R. T. Zahradnik, Fluoridated hydroxyapatite solubility and caries formation. *Nature* 1974, 247, 64–65.

[253] L. Heling, R. Heindel, B. Merin, Calcium-fluorapatite. A new material for bone implants. *J. Oral Implantol.* 1981, 9, 548–555.

[254] J. K. Bibby, N. L. Bubb, D. J. Wood, P. M. Mummery, Fluorapatite-mullite glass sputter coated Ti6Al4V for biomedical applications. *J. Mater. Sci. Mater. Med.* 2005, 16, 379-385.

[255] B. H. Yoon, H. W. Kim, S. H. Lee, C. J. Bae, Y. H. Koh, Y. M. Kong, H. E. Kim, Stability and cellular responses to fluorapatite–collagen composites. *Biomaterials* 2005, 26, 2957-2963.

[256] L. Gineste, M. Gineste, X. Ranz, A. Ellefterion, A. Guilhem, N. Rouquet, P. Frayssinet, Degradation of hydroxylapatite, fluorapatite and fluorhydroxyapatite coatings of dental implants in dogs. *J. Biomed. Mater. Res.* 1999, 48, 224-234.

[257] K. A. Bhadang, K. A. Gross, Influence of fluorapatite on the properties of thermally sprayed hydroxyapatite coatings. *Biomaterials* 2004, 25, 4935-4945.

[258] K. A. Gross, K. A. Bhadang, Sintered hydroxyfluorapatites. Part III: Sintering and resultant mechanical properties of sintered blends of hydroxyapatite and fluorapatite. *Biomaterials* 2004, 25, 1395-1405.

[259] S. M. Barinov, F. Rustichelli, V. P. Orlovskii, A. Lodini, S. Oscarsson, S. A. Firstov, S. V. Tumanov, P. Millet, A. Rosengren, Influence of fluorapatite minor additions on behavior of hydroxyapatite ceramics. *J. Mater. Sci. Mater. Med.*, 2004, 15, 291-296.

[260] S. Agathopoulos, D. U. Tulyaganov, P. A. A. P. Marques, M. C. Ferro, M. H. Fernandes, R. N. Correia, The fluorapatite–anorthite system in biomedicine. *Biomaterials* 2003, 24, 1317-1331.

[261] H. Qu, M. Wei, The effect of fluoride contents in fluoridated hydroxyapatite on osteoblast behavior. *Acta Biomater.* 2006, 2, 113-119.

[262] M. Theiszova, S. Jantova, S. Letasiova, M. Palou, L. Cipak, Cytotoxicity of hydroxyapatite, fluorapatite and fluor-hydroxyapatite: a comparative *in vitro* study. *Neoplasma* (Bratislava) 2008, 55, 312-316.

[263] G. Hilgenstock, Stahl und Eisen, 1883, 3, 498.

[264] G. Hilgenstock, Tetrabasic calcium phosphate and the basicity of the silicate in basic cinder. Chem. Centr. 1887, 1097-1098, from Stahl und Eisen, 1887, 557-560. Cited from: J. Chem. Soc., Abstr., *Inorganic chemistry.* 1888, 54, 219-231.

[265] W. E. Brown, E. F. Epstein, Crystallography of tetracalcium phosphate. J. *Res. Nat. Bur. Stand.* A 1965, 69A, 547-551.

[266] E. Fernandez, F. J. Gil, M. P. Ginebra, F. C. M. Driessens, J. A. Planell, S. M. Best, Calcium phosphate bone cements for clinical applications. Part II: precipitate formation during setting reactions. *J. Mater. Sci. Mater. Med.* 1999, 10, 177-183.

[267] D. McConnell, A. S. Posner, Carbonate in apatites. *Science* 1961, 134, 213-215.

[268] R. Z. LeGeros, Effect of carbonate on the lattice parameters of apatite. *Nature* 1965, 206, 403-404.

[269] R. Z. LeGeros, O. R. Trautz, J, P. LeGeros, E. Klein, W. P. Shirra, Apatite crystallites: effects of carbonate on morphology. *Science* 1967, 155, 1409 – 1411.

[270] R. Astala, M. J. Stott, First principles investigation of mineral component of bone: CO_3 substitutions in hydroxyapatite. *Chem. Mater*. 2005, 17, 4125-4133.

[271] J. P. Lafon, E. Champion, D. Bernache-Assollant, Processing of AB-type carbonated hydroxyapatite $Ca_{10-x}(PO_4)_{(6-x)}(CO_3)_{(x)}(OH)_{(2-x-2y)}(CO_3)_{(y)}$ ceramics with controlled composition. *J. Eur. Ceram. Soc*. 2008, 28, 139-147.

[272] S. Kannan, A. Rebelo, A. F. Lemos, A. Barba, J. M. F. Ferreira, Synthesis and mechanical behaviour of chlorapatite and chlorapatite/β-TCP composites. *J. Eur. Ceram. Soc*. 2007, 27, 2287-2294.

[273] K. Teshima, K. Yubuta, S. Ooi, T. Suzuki, T. Shishido, S. Oishi, Environmentally friendly growth of calcium chlorapatite whiskers from a sodium chloride flux. *Cryst. Growth Des*. 2006, 6, 2538-2542.

[274] S. Pushpakanth, B. Srinivasan, T. P. Sastry, A. B. Mandal, Biocompatible and antibacterial properties of silver-doped hydroxyapatite. *J. Biomed. Nanotechnol.* 2008, 4, 62-66.

[275] T. N. Kim, Q. L. Feng, J. O. Kim, J. Wu, H. Wang, G. C. Chen, F. Z. Cui, Antimicrobial effects of metal ions (Ag^+, Cu^{2+}, Zn^{2+}) in hydroxyapatite. *J. Mater. Sci. Mater. Med.* 1998, 9, 129-134.

[276] S. Thomas, P. Assi, B. Marycel, M. Correa, W. Liberato, V. Brito, Yttrium 90-hydroxyapatite, a new radioisotope for chronic synovitis in hemophilia. *Haemophilia* 2008, 14, 77.

[277] M. Chinol, S. Vallabhajosula, S. J. Goldsmith, M. J. Klein, K. F. Deutsch, L. K. Chinen, J. W. Brodack, E. A. Deutsch, B. A. Watson, A. J. Tofe, Chemistry and biological behavior of samarium-153 and rhenium-186-labeled hydroxyapatite particles: potential radiopharmaceuticals for radiation synovectomy. *J. Nucl. Med.* 1993, 34, 1536-1542.

[278] M. G. Argüelles, I. S. Luppi Berlanga, E. A. Torres, Preparation of ^{153}Sm-particles for radiosynovectomy. *J. Radioanalytical Nuclear Chem*. 1999, 240, 509-511.

[279] E. O'Duffy, G. Clunie, D. Lui, J. Edwards, P. Ell, Double blind glucocorticoid controlled trial of samarium-153 particulate hydroxyapatite radiation synovectomy for chronic knee synovitis. *Ann. Rheum. Dis*. 1999, 58, 554–558.

[280] A. L. Boskey, Assessment of bone mineral and matrix using backscatter electron imaging and FTIR imaging. *Curr. Osteoporosis Reports* 2006, 4, 71-75.

[281] M. Vallet-Regi, J. M. González-Calbet, Calcium phosphates as substitution of bone tissues. *Progr. Solid State Chem*. 2004, 32, 1–31.

[282] W. F. de Jong, La substance minérale dans les os. Recueil des Travaux Chimiques des Pays-Bas 1926, 45, 445-449.

[283] S. Weiner, H. D. Wagner, Material bone: structure-mechanical function relations. *Ann. Rev. Mater. Sci.* 1998, 28, 271-298.

[284] S. Weiner, W. Traub, H. D. Wagner, Lamellar bone: structure-function relations. *J. Struct. Biol.* 1999, 126, 241-255.

[285] H. Limeback, Molecular mechanisms in dental hard tissue mineralization. *Curr. Opin. Dent.* 1991, 1, 826-835.

[286] V. Matkovic, Calcium metabolism and calcium requirements during skeletal modeling and consolidation of bone mass. *Amer. J. Clin. Nutr.* 1991, 54, 245S-260S.

[287] M. L. Power, R. P. Heaney, H. J. Kalkwarf, R. M. Pitkin, J. T. Repke, R. C. Tsang, J. Schulkin, The role of calcium in health and disease. *Amer. J. Obstetrics Gynecol.* 1999, 181, 1560-1569.

[288] J. C. Elliott, Calcium phosphate biominerals. In: *Phosphates: geochemical, geobiological and materials importance. Series: Reviews in Mineralogy and Geochemistry.* Vol. 48, J. M. Hughes, M. Kohn, J. Rakovan (Eds.). Mineralogical Society of America, Washington, D.C. 2002, pp. 427-453.

[289] F. H. Jones, Teeth and bones: application of surface science to dental materials and related biomaterials. *Surface Sci. Reports*, 2001, 42, 75-205.

[290] N. Loveridge, Bone: more than a stick. *J. Anim. Sci.* 1999, 77, Suppl. 2, 190-196.

[291] J. P. Nightingale, D. Lewis, Pole figures of the orientation of apatite in bones. *Nature* 1971, 232, 334-335.

[292] J. D. Currey, *Bones: structure and mechanics*. Princeton Univ. Press. Princeton, 2002, 456 pp.

[293] J. Y. Rho, L. Kuhn-Spearing, P. Zioupos, Mechanical properties and the hierarchical structure of bone. *Med. Eng. Phys.* 1998, 20, 92–102.

[294] S. Mann, *Biomimetic materials chemistry*, VCH, Weinheim, 1996, 400 pp.

[295] N. M. Hancox, *Biology of bone*, Cambridge University Press, Cambridge, 1972, 199 pp.

[296] R. B. Martin, Bone as a ceramic composite material. *Mater. Sci. Forum* 1999, 7, 5-16.

[297] K. S. Davison, K. Siminoski, J. D. Adachi, D. A. Hanley, D. Goltzman, A. B. Hodsman, R. Josse, S. Kaiser, W. P. Olszynski, A. Papaioannou, L. G. Ste-Marie, D. L. Kendler, A. Tenenhouse, J. P. Brown, Bone strength: the whole is greater than the sum of its parts. *Semin. Arthritis Rheum.* 2006, 36, 22-31.

[298] C. H. Turner, D. B. Burr, Basic biomechanical measurements of bone: a tutorial. *Bone* 1993, 14, 595–608.

[299] J. D. Currey, Tensile yield in compact bone is determined by strain, post-yield behaviour by mineral content. *J. Biomechanics* 2004, 37, 549-556.

[300] J. D. Currey, K. Brear, P. Zioupos, Notch sensitivity of mammalian mineralized tissues in impact. *Proc. R. Soc.* London B 2004, 217, 517-522.

[301] J. C. Anderson, C. Eriksson, Piezoelectric properties of dry and wet bone. *Nature* 1970, 227, 491-492.

[302] S. B. Lang, Pyroelectric effect in bone and tendon. *Nature* 1966, 212, 704-705.

[303] V. Haynes, Radiocarbon: analysis of inorganic carbon of fossil bone and enamel. *Science* 1968, 161, 687-688.

[304] J. M. Rensberger, M. Watabe, Fine structure of bone in dinosaurs, birds and mammals. *Nature* 2000, 406, 619-622.

[305] Y. Kolodny, B. Luz, M. Sander, W. A. Clemens, Dinosaur bones: fossils or pseudomorphs? The pitfalls of physiology reconstruction from apatitic fossils. *Palaeo* 1996, 126, 161-171.

[306] C. N. Trueman, N. Tuross, Trace elements in recent and fossil bone apatite. In: *Phosphates: geochemical, geobiological and materials importance. Series: Reviews in Mineralogy and Geochemistry*. Vol. 48, J. M. Hughes, M. Kohn, J. Rakovan (Eds.). Mineralogical Society of America, Washington, D.C. 2002, 489-522.

[307] J. D. Currey, K. Brear, Hardness, Young's modulus and yield stress in mammalian mineralized tissues. *J. Mater. Sci. Mater*. Med. 1990, 1, 14–20.

[308] W. E. Brown, L. C. Chow, Chemical properties of bone mineral. *Ann. Rev. Mater. Sci.* 1976, 6, 213-236.

[309] R. Lakes, Materials with structural hierarchy. *Nature* 1993, 361, 511-515.

[310] M. A. Meyers, A. Y. M. Lin, Y. Seki, Po-Yu Chen, B. K. Kad, S. Bodde, Structural biological composites: an overview. *JOM*, 2006, 58, 36-43.

[311] D. A. Wahl, J. T. Czernuszka, Collagen-hydroxyapatite composites for hard tissue repair. *Eur. Cell Mater*. 2006, 11, 43-56.

[312] M. J. Olszta, X. Cheng, S. S. Jee, R. Kumar, Y. Y. Kim, M. J. Kaufman, E. P. Douglas, L. B. Gower, Bone structure and formation: a new perspective. *Mater. Sci. Engin. R* 2007, 58, 77-116.

[313] A. L. Boskey, Mineralization of bones and teeth. *Elements* 2007, 3, 385-391.

[314] M. J. Glimcher, Bone: nature of the calcium phosphate crystals and cellular, structural and physical chemical mechanisms in their formation. In: *Medical Mineralogy and Geochemistry. Series: Reviews in Mineralogy and Geochemistry.* Vol. 64, N. Sahai, M. A. A. Schoonen (Eds.). Mineralogical Society of America, Washington, D.C. 2006, pp. 223-282.

[315] M. D. McKee, W. N. Addison, M. T. Kaartinen, Hierarchies of extracellular matrix and mineral organization in bone of the craniofacial complex and skeleton. *Cells Tissues Organs* 2005, 181, 176-188.

[316] J. D. Currey, Hierarchies in biomineral structures. *Science* 2005, 309, 253-254.

[317] G. E. Fantner, O. Rabinovych, G. Schitter, P. Thurner, J. H. Kindt, M. M. Finch, J. C. Weaver, L. S. Golde, D. E. Morse, E. A. Lipman, I. W. Rangelow, P. K. Hansma, Hierarchical interconnections in the nano-composite material bone: fibrillar cross-links resist fracture on several length scales. *Composites Sci. Technol*. 2006, 66, 1202-1208.

[318] K. A. Athanasiou, C. Zhu, D. R. Lanctot, C. M. Agrawal, X. Wang, Fundamentals of biomechanics in tissue engineering of bone. *Tissue Eng*. 2000, 6, 361–381.

[319] S. Nikolov, D. Raabe, Hierarchical modeling of the elastic properties of bone at submicron scales: the role of extrafibrillar mineralization. *Biophysical J.* 2008, 94, 4220-4232.

[320] H. S. Gupta, W. Wagermaier, G. A. Zickler, D. R. B. Aroush, S. S. Funari, P. Roschger, H. D. Wagner, P. Fratzl, Nanoscale deformation mechanisms in bone. *Nano Lett.* 2005, 5, 2108-2111.

[321] H. Peterlik, P. Roschger, K. Klaushofer, P. Fratzl, From brittle to ductile fracture of bone, *Nature Mater*. 2006, 5, 52-55.

[322] P. Fratzl, H. S. Gupta, E. P. Paschalis, P. Roschger, Structure and mechanical quality of the collagen-mineral nano-composite in bone. *J. Mater. Chem*. 2004, 14, 2115– 2123.

[323] A. A. Marino, R. O. Becker, Evidence for direct physical bonding between the collagen fibres and apatite crystals in bone. *Nature* 1967, 213, 697–698.

[324] S. J. Eppell, W. Tong, J. L. Katz, L. Kuhn, M. J. Glimcher, Shape and size of isolated bone mineralites measured using atomic force microscopy. *J. Orthopaedic Res*. 2001, 19, 1027-1034.

[325] S. M. Clark, J. Iball, Orientation of apatite crystals in bone. *Nature* 1954, 174, 399–400.

[326] M. A. Rubin, I. Jasiuk, J. Taylor, J. Rubin, T. Ganey, R. P. Apkarian, TEM analysis of the nanostructure of normal and osteoporotic human trabecular bone. *Bone* 2003, 33, 270-282.

[327] X. Su, K. Sun, F. Z. Cui, W. J. Landis, Organization of apatite crystals in human woven bone. *Bone* 2003, 32; 150-162.

[328] G. M. Whitesides, B. Grzybowski, Self-assembly at all scales. *Science* 2002, 295, 2418-2421.

[329] P. Fratzl, N. Fratzl-Zelman, K. Klaushofer, G. Vogl, K. Koller, Nucleation and growth of mineral crystals in bone studied by small-angle X-ray scattering. *Calcif. Tissue Int.* 1991, 48, 407-413.

[330] W. J. Landis, K. J. Hodgens, J. Arena, M. J. Song, B. F. McEwen, Structural relations between collagen and mineral in bone as determined by high voltage electron microscopic tomography. *Microscopy Res. Technique* 1996, 33, 192-202.

[331] V. B. Rosen, L. W. Hobbs, M. Spector, The ultrastructure of anorganic bovine bone and selected synthetic hyroxyapatites used as bone graft substitute materials. *Biomaterials* 2002, 23, 921-928.

[332] F. Z. Cui, Y. Li, J. Ge, Self-assembly of mineralized collagen composites. *Mater. Sci. Engin. R* 2007, 57, 1–27.

[333] K. Sato, Inorganic-organic interfacial interactions in hydroxyapatite mineralization processes. *Topics in Current Chemistry* 2006, 270, 127-153.

[334] J. D. Hartgerink, E. Beniash, S. I. Stupp, Self-assembly and mineralization of peptide-amphiphile nanofibers. *Science* 2001, 294, 1684-1688.

[335] B. K. Hall, (Ed.) *Cartilage: structure, function and biochemistry*, Academic Press, New York, 1983, 385 pp.

[336] S. P. Robins, J. P. Bilezikian, M. J. Seibel. *Dynamics of bone and cartilage metabolism*. Academic Press, New York, 1999, 672 pp.

[337] B. K. Hall (Ed.), *Bones and cartilage: developmental skeletal biology*. Academic Press, New York, 2005, 792 pp.

[338] A. A. Marino, R. O. Becker, Evidence for epitaxy in the formation of collagen and apatite. *Nature* 1970, 226, 652-653.

[339] A. Jodaikin, S. Weiner, Y. Talmon, E. Grossman, W. Traub, Mineral-organic matrix relations in tooth enamel. *Int. J. Biol. Macromol.* 1988, 10, 349-352.

[340] A. G. Fincham, J. Moradian-Oldak, T. G. H. Diekwisch, D. M. Lyaruu, J. T. Wright, P. Bringas, H. C. Slavkin, Evidence for amelogenin "nanospheres" as functional components of secretory-stage enamel matrix. *J. Struct. Biol.* 1995, 115, 50-59.

[341] R. Z. LeGeros, C. M. Pan, S. Suga, N. Watabe, Crystallo-chemical properties of apatite in atremate brachiopod shells. *Calcif. Tissue Int.* 1985, 37, 98-100.

[342] M. Iijima, Y. Moriwaki, Orientation of apatite and organic matrix in *Lingula unguis* shell. *Calcif. Tissue Int.* 1990, 47, 237-242.

[343] A. Williams, M. Cusack, J. O. Buckman, T. Stachel, Siliceous tablets in the larval shells of apatitic discinid Brachiopods. *Science* 1998, 297, 2094-2096.

[344] T. Nakano, T. Ishimoto, J. W. Lee, Y. Umakoshi, Preferential orientation of biological apatite crystallite in original, regenerated and diseased cortical bones. *J. Ceram. Soc.* Japan 2008, 116, 313-315.

[345] T. Nakano, T. Ishimoto, Y. Umakoshi, Y. Tabata, Variation in bone quality during regenerative process. *Mater. Sci. Forum* 2007, 539-543, 675-680.

[346] E. I. Suvorova, P. P. Petrenko, P. A. Buffat, Scanning and transmission electron microscopy for evaluation of order/disorder in bone structure. *Scanning* 2007, 29, 162-170.

[347] S. L. Teitelbaum, Bone resorption by osteoclasts. *Science* 2000, 289, 1504-1508.

[348] G. A. Rodan, T. J. Martin, Therapeutic approaches to bone diseases. *Science* 2000, 289, 1508-1514.

[349] A. F. Schilling, S. Filke, S. Brink, H. Korbmacher, M. Amling, J. M. Rueger, Osteoclasts and biomaterials. *Eur. J. Trauma* 2006, 32, 107-113.

[350] L. C. Bonar, M. Shimizu, J. E. Roberts, R. G. Griffin, M. J. Glimcher, Structural and composition studies on the mineral of newly formed dental enamel: a chemical, X-ray diffraction, and ^{31}P and proton nuclear magnetic resonance study. *J. Bone Miner. Res.* 1991, 6, 1167-1176.

[351] R. M. Biltz, E. D. Pellegrino, The hydroxyl content of calcified tissue mineral. *Calcif. Tissue Res.* 1971, 7, 259-263.

[352] C. Rey, V. Renugopalakrishnan, B. Collins, M. J. Glimcher, Fourier transform infrared spectroscopic study of the carbonate ions in bone mineral during aging. *Calcif. Tissue* Int. 1991, 49, 251-258.

[353] C. Rey, J. L. Miquel, L. Facchini, A. P. Legrand, M. J. Glimcher, Hydroxyl groups in bone mineral. *Bone* 1995, 16, 583-586.

[354] C. K. Loong, C. Rey, L. T. Kuhn, C. Combes, Y. Wu, S. H. Chen, M. J. Glimcher, Evidence of hydroxyl-ion deficiency in bone apatites: an inelastic neutron scattering study. *Bone* 2000, 26, 599-602.

[355] J. D. Pasteris, B. Wopenka, J. J. Freeman, K. Rogers, E. Valsami-Jones, J. A. M. van der Houwen, M. J. Silva, Lack of OH in nanocrystalline apatite as a function of degree of atomic order: implications for bone and biomaterials. *Biomaterials* 2004, 25, 229-238.

[356] M. D. Grynpas, S. Omelon, Transient precursor strategy or very small biological apatite crystals? *Bone* 2007, 41, 162-164.

[357] M. S. Tung, W. E. Brown, An intermediate state in hydrolysis of amorphous calcium phosphate. *Calcif. Tissue Int.* 1983, 35, 783-790.
[358] M. S. Tung, W. E. Brown, The role of octacalcium phosphate in subcutaneous heterotopic calcification. *Calcif. Tissue Int.* 1985, 37, 329-331.
[359] W. E. Brown, N. Eidelman, B. B. Tomazic, Octacalcium phosphate as a precursor in biomineral formation. *Adv. Dent. Res.* 1987, 1, 306-313.
[360] C. Siew, S. E. Gruninger, L. C. Chow, W. E. Brown, Procedure for the study of acidic calcium phosphate precursor phases in enamel mineral formation. *Calcif. Tissue Int.* 1992, 50, 144-148.
[361] W. E. Brown, J. P. Smith, J. R. Lehr, A. W. Frazier, Crystallographic and chemical relations between octacalcium phosphate and hydroxyapatite. *Nature* 1962, 196, 1048–1050.
[362] Y. H. Tseng, C. Y. Mou, J. C. C. Chan, Solid-state NMR study of the transformation of octacalcium phosphate to hydroxyapatite: A mechanistic model for central dark line formation. *J. Amer. Chem. Soc.* 2006, 128, 6909-6918.
[363] E. D. Eanes, I. H. Gillessen, A. S. Posner, Intermediate states in the precipitation of hydroxyapatite. *Nature* 1965, 208, 365-367.
[364] J. D. Termine, A. S. Posner, Infrared analysis of rat bone: age dependency of amorphous and crystalline mineral fractions. *Science* 1966, 153, 1523-1525.
[365] J. D. Termine, A. S. Posner, Infra-red determination of the percentage of crystallinity in apatitic calcium phosphates. *Nature* 1966, 211, 268-270.
[366] R. A. Harper, A. S. Posner, Measurement of non-crystalline calcium phosphate in bone. mineral. *Proc. Soc. Exptl. Biol. Med.* 1966, 122, 137-142.
[367] A. S. Posner, Crystal chemistry of bone mineral. *Physiol. Rev.* 1969, 49, 760-792.
[368] A. S. Posner, Bone mineral on the molecular level. *Fed. Proc.* 1973, 32, 1933-1937.
[369] A. L. Boskey, A. S. Posner, Formation of hydroxyapatite at low supersaturation. *J. Phys. Chem.* 1976, 80, 40-44.
[370] A. S. Posner, The chemistry of bone mineral. *Bull. Hosp. Joint Dis.* 1978, 39, 126-144.
[371] M. J. Glimcher, L. C. Bonar, M. D. Grynpas, W. J. Landis, A. H. Roufosse, Recent studies of bone mineral: is the amorphous calcium phosphate theory valid? *J. Cryst. Growth* 1981, 53, 100-119.
[372] J. L. Meyer, E. D. Eanes, A thermodynamic analysis of the amorphous to crystalline calcium phosphate transformation. *Calcif. Tissue Res.* 1978, 25, 59–68.
[373] J. L. Meyer, E. D. Eanes, A thermodynamic analysis of the secondary transition in the spontaneous precipitation of calcium phosphate. *Calcif. Tissue Res.* 1978, 25, 209–216.
[374] Y. Politi, T. Arad, E. Klein, S. Weiner, L. Addadi, Sea urchin spine calcite forms via a transient amorphous calcium carbonate phase. *Science* 2004, 306, 1161-1164.
[375] S. Weiner, Transient precursor strategy in mineral formation of bone. *Bone* 2006, 39, 431-433.
[376] Y. Pekounov, O. E. Petrov, Bone resembling apatite by amorphous-to-crystalline transition driven self-organisation. *J. Mater. Sci. Mater. Med.* 2008, 19, 753-759.
[377] N. D. Sahar, S. I. Hong, D. H. Kohn, Micro- and nano-structural analyses of damage in bone. *Micron,* 2005, 36, 617-629.
[378] N. M. Hancox, *Biology of bone.* Cambridge Univ. Press, Cambridge, 1972, pp. 3-48.

[379] J. M. Burnell, E. J. Teubner, A. G. Miller, Normal maturational changes in bone matrix, mineral, and crystal size in the rat. *Calcif. Tissue Int.* 1980, 31, 13-19.

[380] S. Weiner, W. Traub, Organization of hydroxyapatite crystals within collagen fibrils. *FEBS Lett.* 1986, 206, 262-266.

[381] E. D. Pellegrino, R. M. Blitz, Mineralization in the chick embryo I. Monohydrogen phosphate and carbonate relationships during maturation of the bone crystal complex. *Calcif. Tissue Res.* 1972, 10, 128-135.

[382] R. Z. LeGeros, N. Balmain, G. Bonel, Age-related changes in mineral of rat and bovine cortical bone. *Calcif. Tissue Int.* 1987, 41, 137-144.

[383] C. Rey, A. Hina, A. Tofighi, M. J. Glimcher, Maturation of poorly crystalline apatites: chemical and structural aspect *in vivo* and *in vitro* behavior. *Cells Mater.* 1995, 5, 345–356.

[384] K. Verdelis, L. Lukashova, J. T. Wright, R. Mendelsohn, M. G. E. Peterson, S. Doty, A. L. Boskey, Maturational changes in dentin mineral properties. *Bone* 2007, 40, 1399-1407.

[385] U. Plate, T. Tkotz, H. P. Wiesmann, U. Stratmann, U. Joos, H. J. Höhling, Early mineralization of matrix vesicles in the epiphyseal growth plate. *J. Microsc.* 1996, 183, 102-107.

[386] U. Stratmann, K. Schaarschmidt, H. P. Wiesmann, U. Plate, H. J. Höhling, Mineralization during matrix-vesicle-mediated mantle dentine formation in molars of albino rats: a microanalytical and ultrastructural study. *Cell Tissue Res.* 1996, 284, 223-230.

[387] W. Jahnen-Dechent, T. Schinke, A. Trindl, W. Muller-Esterl, F. Sablitzky, S. Kaiser, M. Blessing, Cloning and targeted deletion of the mouse fetuin gene. *J. Biol. Chem.* 1997, 272, 31496-31503.

[388] T. Schinke, M. D. McKnee, G. Karsenty, Extracellular matrix calcification: where is the action? *Nature Genetics* 1999, 21, 150-151.

[389] W. Jahnen-Dechent, G. Schäfer, A. Heiss, J. Grötzinger, Systemic inhibition of spontaneous calcification by the serum protein a_2-HS glycoprotein/fetuin. *Z. Kardiol.* 2001, 90, Suppl. 3, III/47-III/56.

[390] J. K. Avery, *Oral development and histology*. 3rd Ed. Thieme Medical Publishers Inc., New York, 2001, 435 pp.

[391] A. R. ten Cate, *Oral histology: development, structure, and function*. 5th Ed. Mosby-Year Book, Saint Louis, 1998, 497 pp.

[392] J. Xue, L. Zhang, L. Zou, Y. Liao, J. Li, L. Xiao, W. Li, High-resolution X-ray microdiffraction analysis of natural teeth. *J. Synchrotron Rad.* 2008, 15, 235-238.

[393] M. Gaft, S. Shoval, G. Panczer, Y. Nathan, B. Champagnon, C. Garapon, Luminescence of uranium and rare-earth elements in apatite of fossil fish teeth. *Palaeogeography Palaeoclimatology Palaeoecology* 1996, 126, 187-193.

[394] C. M. Huang, Q. Zhang, S. Bai, C. S. Wang, FTIR and XRD analysis of hydroxyapatite from fossil human and animal teeth in Jinsha Relict, Chengdu. *Spectroscopy and Spectral Analysis* 2007, 27, 2448-2452.

[395] H. C. Margolis, E. Beniash, C. E. Fowler, Role of macromolecular assembly of enamel matrix proteins in enamel formation. *J. Dent. Res.* 2006, 86, 775-793.

[396] A. Vieira, R. Hancock, H. Limeback, M. Schwartz, M. Grynpas, How does fluoride concentration in the tooth affect apatite crystal size? *J. Dent. Res.* 2003, 82, 909-913.

[397] F. Z. Cui, J. Ge, New observations of the hierarchical structure of human enamel, from nanoscale to microscale. *J. Tissue Engin. Regenerative Medicine* 2007, 1, 185-191.

[398] K. D. Jandt, Probing the future in functional soft drinks on the nanometre scale - towards tooth friendly soft drinks. *Trends Food Sci. Technol.* 2006, 17, 263-271.

[399] H. Chen, Y. Chen, B. G. Orr, M. Banaszak-Holl, I. Majoros, B. H. Clarkson, Nanoscale probing of the enamel nanorod surface using polyamidoamine dendrimers. *Langmuir* 2004, 20, 4168–4171.

[400] E. Rönnholm, The amelogenesis of human teeth as revealed by electron microscopy. II. The development of the enamel crystallites. *J. Ultrastruct. Res.* 1962, 6, 249-303.

[401] M. U. Nylen, E. D. Evans, K. A. Omnel, Crystal growth in rat enamel. *J. Cell. Biol.* 1963, 18, 109-123.

[402] Y. Miake, S. Shimoda, M. Fukae, T. Aoba, Epitaxial overgrowth of apatite crystals on the thin-ribbon precursor at early stages of porcine enamel mineralization. *Calcif. Tissue Int.* 1993, 53, 249-256.

[403] G. Daculsi, J. Menanteau, L. M. Kerebel, D. Mitre, Length and shape of enamel crystals. *Calcif. Tissue Int.* 1984, 36, 550-555.

[404] A. Jodaikin, W. Traub, S. Weiner, Enamel rod relations in the developing rat incisor. *J. Ultrastruct. Res.* 1984, 89, 324-332.

[405] E. F. Bres, J. L. Hutchison, Surface structure study of biological calcium phosphate apatite crystals from human tooth enamel. *J. Biomed. Mater. Res.* 2002, 63, 433-440.

[406] I. Schroeder, R. M. Frank, High-resolution transmission electron microscopy of adult human peritubular dentine. *Cell. Tissue Res.* 1985, 242, 449-451.

[407] E. F. Brès, J. C. Voegel, R. M. Frank, High-resolution electron microscopy of human enamel crystals. *J. Microsc.* 1990, 160, 183-201.

[408] C. Robinson, S. Connell, J. Kirkham, R. Shorea, A. Smith, Dental enamel - a biological ceramic: regular substructures in enamel hydroxyapatite crystals revealed by atomic force microscopy. *J. Mater. Chem.* 2004, 14, 2242–2248.

[409] R. D. Warf, R. R. Watson, Calcium phosphate - nutrition in prevention of early childhood dental caries. In: *Wild-type food in health promotion and disease prevention: the Columbus concept.* F. DeMeester, R. R. Watson (Eds.). 2008, pp. 343-353.

[410] J. P. Simmer, A. G. Fincham, Molecular mechanisms of dental enamel formation. *Crit. Rev. Oral Biol. Med.* 1995, 6, 84-108.

[411] T. G. Diekwisch, B. J. Berman, S. Genters, H. C. Slavkin, Initial enamel crystals are not spatially associated with mineralized dentine. *Cell. Tissue Res.* 1995, 279, 149-167.

[412] T. Aoba, Recent observations on enamel crystal formation during mammalian amelogenesis. *Anat. Rec.* 1996, 245, 208-218.

[413] C. E. Smith, Cellular and chemical events during enamel maturation. *Crit. Rev. Oral. Biol. Med.* 1998, 9, 128-161.

[414] M. Sydney-Zax, I. Mayer, D. Deutsch, Carbonate content in developing human and bovine enamel. *J. Dent. Res.* 1991, 70, 913-916.

[415] C. Rey, V. Renugopalakrishnan, M. Shimizu, B. Collins, M. J. Glimcher, A resolution-enhanced Fourier Transform Infrared spectroscopic study of the environment of the

CO_3^{2-} ion in the mineral phase of enamel during its formation and maturation. *Calcif. Tissue Int.* 1991, 49, 259-268.

[416] T. Takagi, T. Ogasawara, J. Tagami, M. Akao, Y. Kuboki, N. Nagai, R. Z. LeGeros, pH and carbonate levels in. developing enamel. *Connect. Tissue Res.* 1998, 38, 181-187.

[417] H. A. Lowenstam, S. Weiner, Transformation of amorphous calcium phosphate to crystalline dahillite in the radular teeth of chitons. *Science* 1985, 227, 51-53.

[418] K. A. Selvig, Periodic lattice images of hydroxyapatite crystals in human bone and dental hard tissues. *Calcif. Tissue Res.* 1970, 6, 227-238.

[419] K. A. Selvig, Electron microscopy of dental enamel: analysis of crystal lattice images. *Cell. Tissue Res.* 1973, 137, 271-280.

[420] F. J. G. Cuisinier, P. Steuer, B. Senger, J. C. Voegel, R. M. Frank, Human amelogenesis: high resolution electron microscopy of nanometer-sized particles. *Cell. Tissue Res.* 1993, 273, 175-182.

[421] F. J. G. Cuisinier, P. Steuer, A. Brisson, J. C. Voegel, High resolution electron microscopy study of crystal growth mechanisms in chicken bone composites. *J. Cryst. Growth* 1995, 156, 443-453.

[422] P. Houllé, J. C. Voegel, P. Schultz, P. Steuer, F. J. G. Cuisinier, High resolution electron microscopy: structure and growth mechanisms of human dentin crystals. *J. Dent. Res.* 1997, 76, 895-904.

[423] S. Mann, Molecular tectonics in biomineralization and biomimetic materials chemistry. Nature 1993, 365, 499-505.

[424] J. Kirkham, J. Zhang, S. J. Brookes, R. C. Shore, S. R. Wood, D. A. Smith, M. L. Wallwork, O. H. Ryu, C. Robinson, Evidence for charge domains on developing enamel crystal surfaces. *J. Dent. Res.* 2000, 79, 1943-1947.

[425] H. Warshawsky, A. Nanci, Stereo electron microscopy of enamel crystallites. *J. Dental Res.* 1982, 61, 1504-1514.

[426] H. Warshawsky, Organization of crystals in enamel. *Anat. Rec.* 1989, 224, 242-262.

[427] A. L. Arsenault, B. W. Robinson, The dentino-enamel junction: a structural and microanalytical study of early mineralization. *Calcif. Tissue Int.* 1989, 45, 111-121.

[428] Y. Hayashi, High resolution electron microscopy in the dentino-enamel junction. *J. Electron Microsc.* (Tokyo) 1992, 41, 387-391.

[429] Y. Hayashi, High resolution electron microscopic study on the human dentine crystal. *J. Electron Microsc.* (Tokyo) 1993, 42, 141-146.

[430] P. Bodier-Houllé, P. Steuer, J. M. Meyer, L. Bigeard, F. J. G. Cuisinier, High-resolution electron-microscopic study of the relationship between human enamel and dentin crystals at the dentino-enamel junction. *Cell. Tissue Res.* 2000, 301, 389-395.

[431] Y. Takano, Y. Hanaizumi, H. Oshima, Occurrence of amorphous and crystalline mineral deposits at the epithelial-mesenchymal interface of incisors in the calcium-loaded rat: Implication of novel calcium binding domains. *Anat. Rec.* 1996, 245, 174-185.

[432] W. Dong, H. Warshawsky, Lattice fringe continuity in the absence of crystal continuity in enamel. *Adv. Dent. Res.* 1996, 10, 232-237.

[433] M. Finke, D. M. Parker, K. D. Jandt, Influence of soft drinks on the thickness and morphology of in situ acquired pellicle layer on enamel. *J. Colloid Interf. Sci.* 2002, 251, 263–270.
[434] M. E. Barbour, D. M. Parker, K. D. Jandt, Enamel dissolution as a function of solution degree of saturation with respect to hydroxyapatite: a nanoindentation study. *J. Colloid Interf. Sci.* 2003, 265, 9–14.
[435] F. Lippert, D. M. Parker, K. D. Jandt, Susceptibility of deciduous and permanent enamel to dietary acid-induced erosion studied with atomic force microscopy nanoindentation. *Eur. J. Oral Sci.* 2004, 112, 61–66.
[436] M. E. Barbour, D. M. Parker, G. C. Allen, K. D. Jandt, Human enamel erosion in constant composition citric acid solutions as a function of degree of saturation with respect to hydroxyapatite. *J. Oral Rehabil.* 2005, 32, 16–21.
[437] R. Z. LeGeros, Calcium phosphates in demineralization and remineralization processes. *J. Clin. Dent.* 1999, 10, 65-73.
[438] G. Walker, F. Cai, P. Shen, C. Reynolds, B. Ward, C. Fone, S. Honda, M. Koganei, M. Oda, E. Reynolds, Increased remineralization of tooth enamel by milk containing added casein phosphopeptide-amorphous calcium phosphate. *J. Dairy Res.* 2006, 73, 74-78.
[439] F. Lippert, D. M. Parker, K. D. Jandt, *In situ* remineralisation of surface softened human enamel studied with AFM nanoindentation. *Surface Sci.* 2004, 553, 105-114.
[440] F. Lippert, D. M. Parker, K. D. Jandt, *In vitro* demineralization/remineralization cycles at human tooth enamel surfaces investigated by AFM and nanoindentation. *J. Colloid Interface Sci.* 2004, 280, 442–448.
[441] F. Lippert, D. M. Parker, K. D. Jandt, Toothbrush abrasion of surface softened enamel studied with tapping mode AFM and AFM nanoindentation. *Caries Res.* 2004, 38, 464-472.
[442] K. Onuma, K. Yamagishi, A. Oyane, Nucleation and growth of hydroxyapatite nanocrystals for nondestructive repair of early caries lesions. *J. Cryst. Growth* 2005, 282, 199-207.
[443] N. J. Cochrane, S. Saranathan, F. Cai, K. J. Cross, E. C. Reynolds, Enamel subsurface lesion remineralisation with casein phosphopeptide stabilised solutions of calcium, phosphate and fluoride. *Caries Res.* 2008, 42, 88-97.
[444] J. F. McClendon, Fluorapatite and teeth. *Science* 1966, 151, 151.
[445] J. Price, C. Faucheux, S. Allen, Deer antlers as a model of mammalian regeneration. *Curr. Top. Dev. Biol.* 2005, 67, 2-49.
[446] Z. Yue, X. Deng, H. Feng, The mechanisms of deer antlers development and regeneration. *J. Economic Animal* 2005, 9, 46-49.
[447] L. Zhao, Z. Yue, X. Zhang, X. Deng, The deer antlers endochondral ossification and its regulation mechanisms. *J. Economic Animal* 2006, 10, 238-241.
[448] T. Landete-Castilleijos, A. Garcia, L. Gallego, Body weight, early growth and antler size influence antler bone mineral composition of Iberian Red Deer (*Cervus elaphus hispanicus*). *Bone* 2007, 40, 230–235.
[449] J. Huxley, The relative size of antlers of deer. *Proc. Zool. Soc.* London 1931, 72, 819–864.

[450] P. Zioupos, X. T. Wang, J. D. Currey, Experimental and theoretical quantification of the development of damage in fatigue tests of bone and antler. *J. Biomechanics* 1996, 29, 989-1002.

[451] T. Landete-Castilleijos, J. D. Currey, J. A. Estevez, E. Gaspar-Lopez, A. Garcia, L. Gallego, Influence of physiological effort of growth and chemical composition on antler bone mechanical properties. *Bone* 2007, 41, 794-803.

[452] L. A. Evans, A. L. McCutcheon, G. R. Dennis, R. C. Mulley, M. A. Wilson, Pore size analysis of fallow deer (*Dama dama*) antler bone. *J. Mater. Sci.* 2005, 40, 5733-5739.

[453] R. J. Goss, *Deer antlers regeneration, function and evolution*. Academic Press, New York, 1983, 316 pp.

[454] G. A. Bubenik, A. B. Bubenik, Eds. *Horns, pronghorns, and antlers: evolution, morphology, physiology, and social significance*. Springer, New York, 1990, 562 pp.

[455] U. Kierdorf, H. Kierdorf, Antlers as biomonitors of environmental pollution by lead and fluoride: a review. *Eur. J. Wildlife Res.* 2005, 51, 137-150.

[456] P. M. Barling, D. K. Gupta, C. E. L. Lim, Involvement of phosphodiesterase I in mineralization: histochemical studies using antler from red deer (*Cervus elaphus*) as a model. *Calcif. Tissue Int.* 1999, 65, 384-389.

[457] P. M. Barling, K. W. Chong, *The involvement of phosphohydrolases in mineralization: studies on enzymatic activities extracted from red deer antler*. 1999, 65, 232-236.

[458] U. Kierdorf, H. Kierdorf, The fluoride content of antlers as an indicator of fluoride exposure in red deer (*Cervus elaphus*): a historical biomonitoring study. Fluoride, 2000, 33, 92-94.

[459] N. N. Pathak, A. K. Pattanaik, R. C. Patra, B.M. Arora, Mineral composition of antlers of three deer species reared in captivity. *Small Rumin. Res.* 2001, 42, 61–65.

[460] Y. Yuxia, D. Rui, Y. Wang, S. Wang, Calcium and phosphors contents of three-branched and two-branched antler and ossificational antler from sika deer. *J. Economic Animal* 2002, 6, 6-8.

[461] H. Y. Kim, M. R. Rhyu, Sectional composition of minerals in domestic deer antler. *Korean J. Food Sci. Technol.* 2000, 32, 31-36.

[462] C. Li, J. M. Suttie, D. E. Clarck, Histological examination of antler regeneration in red deer (*Cervus elaphus*). *Anat. Rec.* 2005, 282A, 163-174.

[463] W. Meister, Changes in biological structure of the long bones of white-tailed deer during the growth of antlers. *Anat. Rec.* 1956, 124, 709-721.

[464] P. D. Muir, A. R. Sykes, G. K. Barrell, Calcium metabolism in red deer (*Cervus elaphus*) offered herbages during antlerogenesis: kinetic and stable balance studies. *J. Agric. Sci. Camb.* 1987, 109, 357-364.

[465] B. J. Baxter, R. N. Andrews, G. K. Barrell, Bone turnover associated with antler growth in red deer (*Cervus elaphus*). *Anat. Rec.* 1999, 256, 14-19.

[466] T. Landete-Castilleijos, J. A. Estevez, A Martinez, F. Ceacero, A. Garcia, L. Gallego, Does chemical composition of antler bone reflect the physiological effort made to grow it? *Bone* 2007, 40, 1095-1102.

[467] M. Baciut, G. Baciut, V. Simon, C. Albon, V. Coman, P. Prodan, S. Florian, S. Bran, Investigation of deer antler as a potential bone regenerating biomaterial. *J. Optoelectronics Advanced Materials* 2007, 9, 2547-2550.

[468] J. J. Kazama, N. Amizuka, M. Fukagawa, Ectopic calcification as abnormal biomineralization. *Therapeutic Apheresis and Dialysis* 2006, 10, Suppl. 1, S34-S38.

[469] C. Frondel, E. L. Prien, Deposition of calcium phosphates accompanying senile degeneration and disease. *Science* 1946, 103, 326.

[470] C. Frondel, E. L. Prien, Carbonate-apatite and hydroxylapatite in urinary calculi. *Science* 1942, 95, 431.

[471] D. Brancaccio, M. Cozzolino, The mechanism of calcium deposition in soft tissues. *Contrib. Nephrol.* 2005, 149, 279-286.

[472] A. K. Goff, R. Reichard, A soft-tissue calcification: differential diagnosis and pathogenesis. *J. Forensic Sci.* 2006, 51, 493-497.

[473] S. Bittmann, M. W. Gunther, H. Ulus, Tumoral calcinosis of the gluteal region in a child: case report with overview of different soft-tissue calcifications. *J. Pediatric Surg.* 2003, 38, E4-E7.

[474] E. S. Molloy, G. M. McCarthy, Basic calcium phosphate crystals: pathways to joint degeneration. *Curr. Opin. Rheumatol.* 2006, 18, 187-192.

[475] C. M. Giachelli, Vascular calcification mechanisms. *J. Amer. Soc. Nephrol.* 2004, 15, 2959-2964.

[476] J. J. Kazama, N. Amizuka, M. Fukagawa, The making of a bone in blood vessels: from the soft shell to the hard bone. *Kidney International* 2007, 72, 533-534.

[477] W. Achilles, Crystallization in gel matrices: a new experimental model of calcium stone formation. *Contrib. Nephrol.* 1987, 58, 59-64.

[478] W. Achilles, U. Jockel, A. Schaper, M. Burk, H. Riedmiller, *In vitro* formation of "urinary stones": generation of spherulites of calcium phosphate in gel and overgrowth with calcium oxalate using a new flow model of crystallization. *Scanning Microsc.* 1995, 9, 577-585; discussion 585-586.

[479] J. Hayashizaki, S. Ban, H. Nakagaki, A. Okumura, S. Yoshii, C. Robinson, Site specific mineral composition and microstructure of human supra-gingival dental calculus. *Arch. Oral Biology* 2008, 53, 168-174.

[480] J. R. Ortlepp, F. Schmitz, V. Mevissen, S. Weiß, J. Huster, R. Dronskowski, G. Langebartels, R. Autschbach, K. Zerres, C. Weber, P. Hanrath, R. Hoffmann, The amount of calcium-deficient hexagonal hydroxyapatite in aortic valves is influenced by gender and associated with genetic polymorphisms in patients with severe calcific aortic stenosis. *Eur. Heart J.* 2004, 25, 514-522.

[481] K. M. Kim, Cellular mechanism of calcification and its prevention in glutaraldehyde treated vascular tissue. *Z. Kardiol.* 2001, 90, Suppl. 3, III99-III105.

[482] B. B. Tomazic, Physicochemical principles of cardiovascular calcification. *Z. Kardiol.* 2001, 90, Suppl. 3, III68-III80.

[483] S. P. Marra, C. P. Daghlian, M. F. Fillinger, F. E. Kennedy Elemental composition, morphology and mechanical properties of calcified deposits obtained from abdominal aortic aneurysms. *Acta Biomater.* 2006, 2, 515-520.

[484] L. A. Fitzpatrick, R. T. Turner, E. R. Ritman, Endochondral bone formation in the heart: a possible mechanism of coronary calcification. *Endocrinology* 2003, 144, 2214-2219.

[485] E. I. Suvorova, P. A. Buffat, Pathological mineralization of cardiac valves: causes and mechanism. *J. Long-Term Effects of Medical Implants* 2005, 15, 355-367.

[486] C. Giachelli, Ectopic calcification: new concepts in cellular regulation. *Z. Kardiol.* 2001, 90, Suppl. 3, III31-III37.

[487] B. Glasmacher, E. Nellen, H. Reul, G. Rau, *In vitro* hemocompatibility testing of new materials for mechanical heart valves. Mater.-Wiss. u. *Werkstofftech.* 1999, 30, 806-808.

[488] M. Deiwick, B. Glasmacher, E. Pettenazzo, D. Hammel, W. Castellon, G. Thiene, H. Reul, E. Berendes, H. H. Scheld, Primary tissue failure of bioprostheses: new evidence from *in vitro* tests. *Thorac. Cardiovasc. Surg.* 2001, 49, 78-83.

[489] E. Pettenazzo, M. Deiwick, G. Thiene, G. Molin, B. Glasmacher, F. Martignago, T. Bottio, H. Reul, M. Valente, Dynamic *in vitro* calcification of bioprosthetic porcine valves: evidence of apatite crystallization. *J. Thorac. Cardiovasc. Surg.* 2001, 121, 500-509.

[490] F. J. Schoen, R. J. Levy, Calcification of tissue heart valve substitutes: progress toward understanding and prevention. *Ann. Thorac. Surg.* 2005, 79, 1072-1080.

[491] K. Sensui, S. Saitoh, K. Kametani, K. Makino, M. Ohira, T. Kimura, G. A. Cheng, Y. Hata, Property analysis of ectopic calcification in the carpal tunnel identification of apatite crystals: a case report. *Arch. Orthop. Trauma Surgery* 2003, 123, 442-445.

[492] D. J. McCarty, H. M. Hogan, R. A. Gatter, M. Grossmann, Studies on pathological calcifications in human cartilage. *J. Bone Joint Surgery* 1966, 48, 309-325.

[493] P. J. Maddison, D. A. Isenberg, P. Woo, D. N. Glass (Eds.), *Oxford textbook of rheumatology,* Vol. 2, 2nd Edition, Oxford University Press, 1998, pp. 1567-1581.

[494] S. R. Stock, K. Ignatiev, P. L. Lee, K. Abbott, L. M. Pachman, Pathological calcification in juvenile dermatomyositis (JDM): microCT and synchrotron X-ray diffraction reveal hydroxyapatite with varied microstructures. *Connective Tissue Res.* 2004, 45, 248-256.

[495] L. M. Pachman, A. L. Boskey, Clinical manifestations and pathogenesis of hydroxyapatite crystal deposition in juvenile dermatomyositis. *Curr. Rheumatol. Rep.* 2006, 8, 236-243.

[496] E. K. Hale, Metastatic calcification. Dermatology Online J. 2003, 9, 2 (http://dermatology.cdlib.org/94/NYU/Nov2001/3.html) – accessed in September 2008.

[497] P. Grech, P. J. Ell, T. J. Martin, N. A. Barrington, T. J. Martin, *Diagnosis in metabolic bone disease.* Saunders W B Co. 1986, 374 pp.

[498] W. Mohr, Apatite diseases. The pathological substrate in dependence of tissue processing and in consideration of pathogenesis. *Aktuelle Rheumatologie* 2003, 28, 53-58.

[499] B. B. Tomazic, Characterization of mineral phases in cardiovascular calcification. In: *Hydroxyapatite and related materials* (Eds.: P. W. Brown, B. Constantz), CRC Press, Boca Raton, 1994, pp. 93-116.

[500] R. S. Lee, M. V. Kayser, S. Y. Ali, Calcium phosphate microcrystal deposition in the human intervertebral disc. *J. Anat.* 2006, 208, 13–19.

[501] A. K. Rosenthal, Update in calcium deposition diseases. *Curr. Opin. Rheumatol.* 2007, 19, 158-162.

[502] R. Lagier, C. A. Baud, Magnesium whitlockite, a calcium phosphate crystal of special interest in pathology. *Pathol. Res. Pract.* 2003, 199, 329-335.

[503] J. A. Wesson, M. D. Ward, Pathological biomineralization of kidney stones. *Elements* 2007, 3, 415-421.

[504] R. Z. LeGeros, I. Orly, J. P. LeGeros, C. Gomez, J. Kazimiroff, T. Tarpley, B. Kerebel, Scanning electron microscopy and electron probe microanalyses of the crystalline components of human and animal dental calculi. *Scan. Micros.* 1988, 2, 345–356.

[505] T. Kirsch, Determinants of pathological mineralization. *Curr. Opin. Rheumatol.* 2006, 18, 174–180.

[506] C. M. Giachelli, Ectopic calcification: gathering hard facts about soft tissue mineralization. *Amer. J. Pathology*. 1999, 154, 671-675.

[507] T. Kirsch, Physiological and pathological mineralization: a complex multifactorial process. *Curr. Opin. Orthopaedics* 2007, 18, 425-427.

[508] M. Y. Speer, C. M. Giachelli, Regulation of cardiovascular calcification. *Cardiovasc. Pathol.* 2004, 13, 63–70.

[509] C. M. Giachelli, Inducers and inhibitors of biomineralization: lessons from pathological calcification. Orthod. *Craniofac. Res.* 2005, 8, 229–231.

[510] C. M. Giachelli, M. Y. Speer, X. Li, R. M. Rajachar, H. Yang, Regulation of vascular calcification: roles of phosphate and osteopontin. *Circulation Res*. 2005, 96, 717-722.

[511] C. P. Schmitt, T. Odenwald, E. Ritz, Calcium, calcium regulatory hormones, and calcimimetics: impact on cardiovascular mortality. *J. Amer. Soc. Nephrol.* 2006, 17, 78-80.

[512] F. Azari, H. Vali, J. L. Guerquin-Kern, T. D. Wu, A. Croisy, S. K. Sears, M. Tabrizian, M. D. McKee, Intracellular precipitation of hydroxyapatite mineral and implications for pathologic calcification. *J. Struct. Biology* 2008, 162, 468-479.

[513] P. S. Stayton, G. P. Drobny, W. J. Shaw, J. R. Long, M. Gilbert, Molecular recognition at the protein-hydroxyapatite interface. *Crit. Rev. Oral. Biol. Med.* 2003, 14, 370-376.

[514] T. M. Doherty, L. A. Fitzpatrick, D. Inoue, J. H. Qiao, M. C. Fishbein, R. C. Detrano, P. K. Shah, T. B. Rajavashisth, Molecular, endocrine and genetic mechanisms of arterial calcification. *Endocrine Reviews* 2004, 25, 629-672.

[515] G. A. Lamas, A. Ackermann, Clinical evaluation of chelation therapy: is there any wheat amidst the chaff? *Amer. Heart J.* 2000, 140, 4-5.

[516] M. L. Knudtson, D. G. Wyse, P. D. Galbraith, R. Brant, K. Hildebrand, D. Paterson, D. Richardson, C. Burkart, E. Burgess, Chelation therapy for ischemic heart disease: a randomized controlled trial. *JAMA* 2002, 287, 481-486.

[517] H. Ehrlich, P. G. Koutsoukos, K. D. Demadis, O. S. Pokrovsky, Principles of demineralization: modern strategies for the isolation of organic frameworks. Part I. Common definitions and history. *Micron* 2008, 39, 1062-1091.

[518] H. Ehrlich, P. G. Koutsoukos, K. D. Demadis, O. S. Pokrovsky, Principles of demineralization: modern strategies for the isolation of organic frameworks. Part II. Decalcification. *Micron* 2009, 40, 169-193.

[519] S. M. Best, A. E. Porter, E. S. Thian, J. Huang, Bioceramics: past, present and for the future. *J. Eur. Ceram. Soc.* 2008, 28, 1319–1327.

[520] K. D. Jandt, Evolutions, revolutions and trends in biomaterials science – a perspective. *Adv. Engin. Mater*. 2007, 9, 1035-1050.

[521] A. J. Salinas, M. Vallet-Regí, Evolution of ceramics with medical applications. *Z. Anorg. Allg. Chem*. 2007, 633, 1762-1773.

[522] M. E. Ring, *Dentistry: an illustrated history*. Abradale Press, New York, 1985, pp. 15–36.

[523] F. H. Albee, H. F. Morrison, Studies bone growth-triple calcium phosphate as stimulus to osteogenesis. *Ann. Surg*. 1920, 71, 32-39.

[524] C. Balazsi, F. Weber, Z. Kover, E. Horvath, C. Nemeth, Preparation of calcium-phosphate bioceramics from natural resources. *J. Eur. Ceram. Soc*. 2007, 27, 1601-1606.

[525] R. Murugan, S. Ramakrishna, Crystallographic study of hydroxyapatite bioceramics derived from various sources. *Cryst. Growth Des*. 2005, 5, 111-112.

[526] T. Kokubo, (Ed.), *Bioceramics and their clinical applications*. Woodhead Publishing Ltd., Abington Hall, Abington, Cambridge. 2008, 784 pp.

[527] D. C. Greenspan, Bioactive ceramic implant materials. *Curr. Opin. Solid State Mater. Sci*. 1999, 4, 389-393.

[528] T. J. Blokhuis, M. F. Termaat, F. C. den Boer, P. Patka, F. C. Bakker, H. J. T. M. Haarman, Properties of calcium phosphate ceramics in relation to their *in vivo* behavior. *J. Trauma* 2000, 48, 179-189.

[529] H. M. Kim, Bioactive ceramics: challenges and perspectives. *J. Ceram. Soc. Japan* 2001, 109, S49-S57.

[530] W. Cao, L. L. Hench, Bioactive materials. *Ceramics Intern*. 1996, 22, 493-507.

[531] T. Okuda, K. Ioku, I. Yonezawa, H. Minagi, Y. Gonda, G. Kawachi, M. Kamitakahara, Y. Shibata, H. Murayama, H. Kurosawa, T. Ikeda, The slow resorption with replacement by bone of a hydrothermally synthesized pure calcium-deficient hydroxyapatite. *Biomaterials* 2008, 29, 2719-2728.

[532] Z. Seeley, A. Bandyopadhyay, S. Bose, Tricalcium phosphate based resorbable ceramics: influence of NaF and CaO addition. *Mater. Sci. Engin*. C 2008, 28, 11-17.

[533] E. K. Cushnie, Y. M. Khan, C. T. Laurencin, Amorphous hydroxyapatite-sintered polymeric scaffolds for bone tissue regeneration: physical characterization studies. *J. Biomed. Mater. Res*. A 2008, 84A, 54-62.

[534] W. Linhart, D. Briem, M. Amling, J. M. Rueger, J. Windolf, Mechanical failure of porous hydroxyapatite ceramics 7.5 years after implantation in the proximal tibial. *Unfallchirurg* 2004, 107, 154–157.

[535] L. H. He, O. C. Standard, T. T. Huang, B. A. Latella, M. V. Swain, Mechanical behaviour of porous hydroxyapatite. *Acta Biomater*. 2008, 4, 577-586.

[536] J. Norton, K. R. Malik, J. A. Darr, I. Rehman, Recent developments in processing and surface modification of hydroxyapatite. *Adv. Appl. Ceram*. 2006, 105, 113-139.

[537] R. Z. LeGeros, J. P. LeGeros, Calcium phosphate bioceramics: past, present, future. *Key Engin. Mater*. 2003, 240-242, 3-10.

[538] P. C. McAfee, B. W. Cunningham, D. O. Orbegoso, J. C. Sefter, A. E. Dmitriev, I. L. Fedder, Analysis of porous ingrowth in intervertebral disc prostheses. *Spine* 2003, 28, 332–340.

[539] M. Mastrogiacomo, S. Scaglione, R. Martinetti, L. Dolcini, F. Beltrame, R. Cancedda, R. Quarto, Role of scaffold internal structure on *in vivo* bone formation in macroporous calcium phosphate bioceramics. *Biomaterials* 2006, 27, 3230-3237.

[540] M. Okamoto, Y. Dohi, H. Ohgushi, H. Shimaoka, M. Ikeuchi, A. Matsushima, K. Yonemasu, H. Hosoi, Influence of the porosity of hydroxyapatite ceramics on *in vitro* and *in vivo* bone formation by cultured rat bone marrow stromal cells. *J. Mater. Sci. Mater. Med.* 2006, 17, 327-336.

[541] S. Takagi, L. C. Chow, Formation of macropores in calcium phosphate cement implants. *J. Biomed. Mater. Res.* 2001, 12, 135-139.

[542] D. Walsh, J. Tanaka, Preparation of a bone-like apatite foam cement. *J. Mater. Sci. Mater. Med.* 2001, 12, 339-344.

[543] E. Chevalier, D. Chulia, C. Pouget, M. Viana, Fabrication of porous substrates: a review of processes using pore forming agents in the biomaterial field. *J. Pharmaceutical Sci.* 2008, 97, 1135-1154.

[544] V. S. Komlev, S. M. Barinov, Porous hydroxyapatite ceramics of bi-modal pore size distribution. *J. Mater. Sci. Mater. Med.* 2002, 13, 295–299.

[545] Y. H. Hsu, I. G. Turner, A. W. Miles, Mechanical characterization of dense calcium phosphate bioceramics with interconnected porosity. *J. Mater. Sci. Mater. Med.* 2007, 18, 2319-2329.

[546] Y. Ota, T. Kasuga, Y. Abe, Preparation and compressive strength behaviour of porous ceramics with β-$Ca_3(PO_3)_2$ fiber skeletons. *J. Amer. Ceram. Soc.* 1997, 80, 225–231.

[547] M. C. von Doernberg, B. von Rechenberg, M. Bohner, S. Grünenfelder, G. H. van Lenthe, R. Müller, B. Gasser, R. Mathys, G. Baroud, J. Auer, *In vivo* behavior of calcium phosphate scaffolds with four different pore sizes. *Biomaterials* 2006, 27, 5186-5198.

[548] D. Walsh, J. D. Hopwood, S. Mann, Crystal tectonics: construction of reticulated calcium phosphate frameworks in bicontinuous reverse microemulsions. *Science* 1994, 264, 1576-1578.

[549] X. Yao, S. Tan, D. Jiang, Improving the properties of porous hydroxyapatite ceramics by fabricating methods. *J. Mater. Sci.* 2005, 40, 4939-4942.

[550] J. Zhang, M. Fujiwara, Q. Xu, Y. Zhu, M. Iwasa, D. Jiang, Synthesis of mesoporous calcium phosphate using hybrid templates. *Microporous and Mesoporous Materials*, 2008, 111, 411-416.

[551] H. Wang, L. Zhai, Y. Li, T. Shi, Preparation of irregular mesoporous hydroxyapatite. *Mater. Res. Bull.* 2008, 43, 1607-1614.

[552] L. A. Cyster, D. M. Grant, S. M. Howdle, F. R. A. J. Rose, D. J. Irvine, D. Freeman, C. A. Scotchford, K. M. Shakesheff, The influence of dispersant concentration on the pore morphology of hydroxyapatite ceramics for bone tissue engineering. *Biomaterials* 2005, 26, 697-702.

[553] E. J. Lee, Y. H. Koh, B. H. Yoon, H. E. Kim, H. W. Kim, Highly porous hydroxyapatite bioceramics with interconnected pore channels using camphene-based freeze casting. *Mater. Lett.* 2007, 61, 2270-2273.

[554] J. R. Jones, L. L. Hench, Regeneration of trabecular bone using porous ceramics. *Curr. Opin. Solid State Mater. Sci.* 2003, 7, 301–307.

[555] A. C. Tas, Preparation of porous apatite granules from calcium phosphate cement. *J. Mater. Sci. Mater. Med.* 2008, 19, 2231-2239.

[556] Q. Fu, M. N. Rahaman, F. Dogan, B. S. Bal, Freeze casting of porous hydroxyapatite scaffolds. I. Processing and general microstructure. *J. Biomed. Mater. Res. B Appl. Biomater*. 2008, 86B, 125-135.

[557] Y. J. Tang, Y. F. Tang, C. T. Lv, Z. H. Zhou, Preparation of uniform porous hydroxyapatite biomaterials by a new method. *Appl. Surf. Sci*. 2008, 254, 5359-5362.

[558] K. A. Khalil, S. W. Kim, N. Dharmaraj, K. W. Kim, H. Y. Kim, Novel mechanism to improve toughness of the hydroxyapatite bioceramics using high-frequency induction heat sintering. *J. Mater. Process. Technol*. 2007, 187-188, 417-420.

[559] X. Yan, C. Yu, X. Zhou, J. Tang, D. Zhao. Highly ordered mesoporous bioactive glasses with superior in vitro bone-forming bioactivities. *Angew. Chem. Int. Ed. Engl.* 2004, 43, 5980–5984.

[560] I. Izquierdo-Barba, L. Ruiz-González, J. C. Doadrio, J. M. González-Calbet, M. Vallet-Regí, Tissue regeneration: a new property of mesoporous materials. *Solid State Sci.* 2005, 7, 983–989.

[561] R. V. da Silva, C. A. Bertran, E. Y. Kawachi, J. A. Camilli, Repair of cranial bone defects with calcium phosphate ceramic implant or autogenous bone graft. *J. Craniofacial Surgery* 2007, 18, 281-286.

[562] D. R. Jordan, S. Gilberg, A. Bawazeer, Coralline hydroxyapatite orbital implant (Bio-Eye): experience with 158 patients. *Ophthalmic Plastic and Reconstructive Surg*ery 2004, 20, 69-74.

[563] J. S. Yoon, H. Lew, S. J. Kim, S. Y. Lee, Exposure rate of hydroxyapatite orbital implants. *Ophthalmology* 2008, 115, 566-572.

[564] R. Schnettler, J. P. Stahl, V. Alt, T. Pavlidis, E. Dingeldein, S. Wenisch, Calcium phosphat-based bone substitutes. *Eur. J. Trauma* 2004, 4, 219–229.

[565] Z. Zyman, V. Glushko, N. Dedukh, S. Malyshkina, N. Ashukina, Porous calcium phosphate ceramic granules and their behaviour in differently loaded areas of skeleton. *J. Mater. Sci. Mater. Med.* 2008, 19, 2197-2205.

[566] D. Tadic, M. Epple, A thorough physicochemical characterization of 14 calcium phosphate-based bone substitution materials in comparison to natural bone. *Biomaterials*, 2004, 25, 987–994.

[567] R. Z. LeGeros, Properties of osteoconductive biomaterials: calcium phosphates. *Clin. Orthop. Rel. Res*. 2002, 395, 81–98.

[568] J. M. Ruan, J. P. Zou, J. N. Zhou, J. Z. Hu, Porous hydroxyapatite–tricalcium phosphate bioceramics. *Powder Metallurgy*, 2006, 49, 66-69.

[569] M. Bohner, Calcium orthophosphates in medicine: from ceramics to calcium phosphate cements. *Injury* 2000, 31, Suppl. 4, D37-D47.

[570] S. V. Dorozhkin, *Calcium orthophosphate-based biocements and bioconcretes*. (this book).

[571] C. E. Wilson, M. C. Kruyt, J. de Bruijn, C. A. van Blitterswijk, F. C. Oner, A. J. Verbout, W. J. A. Dhert, A new *in vivo* screening model for posterior spinal bone formation: comparison of ten calcium phosphate ceramic material treatments. *Biomaterials* 2006, 27, 302-314.

[572] D. D. Weiss, M. A. Sachs, C. R. Woodard, Calcium phosphate bone cements: a comprehensive review. *J. Long Term Eff. Med. Implants* 2003, 13, 41-47.

[573] A. J. Ambard, L. Mueninghoff, Calcium phosphate cement: review of mechanical and biological properties. *J. Prosthodontics* 2006, 15, 321-328.

[574] P. D. Costantino, C. D. Friedman, K. Jones, L. C. Chow, H. J. Pelzer, G. A. Sisson, Hydroxyapatite cement. I. Basic chemistry and histologic properties. Arch. Otolaryngol. *Head Neck Surg*. 1991, 117, 379-384.

[575] P. D. Costantino, C. D. Friedman, K. Jones, L. C. Chow, H. J. Pelzer, G. A. Sisson, Hydroxyapatite cement. II. Obliteration and reconstruction of the cat frontal sinus. Arch. Otolaryngol. *Head Neck Surg*. 1991, 117, 385-389.

[576] S. J. Hong, Y. K. Park, J. H. Kim, S. H. Lee, K. N. Ryu, C. M. Park, Y. S. Kim, The biomechanical evaluation of calcium phosphate cements for use in vertebroplasty. *J. Neurosurgery Spine* 2006, 4, 154-159.

[577] J. Lin, S. Zhang, T. Chen, C. Liu, S. Lin, X. Tian, Calcium phosphate cement reinforced by polypeptide copolymers. *J. Biomed. Mater. Res. B Appl. Biomater*. 2006, 76B, 432-439.

[578] P. Iooss, A. M. Leray, G. Grimandi, G. Daculsi, C. Merle, A new injectable bone substitute combining poly(ε-caprolactone) microparticles with biphasic calcium phosphate granules. *Biomaterials* 2001, 22, 2785-2794.

[579] O. Gauthier, E. Goyenvalle, J. M. Bouler, J. Guicheux, P. Pilet, P. Weiss, G. Daculsi, Macroporous biphasic calcium phosphate ceramics versus injectable bone substitute: a comparative study 3 and 8 weeks after implantation in rabbit bone. *J. Mater. Sci. Mater. Med.* 2001, 12, 385-390.

[580] M. Schmitt, P. Weiss, X. Bourges, G. Amadordel-Valle, G. Daculsi, Crystallization at the polymer/calcium-phosphate interface in a sterilized injectable bone substitute IBS. *Biomaterials* 2002, 23, 2789-2794.

[581] O. Gauthier, I. Khairoun, J. Bosco, L. Obadia, X. Bourges, C. Rau, D. Magne, J. M. Bouler, E. Aguado, G. Daculsi, Noninvasive bone replacement with a new injectable calcium phosphate biomaterial. *J. Biomed. Mater. Res.* A 2003, 66A, 47-54.

[582] C. Trojani, F. Boukhechba, J. C. Scimeca, F. Vandenbos, J. F. Michiels, G. Daculsi, P. Boileau, P. Weiss, G. F. Carle, N. Rochet, Ectopic bone formation using an injectable biphasic calcium phosphate/Si-HPMC hydrogel composite loaded with undifferentiated bone marrow stromal cells. *Biomaterials* 2006, 27, 3256-3264.

[583] E. Lerouxel, P. Weiss, B. Giumelli, A. Moreau, P. Pilet, J. Guicheux, P. Corre, J. M. Bouler, G. Daculsi, O. Malard, Injectable calcium phosphate scaffold and bone marrow graft for bone reconstruction in irradiated areas: an experimental study in rats. *Biomaterials* 2006, 27, 4566-4572.

[584] S. Blouin, M. F. Moreau, P. Weiss, G. Daculsi, M. F. Basle, D. Chappard, Evaluation of an injectable bone substitute (β-TCP/hydroxyapatite/hydroxy-propyl-methyl-cellulose) in severely osteopenic and aged rats. *J. Biomed. Mater. Res.* A 2006, 78A, 570-580.

[585] S. V. Dorozhkin, Is there a chemical interaction between calcium phosphates and hydroxypropylmethylcellulose (HPMC) in organic/inorganic composites? *J. Biomed. Mater. Res.* 2001, 54, 247–255.

[586] J. J. Chris Arts, N. Verdonschot, B. W. Schreurs, P. Buma, The use of a bioresorbable nano-crystalline hydroxyapatite paste in acetabular bone impaction grafting. *Biomaterials* 2006, 27, 1110–1118.

[587] M. W. Laschke, K. Witt, T. Pohlemann, M. D. Menger, Injectable nanocrystalline hydroxyapatite paste for bone substitution: *in vivo* analysis of biocompatibility and vascularization. *J. Biomed. Mater. Res. B Appl. Biomater*. 2007, 82B, 494–505.

[588] F. X. Huber, I. Berger, N. McArthur, C. Huber, H. P. Kock, J. Hillmeier, P. J. Meeder, Evaluation of a novel nanocrystalline hydroxyapatite paste and a solid hydroxyapatite ceramic for the treatment of critical size bone defects (CSD) in rabbits. *J. Mater. Sci. Mater. Med.* 2008, 19, 33–38.

[589] H. H. Xu, M. D. Weir, E. F. Burguera, A. M. Fraser, Injectable and macroporous calcium phosphate cement scaffold. *Biomaterials* 2006, 27, 4279-4287.

[590] M. C. Kruyt, C. Persson, G. Johansson, W. J. Dhert, J. de Bruijn, Towards injectable cell-based tissue-engineered bone: the effect of different calcium phosphate microparticles and pre-culturing. *Tissue Engin.* 2006, 12, 309-317.

[591] C. Trojani, F. Boukhechba, J. C. Scimeca, F. Vandenbos, J. F. Michiels, G. Daculsi, P. Boileau, P. Weiss, G. F. Carle, N. Rochet, Ectopic bone formation using an injectable biphasic calcium phosphate/Si-HPMC hydrogel composite loaded with undifferentiated bone marrow stromal cells. *Biomaterials* 2006, 27, 3256-3264.

[592] Z. Z. Zyman, I. Ivanov, D. Rochmistrov, V. Glushko, N. Tkachenko, S. Kijko, Sintering peculiarities for hydroxyapatite with different degrees of crystallinity. *J. Biomed. Mater. Res*. 2001, 54, 256-263.

[593] G. Willmann, Coating of implants with hydroxyapatite - material connections between bone and metal. *Adv. Eng. Mater*. 1999, 1, 95-105.

[594] J. A. M. D. Epinette, R. G. T. Geesink, Hydroxyapatite coated hip and knee arthroplasty. Elsevier, Amsterdam, 1995, 394 pp.

[595] H. Schliephake, D. Scharnweber, S. Roesseler, M. Dard, A. Sewing, A. Aref, Biomimetic calcium phosphate composite coating of dental implants. *Int. J. Oral Maxillofac. Implants* 2006, 21, 738-746.

[596] Y. Yang, K. H. Kim, J. L. Ong, A review on calcium phosphate coatings produced using a sputtering process - an alternative to plasma spraying. *Biomaterials* 2005, 26, 327–337.

[597] A. L. Oliveira, J. F. Mano, R. L. Reis, Nature-inspired calcium phosphate coatings: present status and novel advances in the science of mimicry. *Curr. Opin. Solid State Mater. Sci.* 2003, 7, 309–318.

[598] A. Kurella, N. B. Dahotre, Surface modification for bioimplants: the role of laser surface engineering. *J. Biomater. Appl.* 2005, 20, 5-50.

[599] M. C. Kuo, S. K. Yen, The process of electrochemical deposited hydroxyapatite coatings on biomedical titanium at room temperature. *Mater. Sci. Engin*. C 2002, 20, 153-160.

[600] N. Eliaz, T. M. Sridhar, U. K. Mudali, B. Raj, Electrochemical and electrophoretic deposition of hydroxyapatite for orthopaedic applications. *Surface Engineering* 2005, 21, 238-242.

[601] M. Ma, W. Ye, X. X. Wang, Effect of supersaturation on the morphology of hydroxyapatite crystals deposited by electrochemical deposition on titanium. *Mater. Lett.* 2008, 62, 3875-3877.

[602] J. K. Chang, C. H. Chen, K. Y. Huang, G. J. Wang, Eight-year results of hydroxyapatite-coated hip arthroplasty. *J. Arthroplasty*, 2006, 21, 541-546.

[603] R. Slack, A. Tindall, A. A. Shetty, K. D. James, C. Rand, 15-year follow-up results of the hydroxyapatite ceramic-coated femoral stem. *J. Orthopaedic Surgery*, 2006, 14, 151-154.

[604] J. M. Buchanan, 17 year review of hydroxyapatite ceramic coated hip implants - a clinical and histological evaluation. *Key Engin. Mater*. 2006, 309-311, 1341-1344.

[605] J. M. Buchanan, S. Goodfellow, Nineteen years review of hydroxyapatite ceramic coated hip implants: a clinical and histological evaluation. *Key Engin. Mater*. 2008, 361-363, 1315-1318.

[606] A. Binahmed, A. Stoykewych, A. Hussain, B. Love, V. Pruthi, Long-term follow-up of hydroxyapatite-coated dental implants - a clinical trial. *Int. J. Oral Maxillofac. Implan*ts 2007, 22, 963-968.

[607] G. Iezzi, A. Scarano, G. Petrone, A. Piattelli, Two human hydroxyapatite-coated dental implants retrieved after a 14-year loading period: a histologic and histomorphometric case report. *J. Periodontology* 2007, 78, 940-947.

[608] R. G. T. Geesink, Osteoconductive coating for total joint arthroplasty. *Clin. Orthop. Related Res*. 2002, 395, 53–65.

[609] X. Zheng, S. Zhou, X. Li, J. Weng, Shape memory properties of poly(D,L-lactide)/hydroxyapatite composites. *Biomaterials* 2006, 27, 4288-4295.

[610] W. Bonfield, M. D. Grynpas, A. E. Tully, J. Bowman, J Abram, Hydroxyapatite reinforced polyethylene - a mechanically compatible implant material for bone replacement. *Biomaterials* 1981, 2, 185-186.

[611] M. Neumann, M. Epple, Composites of calcium phosphate and polymers as bone substitution materials. *Eur. J. Trauma* 2006, 32, 125-131.

[612] R. A. Mickiewicz, A. M. Mayes, D. Knaack, Polymer-calcium phosphate cement composites for bone substitutes. *J. Biomed. Mater.* Res. 2002, 61, 581-592.

[613] G. Wei, P. X. Ma, Structure and properties of nano-hydroxyapatite/polymer composite scaffolds for bone tissue engineering. *Biomaterials* 2004, 25, 4749-4757.

[614] L. Sun, C. C. Berndt, K. A. Gross, Hydroxyapatite/polymer composite flame sprayed coatings for orthopedic application. *J. Biomater. Sci. Polymer* Ed. 2002, 13, 977-990.

[615] K. U. Lewandrowski, S. P. Bondre, M. Shea, C. M. Untch, W. C. Hayes, D. D. Hile, D. L. Wise, D. J. Trantolo, Composite resorbable polymer/hydroxylapatite composite screws for fixation of osteochondral osteotomies. *Biomed. Mater. Engin*. 2002, 12, 423-438.

[616] E. Salernitano, C. Migliares, Composite materials for biomedical applications: a review. *J. Appl. Biomater. Biomech.* 2003, 1, 3-18.

[617] F. Kusmanto, G. Walker, Q. Gan, P. Walsh, F. Buchanan, G. Dickson, M. McCaigue, C. Maggs, M. Dring, Development of composite tissue scaffolds containing naturally sourced mircoporous hydroxyapatite. *Chem. Engin. J.* 2008, 139, 398-407.

[618] R. K. Roeder, G. L. Converse, R. J. Kane, W. M. Yue, Hydroxyapatite-reinforced polymer biocomposites for synthetic bone substitutes. *JOM*, 2008, 60, 38-45.

[619] J. N. R. O'Donnell, J. M. Antonucci, D. Skrtic, Amorphous calcium phosphate composites with improved mechanical properties. *J. Bioact. Comp. Polym*. 2006, 21, 169-184.

[620] A. Baji, S. C. Wong, T. S. Srivatsan, G. O. Njus, G. Mathur, Processing methodologies for polycaprolactone-hydroxyapatite composites: a review. *Mater. Manufact. Processes* 2006, 21, 211-218.

[621] P. Q. Ruhe, E. L. Hedberg-Dirk, N. T. Padron, P. H. Spauwen, J. A. Jansen, A. G. Mikos, Porous poly(DL-lactic-*co*-glycolic acid)/calcium phosphate cement composite for reconstruction of bone defects. *Tissue Engin*. 2006, 12, 789-800.

[622] S. Nath, B. Basu, Designing materials for hard tissue replacement. *J. Korean Ceram. Soc.* 2008, 45, 1-29.

[623] I. Orly, M. Gregoire, J. Menanteau, M. Heughebaert, B. Kerebel, Chemical changes in hydroxyapatite biomaterial under *in vivo* and *in vitro* biological conditions. *Calcif. Tissue Int.* 1989, 45, 20-26.

[624] J. M. Benyus, *Biomimicry: innovation inspired by nature*. William Morrow, New York, 1997, 308 pp.

[625] S. V. Dorozhkin, E. I. Dorozhkina, M. Epple, A model system to provide a good *in vitro* simulation of biological mineralization. *Cryst. Growth Des*. 2004, 4, 389–395.

[626] I. Izquierdo-Barba, A. J. Salinas, M. Vallet-Regi, Effect of the continuous solution exchange on the in vitro reactivity of a CaO-SiO_2 sol-gel glass. *J. Biomed. Mater. Res.* 2000, 51, 191-199.

[627] M. Vallet-Regi, J. Pėrez-Pariente, I. Izquierdo-Barba, A. J. Salinas, Compositional variations in the calcium phosphate layer growth on gel glasses soaked in a simulated body fluid. *Chem. Mater.* 2000, 12, 3770-3775.

[628] P. Koutsoukos, Z. Amjad, M. B. Tomson, G. H. Nancollas, Crystallization of calcium phosphates: a constant composition study. *J. Amer. Chem. Soc*. 1980, 102, 1553-1557.

[629] M. B. Tomson, G. H. Nancollas, Mineralization kinetics: a constant composition approach. *Science* 1978, 200, 1059-1060.

[630] I. Manjubala, S. Scheler, J. Bössert, K. D. Jandt, Mineralisation of chitosan scaffolds with nano-apatite formation by double diffusion technique. *Acta Biomater*. 2006, 2, 75-84.

[631] S. V. Dorozhkin, E. I. Dorozhkina, The influence of bovine serum albumin on the crystallization of calcium phosphates from a revised simulated body fluid. *Colloids and Surfaces A: Physiochem. Eng. Aspects* 2003, 215, 191–199.

[632] E. I. Dorozhkina, S. V. Dorozhkin, *In vitro* crystallization of carbonateapatite on cholesterol from a modified simulated body fluid. *Colloids and Surfaces A: Physiochem. Eng. Aspects* 2003, 223, 231–237.

[633] S. V. Dorozhkin, E. I. Dorozhkina, M. Epple, Precipitation of carbonateapatite from a revised simulated body fluid in the presence of glucose. *J. Appl. Biomater. Biomech.* 2003, 1, 200–208.

[634] S. V. Dorozhkin, E. I. Dorozhkina, *In vitro* simulation of vascular calcification by the controlled crystallization of amorphous calcium phosphates onto porous cholesterol. J. *Mater. Sci.* 2005, 40, 6417–6422.

[635] S. V. Dorozhkin, *In vitro* mineralization of silicon containing calcium phosphate bioceramics. *J. Amer. Ceram. Soc.* 2007, 90, 244–249.

[636] A. Becker, M. Epple, A high-throughput crystallisation device to study biomineralisation *in vitro*. *Mater. Res. Soc. Symp. Proc.* 2005, 873E, K12.1.1-K12.1.10.

[637] M. Krings, D. Kanellopoulou, D. Mavrilas, B. Glasmacher, *In vitro* pH-controlled calcification of biological heart valve prostheses. *Mater.-Wiss. u. Werkstofftech.* 2006, 37, 432-435.

[638] L. J. Wang, X. Y. Guan, H. Y. Yin, J. Moradian-Oldak, G. H. Nancollas, Mimicking the self-organized microstructure of tooth enamel. *J. Phys. Chem.* C 2008, 112, 5892-5899.

[639] J. H. Hanks, R. E. Wallace, Relation of oxygen and temperature in the preservation of tissues by refrigeration. *Proc. Soc. Exp. Biol. Med.* 1949, 71, 196-200.

[640] Y. Shibata, H. Takashima, H. Yamamoto, T. Miyazaki, Functionally gradient bonelike hydroxyapatite coating on a titanium metal substrate created by a discharging method in HBSS without organic molecules. *Int. J. Oral Maxillofac. Implants* 2004, 19, 177-183.

[641] P. A. A. P. Marques, A. P. Serro, B. J. Saramago, A. C. Fernandes, M. C. F. Magalhães, R. N. Correia, Mineralisation of two phosphate ceramics in HBSS: role of albumin. *Biomaterials* 2003, 24, 451-460.

[642] V. Gopikrishna, P. S. Baweja, N. Venkateshbabu, T. Thomas, D. Kandaswamy, Comparison of coconut water, propolis, HBSS, and milk on PDL cell survival. *J. Endodontics* 2008, 34, 587-589.

[643] T. Hanawa, K. Asami, K. Asaoka, Repassivation of titanium and surface oxide film regenerated in simulated bioliquid. *J. Biomed. Mater. Res.* 1998, 40, 530-538.

[644] L. A. Rocha, E. Anza, A. M. Costa, F. J. Oliveira, R. F. Silva, Electrochemical behavior of Ti/Al_2O_3 interfaces produced by diffusion bonding. *Mater. Res.* 2003, 6, 439-444.

[645] N. Meuleman, T. Tondreau, A. Delforge, M. Dejeneffe, M. Massy, M. Libertalis, D. Bron, L. Lagneaux, Human marrow mesenchymal stem cell culture: serum-free medium allows better expansion than classical α-MEM medium. *Eur. J. Haematology* 2006, 76, 309-316.

[646] Y. Okazaki, E. Gotoh, Corrosion fatigue properties of metallic biomaterials in Eagle's medium. *Materials Transactions* 2002, 43, 2949-2955.

[647] M. J. Coelho, A. T. Cabral, M. H. Fernandes, Human bone cell cultures in biocompatibility testing. Part I: Osteoblastic differentiation of serially passaged human bone marrow cells cultured in α-MEM and in DMEM. *Biomaterials* 2000, 21, 1087-1094.

[648] Y. B. Gao, W. J. Weng, X. L. Deng, K. Cheng, X. G. Liu, P. Y. Du, G. Shen, G. R. Han, Surface morphology variations of porous nano-calcium phosphate/poly(L-lactic acid) composites in PBS. *Key Engin. Mater.* 2006, 309-311, 569-572.

[649] A. C. Lewis, M. R. Kilburn, I. Papageorgiou, G. C. Allen, C. P. Case, Effect of synovial fluid, phosphate-buffered saline solution, and water on the dissolution and corrosion properties of CoCrMo alloys as used in orthopedic implants. *J. Biomed. Mater. Res.* A 2005, 73A, 456-467.

[650] S. P. Humphrey, R. T. Williamson, A review of saliva: normal composition, flow, and function. *J. Prosthetic Dentistry*, 2001, 85, 162-169.

[651] A. Preetha, R. Banerjee, Comparison of artificial saliva substitutes. *Trends Biomater. Artif. Organs* 2005, 18, 178-186.

[652] T. Kokubo, H. Kushitani, S. Sakka, T. Kitsugi, T. Yamamuro, Solutions able to reproduce in vivo surface-structure changes in bioactive glass-ceramic A-W3. *J. Biomed. Mater. Res.* 1990, 24, 721-734.

[653] A. C. Tas, Synthesis of biomimetic Ca-hydroxyapatite powders at 37°C in synthetic body fluids. *Biomaterials* 2000, 21, 1429-1438.

[654] E. Landi, A. Tampieri, G. Celotti, R. Langenati, M. Sandri, S. Sprio, Nucleation of biomimetic apatite in synthetic body fluids: dense and porous scaffold development. *Biomaterials* 2005, 26, 2835-2845.

[655] S. Jalota, S. B. Bhaduri, A. C. Tas, Using a synthetic body fluid (SBF) solution of 27 mM HCO_3^- to make bone substitutes more osteointegrative. *Mater. Sci. Engin.* C 2008, 28, 129-140.

[656] H. M. Kim, T. Miyazaki, T. Kokubo, T. Nakamura, Revised simulated body fluid. In: *Bioceramics* 13; S. Giannini, A. Moroni, Eds.; Trans Tech Publ.: Switzerland, 2001, 192-195, pp. 47-50.

[657] A. Oyane, H. M. Kim, T. Furuya, T. Kokubo, T. Miyazaki, T. Nakamura, Preparation and assessment of revised simulated body fluids. *J. Biomed. Mater. Res.* A 2003, 65A, 188–195.

[658] T. Kokubo, H. Takadama, How useful is SBF in predicting *in vivo* bone bioactivity? *Biomaterials* 2006, 27, 2907-2915.

[659] H. M. Kim, Ceramic bioactivity and related biomimetic strategy. *Curr. Opin. Solid State Mater. Sci.* 2003, 7, 289-299.

[660] X. Lu, Y. Leng, Theoretical analysis of calcium phosphate precipitation in simulated body fluid. *Biomaterials* 2005, 26, 1097–1108.

[661] P. A. A. P. Marques, M. C. F. Magalhães, R. N. Correia, Inorganic plasma with physiological CO_2/HCO_3^- buffer. *Biomaterials* 2003, 24, 1541-1548.

[662] E. I. Dorozhkina, S. V. Dorozhkin, Surface mineralisation of hydroxyapatite in modified simulated body fluid (mSBF) with higher amounts of hydrogencarbonate ions. *Colloids and Surfaces A: Physiochem. Eng. Aspects* 2002, 210, 41–48.

[663] F. Miyaji, H. M. Kim, S. Handa, T. Kokubo, T. Nakamura, Bonelike apatite coating on organic polymers: novel nucleation process using sodium silicate solution. *Biomaterials* 1999, 20, 913–919.

[664] H. M. Kim, K. Kishimoto, F. Miyaji, T. Kokubo, T. Yao, Y. Suetsugu, J. Tanaka, T. Nakamura, Composition and structure of apatite formed on organic polymer in simulated body fluid with a high content of carbonate ion. *J. Mater. Sci. Mater. Med.* 2000, 11, 421–426.

[665] F. Barrere, C. A. van Blitterswijk, K. de Groot, P. Layrolle, Influence of ionic strength and carbonate on the Ca-P coating formation from SBF×5 solution. *Biomaterials* 2002, 23, 1921–1930.

[666] F. Barrere, C. A. van Blitterswijk, K. de Groot, P. Layrolle, Nucleation of biomimetic Ca–P coatings on Ti6Al4V from a SBF×5 solution: influence of magnesium. *Biomaterials* 2002, 23, 2211–2220.

[667] A. C. Tas, S. B. Bhaduri, Rapid coating of Ti6Al4V at room temperature with a calcium phosphate solution similar to 10x simulated body fluid. *J. Mater. Res.* 2004, 19, 2742-2749.

[668] E. I. Dorozhkina, S. V. Dorozhkin, Structure and properties of the precipitates formed from condensed solutions of the revised simulated body fluid. *J. Biomed. Mater. Res. A* 2003, 67A, 578–581.

[669] W. Pompe, S. Lampenscherf, S. Rößler, D. Scharnweber, K. Weis, H. Worch, J. Hofinger, Functionally graded bioceramics. *Mater. Sci. Forum* 1999, 308-311, 325-330.

[670] Y. Fan, K, Duan, R. Wang, A composite coating by electrolysis-induced collagen self-assembly and calcium phosphate mineralization. *Biomaterials* 2005, 26, 1623-1632.

[671] K. Yamauchi, T. Goda, N. Takeuchi, H. Einaga, T. Tanabe, Preparation of collagen/calcium phosphate multilayer sheet using enzymatic mineralization. *Biomaterials*, 2004, 25, 5481-5489.

[672] W. Zhang, Z. L. Huang, S. S. Liao, F. Z. Cui, Nucleation sites of calcium phosphate crystals during collagen mineralization. *J. Amer. Ceram. Soc.* 2003, 86, 1052-1054.

[673] Y. Wang, C. Yang, X. Chen, N. Zhao, Biomimetic formation of hydroxyapatite/collagen matrix composite. *Adv. Eng. Mater.* 2006, 8, 97-100.

[674] D. Lickorish, J. A. M. Ramshaw, J. A. Werkmeister, V. Glattauer, C. R. Howlett, Collagen-hydroxyapatite composite prepared by biomimetic process. *J. Biomed. Mater. Res.* A 2004, 68A, 19-27.

[675] F. Zhao, Y. Yin, W. W. Lu, J. C. Leong, W. Zhang, J. Zhang, M. Zhang, K. Yao, Preparation and histological evaluation of biomimetic three-dimensional hydroxyapatite/chitosan-gelatin network composite scaffolds. *Biomaterials* 2002, 23, 3227-3234.

[676] H. W. Kim, H. E. Kim, V. Salih, Stimulation of osteoblast responses to biomimetic nanocomposites of gelatin–hydroxyapatite for tissue engineering scaffolds. *Biomaterials* 2005, 26, 5221-5230.

[677] H. W. Kim, J. C. Knowles, H. E. Kim, Porous scaffolds of gelatin-hydroxyapatite nanocomposites obtained by biomimetic approach: Characterization and antibiotic drug release. *J. Biomed. Mater. Res. B Appl. Biomater.* 2005, 74B, 686-698.

[678] Z. Chen, Q. L. Li, Q. Zen, G. Li, H. Jiang, L. Liu, B. W. Darvell, Biomimetic mineralization and bioactivity of phosphorylated chitosan. *Key Engin. Mater.* 2005, 288-289, 429-432.

[679] Q. L. Li, Z. Chen, G. Ou, L. Liu, H. Jiang, Q. Zeng, G. Li, G. He, A. Mo, B. W. Darvell, Biomimetic synthesis of apatite - polyelectrolyte complex (chitosan -. phosphorylated chitosan) hydrogel as an osteoblast carrier. *Key Engin. Mater.* 2005, 288-289, 75-78.

[680] S. I. Stupp, G. W. Ciegler, Organoapatites: materials for artificial bone. I. Synthesis and microstructure. *J. Biomed. Mater. Res.* 1992, 26, 169-183.

[681] S. I. Stupp, P. V. Braun, Molecular manipulation of microstructures: biomaterials, ceramics, and semiconductors. *Science* 1997, 277, 1242-1248.

[682] S. I. Stupp, G. C. Mejicano, J. A. Hanson, Organoapatites: materials for artificial bone. II. Hardening reactions and properties. *J. Biomed. Mater. Res.* 1993, 27, 289-299.

[683] S. I. Stupp, J. A. Hanson, J. A. Eurell, G. W. Ciegler, A. Johnson, Organoapatites: materials for artificial bone. III. Biological testing. *J. Biomed. Mater. Res.* 1993, 27, 301-311.

[684] Y. Liu, P. Layrolle, J. de Bruijn, C. van Blitterswijk, K. de Groot, Biomimetic coprecipitation of calcium phosphate and bovine serum albumin on titanium alloy. *J. Biomed. Mater. Res.* 2001, 57, 327-335.

[685] J. Wang, P. Layrolle, M. Stigter, K. de Groot, Biomimetic and electrolytic calcium phosphate coatings on titanium alloy: physicochemical characteristics and cell attachment. *Biomaterials* 2004, 25, 583-592.

[686] Q. Zhang, Y. Leng, Electrochemical activation of titanium for biomimetic coating of calcium phosphate. *Biomaterials* 2005, 26, 3853-3859.

[687] A. Bigi, E. Boanini, B. Bracci, A. Facchini, S. Panzavolta, F. Segatti, L. Sturba, Nanocrystalline hydroxyapatite coatings on titanium: a new fast biomimetic method. *Biomaterials* 2005, 26, 4085-4089.

[688] H. M. Kim, T. Himeno, M. Kawashita, J. H. Lee, T. Kokubo, T. Nakamura, Surface potential change in bioactive titanium metal during the process of apatite formation in simulated body fluid. *J. Biomed. Mater. Res.* A 2003, 67A, 1305–1309.

[689] S. Allegrini, E. Rumpel, E. Kauschke, J. Fanghänel, B. König, Hydroxyapatite grafting promotes new bone formation and osseointegration of smooth titanium implants. *Annals of Anatomy* 2006, 188, 143-151.

[690] C. Arnould, J. Delhalle, Z. Mekhalif, Multifunctional hybrid coating on titanium towards hydroxyapatite growth: electrodeposition of tantalum and its molecular functionalization with organophosphonic acids films. *Electrochimica Acta* 2008, 53, 5632-5638.

[691] T. Iwatsubo, S. P. Kusumocahyo, T. Kanamori, T. Shinbo, Mineralization of hydroxyapatite on a polymer substrate in a solution supersaturated by polyelectrolyte. *J. Appl. Polymer Sci.* 2006, 100, 1465-1470.

[692] A. Bodin, L. Gustafsson, P. Gatenholm, Surface-engineered bacterial cellulose as template for crystallization of calcium phosphate. *J. Biomater. Sci. Polymer* Ed. 2006, 17, 435-447.

[693] G. K. Toworfe, R. J. Composto, I. M. Shapiro, P. Ducheyne, Nucleation and growth of calcium phosphate on amine-, carboxyl- and hydroxyl-silane self-assembled monolayers. *Biomaterials* 2006, 27, 631-642.

[694] L. G. Griffith, G. Naughton, Tissue engineering - current challenges and expanding opportunities. *Science* 2002, 295, 1009-1014.

[695] http://www.nsf.gov/pubs/2004/nsf0450/start.htm (accessed in September 2008).

[696] R. Langer, J. P. Vacanti, Tissue engineering. *Science* 1993, 260, 920-926.

[697] M. Schieker, H. Seitz, I. Drosse, S. Seitz, W. Mutschler, Biomaterials as scaffold for bone tissue engineering. *Eur. J. Trauma* 2006, 32, 114-124.

[698] M. Fini, R. Giardino, V. Borsari, P. Torricelli, L. Rimondini, G. Giavaresi, N. N. Aldini, *In vitro* behaviour of osteoblasts cultured on orthopaedic biomaterials with different surface roughness, uncoated and fluorohydroxyapatite-coated, relative to the *in vivo* osteointegration rate. *Int. J. Artificial Organs* 2003, 26, 520-528.

[699] R. Zimmerman, D. Ila, C. Muntele, M. Rodrigues, D. B. Poker, D. Hensley, Enhanced tissue adhesion by increased porosity and surface roughness of carbon based biomaterials. *Nuclear Instruments and Methods in Physics Research Section B*, 2002, 191, 825-829.

[700] M. Sato, T. J. Webster, Designing orthopedic implant surfaces: harmonization of nanotopographical and chemical aspects. *Nanomedicine*, 2006, 1, 351-354.

[701] M. Okamoto, Y. Dohi, H. Ohgushi, H. Shimaoka, M. Ikeuchi, A. Matsushima, K. Yonemasu, H. Hosoi, Influence of the porosity of hydroxyapatite ceramics on *in vitro* and *in vivo* bone formation by cultured rat bone marrow stromal cells. *J. Mater. Sci. Mater. Med.* 2006, 17, 327-336.

[702] B. Annaz, K. A. Hing, M. Kayser, T. Buckland, L. di Silvio, Porosity in phase-pure hydroxyapatite. *J. Microscopy* 2004, 216, 97-109.

[703] E. Ebaretonbofa, J. R. Evans, High porosity hydroxyapatite foam scaffolds for bone substitute. *J. Porous Mater*. 2002, 9, 257-263.

[704] N. Specchia, A. Pagnotta, M. Cappella, A. Tampieri, F. Greco, Effect of hydroxyapatite porosity on growth and differentiation of human osteoblast-like cells. *J. Mater. Sci.* 2002, 37, 577-584.

[705] C. C. Teixeira, Y. Nemelivsky, C. Karkia, R. Z. LeGeros, Biphasic calcium phosphate: a scaffold for growth plate chondrocyte maturation. *Tissue Engin*. 2006, 12, 2283-2289.

[706] Z. Artzi, M. Weinreb, N. Givol, M. D. Rohrer, C. E. Nemcovsky, H. S. Prasad, H. Tal, Biomaterial resorbability and healing site morphology of inorganic bovine bone and beta tricalcium phosphate in the canine. A 24-month longitudinal histologic study and morphometric analysis. *Int. J. Oral Maxillofac. Implants* 2004, 19, 357-368.

[707] L. G. Griffith, Polymeric biomaterials. *Acta Mater*. 2000, 48, 263-277.

[708] J. G. Dellinger, J. A. C. Eurell, R. D. Jamison, Bone response to 3D periodic hydroxyapatite scaffolds with and without tailored microporosity to deliver bone morphogenetic protein 2. *J. Biomed. Mater. Res*. A 2006, 76A, 366-376.

[709] K. Pal, S. Pal, Development of porous hydroxyapatite scaffolds. *Mater. Manuf. Process.* 2006, 21, 325-328.

[710] C. J. Bae, H. W. Kim, Y. H. Koh, H. E. Kim, Hydroxyapatite (HA) bone scaffolds with controlled macrochannel pores. J. *Mater. Sci. Mater. Med.* 2006, 17, 517-521.

[711] H. Liu, T. J. Webster, Nanomedicine for implants: a review of studies and necessary experimental tools. *Biomaterials* 2007, 28, 354-369.

[712] T. Matsumoto, M. Okazaki, A. Nakahira, J. Sasaki, H. Egusa, T. Sohmura, Modification of apatite materials for bone tissue engineering and drug delivery carriers. *Curr. Medicinal Chem*. 2007, 14, 2726-2733.

[713] H. W. Kim, Y. H. Koh, Y. M. Kong, J. G. Kang, H. E. Kim, Strontium substituted calcium phosphate biphasic ceramics obtained by a powder precipitation method. *J. Mater. Sci. Mater. Med.* 2004, 15, 1129-1134.

[714] M. Vallet-Regi, D. Arcos, Silicon substituted hydroxyapatites. A method to upgrade calcium phosphate based implants. *J. Mater. Chem.* 2005, 15, 1509-1516.

[715] U. Gbureck, R. Thull, J. E. Barralet, Alkali ion substituted calcium phosphate cement formation from mechanically activated reactants. *J. Mater. Sci. Mater. Med.* 2005, 16, 423-427.

[716] S. Kannan, J. M. Ventura, J. M. F. Ferreira, *In situ* formation and characterization of flourine-substituted biphasic calcium phosphate ceramics of varied F-HAP/β-TCP ratios. *Chem. Mater.* 2005, 17, 3065-3068.

[717] U. Gbureck, O. Knappe, L. M. Grover, J. E. Barralet, Antimicrobial potency of alkali ion substituted calcium phosphate cements. *Biomaterials,* 2005, 26, 6880-6886.

[718] A. M. Pietak, J. W. Reid, M. J. Stott, M. Sayer, Silicon substitution in the calcium phosphate bioceramics. *Biomaterials* 2007, 28, 4023-4032.

[719] D. Tadic, A. Veresov, V. I. Putlayev, M. Epple, *In vitro* preparation of nanocrystalline calcium phosphates as bone substitution materials in surgery. *Mater.-Wiss. u. Werkstofftech.* 2003, 34, 1048-1051.

[720] K. J. Lilley, U. Gbureck, A. J. Wright, D. F. Farrar, J. E. Barralet, Cement from nanocrystalline hydroxyapatite: effect of calcium phosphate ratio. *J. Mater. Sci. Mater. Med.* 2005, 16, 1185-1190.

[721] S. Meejoo, W. Maneeprakorn, P. Winotai, Phase and thermal stability of nanocrystalline hydroxyapatite prepared via microwave heating. *Thermochimica Acta* 2006, 447, 115-120.

[722] X. Zhu, O. Eibl, C. Berthold, L. Scheideler, J. Geis-Gerstorfer, Structural characterization of nanocrystalline hydroxyapatite and adhesion of pre-osteoblast cells. *Nanotechnology* 2006, 17, 2711-2721.

[723] H. Li, M. Y. Zhu, L. H. Li, C. R. Zhou, Processing of nanocrystalline hydroxyapatite particles via reverse microemulsions. *J. Mater. Sci.* 2008, 43, 384-389.

[724] A. Banerjee, S. Bose, Effect of dopants on the properties of nanocrystalline hydroxyapatite. *Ceramic Transact.* 2005, 164, 91-99.

[725] W. Feng, L. M. Sen, L. Y. Peng, G. S. Song, Synthesis of nanocrystalline hydroxyapatite powders in stimulated body fluid. *J. Mater. Sci.* 2005, 40, 2073-2076.

[726] H. Ito, Y. Oaki, H. Imai, Selective synthesis of various nanoscale morphologies of hydroxyapatite via an intermediate phase. *Cryst. Growth Des.* 2008, 8, 1055-1059.

[727] M. H. Fathi, A. Hanifi, V. Mortazavi, Preparation and bioactivity evaluation of bone-like hydroxyapatite nanopowder. *J. Mater. Process. Technol.* 2008, 202, 536-542.

[728] J. Li, Y. Chen, Y. Yin, F. Yao, K. Yao, Modulation of nano-hydroxyapatite size via formation on chitosan–gelatin network film *in situ. Biomaterials* 2007, 28, 781-790.

[729] Q. He, Z. Huang, Y. Liu, W. Chen, T. Xu, Template-directed one-step synthesis of flowerlike porous carbonated hydroxyapatite spheres. *Mater. Lett.* 2007, 61, 141-143.

[730] C. You, T. Miyazaki, E. Ishida, M. Ashizuka, C. Ohtsuki, M. Tanihara, Fabrication of poly(vinyl alcohol)-apatite hybrids through biomimetic process. *J. Eur. Ceram. Soc.* 2007, 27, 1585-1588.

[731] M. Aizawa, A. E. Porter, S. M. Best, W. Bonfield, Ultrastructural observation of single-crystal apatite fibres. *Biomaterials* 2005, 26, 3427-3433.
[732] Y. M. Park, S. C. Ryu, S. Y. Yoon, R. Stevens, H. C. Park, Preparation of whisker-shaped hydroxyapatite/β-tricalcium phosphate composite. *Mater. Chem. Phys.* 2008, 109, 440-447.
[733] H. Morisue, M. Matsumoto, K. Chiba, H. Matsumoto, Y. Toyama, M. Aizawa, N. Kanzawa, T. J. Fujimi, H. Uchida, I. Okada, A novel hydroxyapatite fiber mesh as a carrier for recombinant human bone morphogenetic protein-2 enhances bone union in rat posterolateral fusion model. *Spine* 2006, 31, 1194-1200.
[734] A. Matsuda, T. Ikoma, H. Kobayashi, J. Tanaka, Preparation and mechanical property of core-shell type chitosan/calcium phosphate composite fiber. *Mater. Sci. Engin. C* 2004, 24, 723-728.
[735] Y. Wu, L. L. Hench, J. Du, K. L. Choy, J. Guo, Preparation of hydroxyapatite fibers by electrospinning technique. *J. Amer. Ceram. Soc.* 2004, 87, 1988-1991.
[736] S. R. Ramanan, R. Venkatesh, A study of hydroxyapatite fibers prepared via sol–gel route. *Mater. Lett.* 2004, 58, 3320-3323.
[737] D. S. Seo, J. K. Lee, Synthesis of hydroxyapatite whiskers through dissolution-reprecipitation process using EDTA. *J. Cryst. Growth* 2008, 310, 2162-2167.
[738] I. S. Neira, F. Guitián, T. Taniguchi, T. Watanabe, M. Yoshimura, Hydrothermal synthesis of hydroxyapatite whiskers with sharp faceted hexagonal morphology. *J. Mater. Sci.* 2008, 43, 2171-2178.
[739] C. C. Ribeiro, C. C. Barrias, M. A. Barbosa, Preparation and characterisation of calcium-phosphate porous microspheres with a uniform size for biomedical applications. *J. Mater. Sci. Mater. Med.* 2006, 17, 455-463.
[740] C. C. Ribeiro, C. C. Barrias, M. A. Barbosa, Calcium phosphate-alginate microspheres as enzyme delivery matrices. *Biomaterials* 2004, 25, 4363-4373.
[741] W. Y. Zhou, M. Wang, W. L. Cheung, B. C. Guo, D. M. Jia, Synthesis of carbonated hydroxyapatite nanospheres through nanoemulsion. *J. Mater. Sci. Mater. Med.* 2008, 19, 103-110.
[742] H. W. Kim, H. J. Gu, H. H. Lee, Microspheres of collagen-apatite nanocomposites with osteogenic potential for tissue engineering. *Tissue Eng.* 2007, 13, 965-973.
[743] S. Deville, E. Saiz, A. P. Tomsia, Freeze casting of hydroxyapatite scaffolds for bone tissue engineering. *Biomaterials* 2006, 27, 5480-5489.
[744] S. H. Min, H. H. Jin, H. Y. Park, I. M. Park, H. C. Park, S. Y. Yoon, Preparation of porous hydroxyapatite scaffolds for bone tissue engineering. *Mater. Sci. Forum* 2006, 510-511, 754-757.
[745] B. Leukers, H. Gülkan, S. H. Irsen, S. Milz, C. Tille, M. Schieker, H. Seitz, Hydroxyapatite scaffolds for bone tissue engineering made by 3D printing. *J. Mater. Sci. Mater. Med.* 2005, 16, 1121-1124.
[746] S. Deville, E. Saiz, R. K. Nalla, A. P. Tomsia, Strong biomimetic hydroxyapatite scaffolds. *Advances in Science and Technology* 2006, 49, 148-152.
[747] W. Yang, D. Zhou, G. Yin, H. Chen, Progress of biphasic calcium phosphate bioceramic as scaffold materials of bone tissue engineering. *J. Chinese Ceram. Soc.* 2004, 32, 1143-1149.

[748] A. Tampieri, G. Celotti, S. Sprio, A. Delcogliano, S. Franzese, Porosity-graded hydroxyapatite ceramics to replace natural bone. *Biomaterials* 2001, 22, 1365-1370.

[749] K. Furuichi, Y. Oaki, H. Ichimiya, J. Komotori, H. Imai, Preparation of hierarchically organized calcium phosphate–organic polymer composites by calcification of hydrogel. *Science and Technology of Advanced Materials* 2006, 7, 219-225.

[750] M. Okamoto, Y. Dohi, H. Ohgushi, H. Shimaoka, M. Ikeuchi, A. Matsushima, K. Yonemasu, H. Hosoi, Influence of the porosity of hydroxyapatite ceramics on in vitro and in vivo bone formation by cultured rat bone marrow stromal cells. *J. Mater. Sci. Mater. Med.* 2006, 17, 327-336.

[751] L. L. Hench, J. M. Polak, Third-generation biomedical materials. *Science* 2002, 295, 1014-1017.

[752] A. S. Blawas, W. M. Reichert, Protein patterning. *Biomaterials* 1998, 19, 595-609.

[753] S. S. Kim, M. S. Park, O. Jeon, C. Y. Choi, B. S. Kim, Poly(lactide-*co*-glycolide)/hydroxyapatite composite scaffolds for bone tissue engineering. *Biomaterials* 2006, 27, 1399-1409.

[754] M. J. Mondrinos, R. Dembzynski, L. Lu, V. K. C. Byrapogu, D. M. Wootton, P. I. Lelkes, J. Zhou, Porogen-based solid freeform fabrication of polycaprolactone–calcium phosphate scaffolds for tissue engineering. *Biomaterials* 2006, 27, 4399-4408.

[755] S. S. Kim, K. M. Ahn, M. S. Park, J. H. Lee, C. Y. Choi, B. S. Kim, A poly(lactide-*co*-glycolide)/hydroxyapatite composite scaffold with enhanced osteoconductivity. *J. Biomed. Mater. Res.* A 2007, 80A, 206-215.

[756] J. Li, A. Beaussart, Y. Chen, A. F. T. Mak, Transfer of apatite coating from porogens to scaffolds: uniform apatite coating within porous poly(DL-lactic-*co*-glycolic acid) scaffold *in vitro*. *J. Biomed. Mater. Res.* A 2007, 80A, 226-233.

[757] S. Sanchez-Salcedo, I. Izquierdo-Barba, D. Arcos, M. Vallet-Regi, *In vitro* evaluation of potential calcium phosphate scaffolds for tissue engineering. *Tissue Engin.* 2006, 12, 279-290.

[758] J. A. Meganck, M. J. Baumann, E. D. Case, L. R. McCabe, J. N. Allar, Biaxial flexure testing of calcium phosphate bioceramics for use in tissue engineering. *J. Biomed. Mater. Res.* A 2005, 72A, 115-126.

[759] E. D. Case, I. O. Smith, M. J. Baumann, Microcracking and porosity in calcium phosphates and the implications for bone tissue engineering. *Mater. Sci. Engin. A,* 2005, 390, 246-254.

[760] P. Sibilla, A. Sereni, G. Aguiari, M. Banzi, E. Manzati, C. Mischiati, L. Trombelli, L. del Senno, Effects of a hydroxyapatite-based biomaterial on gene expression in osteoblast-like cells. *J. Dent. Res.* 2006, 85, 354-358.

[761] A. A. Sawyer, K. M. Hennessy, S. L. Bellis, The effect of adsorbed serum proteins, RGD and proteoglycan-binding peptides on the adhesion of mesenchymal stem cells to hydroxyapatite. *Biomaterials* 2007, 28, 383-392.

[762] M. Mastrogiacomo, A. Muraglia, V. Komlev, F. Peyrin, F. Rustichelli, A. Crovace, R. Cancedda, Tissue engineering of bone: search for a better scaffold. Orthod. *Craniofacial Res.* 2005, 8, 277–284.

[763] R. M. Schek, J. M. Taboas, S. J. Hollister, P. H. Krebsbach, Tissue engineering osteochondral implants for temporomandibular joint repair. *Orthod. Craniofacial Res.* 2005, 8, 313–319.

[764] E. A. Krylova, A. A. Ivanov, S. E. Krylov, I. G. Plashchina, A. S. Grigorjan, D. V. Goldstein, A. A. Pulin, T. H. Fatkhudinov, Hydroxyapatite-alginate structure as living cells supporting system. *Minerva Biotecnologica* 2006, 18, 17-22.

[765] L. L. Hench, Biomaterials: a forecast for the future. *Biomaterials* 1998, 19, 1419-1423.

[766] B. D. Ratner, S. J. Bryant, Biomaterials: where we have been and where we are going. *Annual Review of Biomedical Engineering* 2004, 6, 41-75.

[767] C. Drouet, C. Largeot, G. Raimbeaux, C. Estournès, G. Dechambre, C. Combes, C. Rey, Bioceramics: spark plasma sintering (SPS) of calcium phosphates. *Advances in Science and Technology* 2006, 49, 45-50.

[768] A. A. White, S. M. Best, I. A. Kinloch, Hydroxyapatite-carbon nanotube composites for biomedical applications: a review. *Int. J. Appl. Ceram. Technol.* 2007, 4, 1-13.

[769] C. Kealley, M. Elcombe, A. van Riessen, B. Ben-Nissan, Development of carbon nanotube-reinforced hydroxyapatite bioceramics. *Physica* B 2006, 385-386, 496-498.

[770] K. Balani, R. Anderson, T. Laha, M. Andara, J. Tercero, E. Crumpler, A. Agarwal, Plasma-sprayed carbon nanotube reinforced hydroxyapatite coatings and their interaction with human osteoblasts *in vitro*. *Biomaterials* 2007, 28, 618-624.

[771] J. W. Reid, J. A. Hendry, Rapid, accurate phase quantification of multiphase calcium phosphate materials using Rietveld refinement. *J. Appl. Cryst.* 2006, 39, 536-543.

[772] S. V. Dorozhkin, Green chemical synthesis of calcium phosphate bioceramics. *J. Appl. Biomater. Biomech.* 2008, 6, 104-109.

[773] Y. Mizushima, T. Ikoma, J. Tanaka, K. Hoshi, T. Ishihara, Y. Ogawa, A. Ueno, Injectable porous hydroxyapatite microparticles as a new carrier for protein and lipophilic drugs. *J. Controlled Release* 2006, 110, 260-265.

[774] M. P. Ginebra, T. Traykova, J. A. Planell, Calcium phosphate cements as bone drug delivery systems: a review. *J. Controlled Release* 2006, 113, 102-110.

[775] M. P. Ginebra, T. Traykova, J. A. Planell, Calcium phosphate cements: competitive drug carriers for the musculoskeletal system? *Biomaterials* 2006, 27, 2171-2177.

[776] J. Fan, J. Lei, C. Yu, B. Tu, D. Zhao, Hard-templating synthesis of a novel rod-like nanoporous calcium phosphate bioceramics and their capacity as antibiotic carriers. *Mater. Chem. Phys.* 2007, 103, 489-493.

[777] F. Barrère, T. A. Mahmood, K. de Groot, C. A. van Blitterswijk, Advanced biomaterials for skeletal tissue regeneration: instructive and smart functions. *Mater. Sci. Engin. R: Reports* 2008, 59, 38-71.

[778] A. Sudo, M. Hasegawa, A. Fukuda, A. Uchida, Treatment of infected hip arthroplasty with antibiotic-impregnated calcium hydroxyapatite. *J. Arthroplasty* 2008, 23, 145-150.

In: Bioceramics: Properties, Preparations and Applications ISBN: 978-1-60741-056-0
Editors: W. Kossler, J. Fuchs, pp. 163-200

Chapter III

Novel Insights into Ordered Mesoporous Materials for Biomedical Applications

Montserrat Colilla and María Vallet-Regí*
Departamento de Química Inorgánica y Bioinorgánica, Facultad de Farmacia, Universidad Complutense de Madrid, E-28040-Madrid, Spain
Centro de Investigación Biomédica en Red. Bioingeniería, Biomateriales y Nanomedicina, CIBER-BBN, Spain

Abstract

Biomedical scientific community is currently demanding new nanotechnological advances for the development of third generation bioceramics that promote bone tissue regeneration. Much effort is being devoted to the design of scaffolds with three-dimensional (3D) interconnected hierarchical porosity that allows new bone in-growth.

Recently, silica-based ordered mesoporous materials have been proposed as starting materials for the manufacture of 3D scaffolds for bone tissue engineering. The outstanding textural properties of mesoporous materials, such as high surface areas and pore volumes and narrow pore size distributions, make these matrices excellent candidates for local controlled delivery systems of biologically active molecules. These molecules include different drugs to treat bone infection, inflammation or diseases and diverse osteogenic agents such as amino acids, peptides, proteins or growth factors, which can promote new bone formation. The structural and textural properties of host mesoporous matrices can be tailored depending on the targeted guest-molecule. Moreover, their silanol-rich surfaces can undergo chemical functionalization with different organic groups, allowing a better control over molecule loading and release kinetics.

On the other hand, the *in vitro* bioactive behavior of mesoporous silicas has been demonstrated; since the growth of an apatite-like layer onto their surfaces is observed when they are in contact with simulate body fluids. This apatite is quite similar to the

* Tel: +34-913941843; Fax: +34-913941786; E-mail: vallet@farm.ucm.es

mineral phase of bone, leading to a bioactive bond that would ensure the implant-tissue integration. Recently, in an effort to accelerate bioactive responses, the synthesis of mesoporous glasses, which exhibit the excellent textural properties of mesoporous materials and chemical compositions similar to those of bioactive sol-gel glasses, has been reported. Mesoporous glasses have shown extraordinary *in vitro* behaviors, such as biomimetic bone mineralization and the fastest bioactive response reported so far.

The recent advances in mesoporous materials as bioceramics for bone tissue regeneration are reviewed in this chapter. Moreover, a critical discussion of the current possibilities of these materials for biomedical purposes together with the future perspectives is also carried out.

This chapter describes the general properties and the different synthesis methods of mesoporous materials. Moreover, the recent nanotechnological advances to enhance the bioactive behavior and controlled delivery capability of mesoporous matrices for bone tissue regeneration applications are also tackled. In addition, the recently developed strategies to design 3D scaffolds starting from mesoporous materials for bone tissue engineering are reviewed. Finally, a critical discussion of the current possibilities of these materials for biomedical purposes together with their future perspectives is also carried out.

1. Introduction

Bioceramics have been widely employed as bone implants by the biomedical scientific community due to their high biocompatible character and their capability to be designed and manufactured with tailored biostable, bioactive or bioresorbable properties [1,2]. The first generation of bioceramics consisted in the so-called *inert* ceramics, such as alumina, zirconia and carbon [3,4], which played an important role for substitution purposes due to their low reactivity.

The scenario significantly changed with the introduction of second generation ceramics by Larry Hench in the early 1970s, who evidenced that certain glasses in contact with living tissues formed mechanically strongly bioactive bond when implanted [5,6]. The bond forming mechanism involves a series of surface reactions that lead to the growth onto the material surfaces of nanocrystalline non-stoichiometric carbonate hydroxyapatite (CHA) similar to the biological ones [2,7-9]. This CHA layer, which is produced from species lixiviated from the glass and/or contained in the surrounding fluids, acts as bonding site between the glass and the bone. Therefore, this apatite layer in the presence of cells and proteins of the surrounding fluids ensures bone-implant fixation [10-12]. Among these ceramics we can mention calcium phosphates, and several compositions of glasses and ceramic glasses [1,2,13-17]. For biomedical applications, bioactive ceramics are provided as powder, porous pieces, dense pieces, injectable mixtures and coatings. They exhibit outstanding features concerning biocompatible and bioactive behavior, but their brittleness could limit their application in the repair of large bone defects. To solve this drawback, recent advances have been made throughout the synthesis of bioactive organic-inorganic hybrids [18,19]. In fact, it is possible to obtain organic-inorganic hybrids with mechanical features similar to those of natural bone [20].

However, the present scientific efforts go further than just ensuring bioactive bond and currently, third generation bioceramics are demanded [21]. Therefore, much attention is being dedicated to the research on bioceramics able to stimulate the regeneration of living bone, as well as to be shaped into scaffolds for bone tissue engineering. The concept is to incorporate biologically active molecules, such as drugs, peptides, proteins, growth factors and so forth, which are used to stimulate tissue regeneration, within a porous-degradable material known as scaffold [22].

When the growth of new bone is targeted, it is essential to understand the structure of natural hard tissues (Figure 1). Natural hard tissues in vertebrates are natural organic inorganic composite materials [23-25]. The inorganic component consists of CHA of nanometric size, ranging from 25 to 50 nm. Vertebrates fabricate natural bone by scattering these inorganic apatites into an organic matrix mainly consisting of type I collagen, a structural protein associated with a smaller fraction of other non-collagenous proteins. The inorganic phase of natural bone represents the 45% of the total mass of bone, organic matter constitutes the 30% and the 25% remaining is water. The type I collagen proteins are bonded forming linear chains that are self-arranged in fibers, giving rise to various macroscopic structures and leaving small empty interstitial empty compartments where apatite nanocrystals are deposited during a controlled biomineralization process [24]. Therefore, pore sizes in cortical bone range from 1 μ to 100 μm, being 200 μm to 400μm in trabecular bone. In addition, trabecular bone presents 50-95% of porosity, where 55-70% of such pores are interconnected [26]. This hierarchical organization of bone at many levels of scale is crucial to permit an appropriate physiological performance [27].

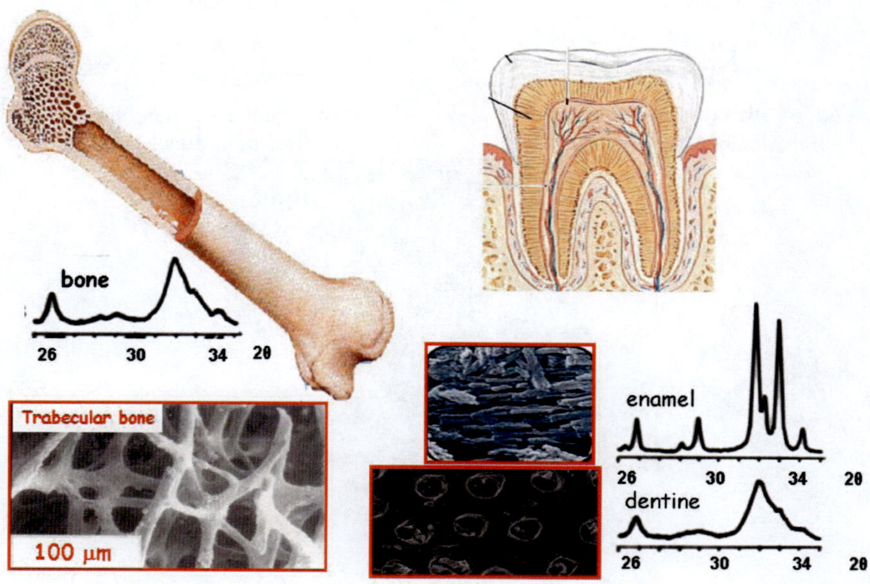

$$Ca_{8.3}\,\square_{0.7}(PO_4)_{4.3}(HPO_4,CO_3)_{1.7}(2OH,CO_3)_{0.15}\,\square_{1.7}$$

Figure 1. Structure of natural hard tissues (bones and teeth) in vertebrates. Scanning electron microscopy (SEM) studies reveal that bone pores are at the micrometric scale. Moreover, X-ray diffraction (XRD) patterns evidence that biological apatites are formed by nanometric crystals.

Synthetic scaffolds are matrices for bone growth that provides specific environment and architecture to promote cellular attachment, growth and differentiation. These scaffolds should exhibit a wide range of pore sizes and 3D interconnected porosity with certain values of porosity that should be in agreement with natural biological requirements of natural bone [28]. According to the porosity of natural bone, bone scaffolds should exhibit hierarchical pore structures, with pore sizes ranging from 1 μm to 1000 μm. However there is still a lack of unanimity concerning the ideal porosity required for appropriate bone in-growth [29].

Bioceramics have been widely employed in the development of bone implants and they have been proposed as starting materials for the manufacture of scaffolds for bone tissue engineering [30]. Among bioceramics, silica-based ordered mesoporous materials (SMMs) open promising expectations in the bioclinical field (Figure 2). The biocompatibility of silica-based materials has been probed [31-34]. Moreover, the *in vitro* bioactive behavior of SMMs has been demonstrated [9,35]. Recently, the synthesis of mesoporous bioactive glasses (MBGs), with chemical compositions similar to those of conventional bioactive sol-gel glasses (BGs) and the textural properties and ordered mesopore arrangement of SMMs has been reported [36,37]. MBGs exhibit outstanding features such as the fastest bioactive response reported up to date for bioceramic materials or biomimetic behavior similar to the *in vivo* bone mineralization process [38].

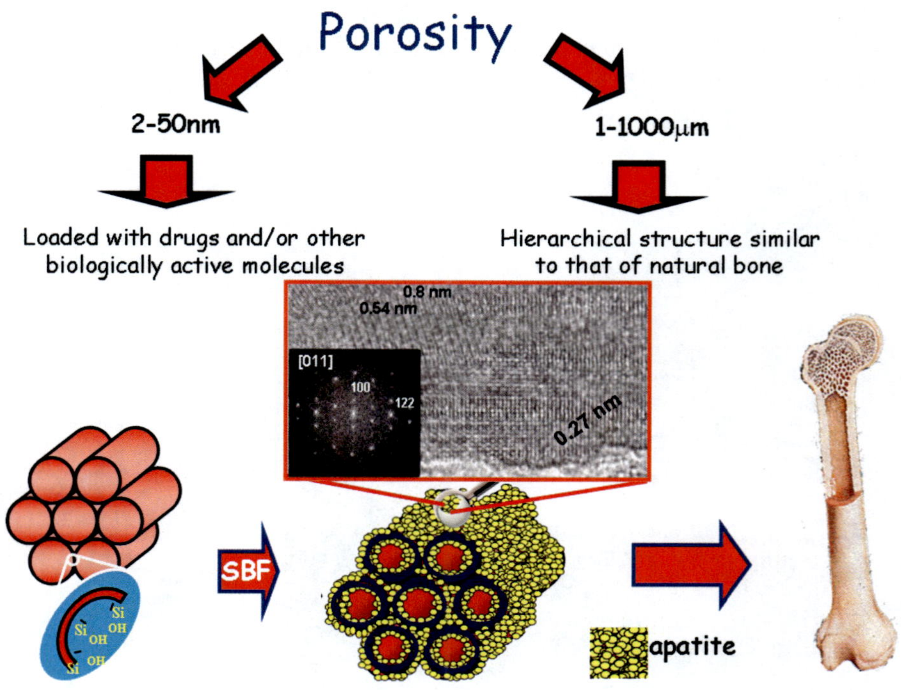

Figure 2. Porosity necessary in an ideal bone-scaffold for bone tissue engineering. Macroporosity in the 1-1000 μm range with hierarchical structure provides the implant of the appropriate functionality. The employment of ordered mesoporous materials allows the confinement of biologically active molecules that promote bone tissue regeneration. Moreover, mesoporous silica, in contact with physiological fluids produces a nanocrystalline apatite layer similar to those of natural bone, as confirmed by electron diffraction (ED) and high resolution transmission electron microscopy (TEM).

The outstanding structural and textural properties of mesoporous matrices make them suitable to act as host systems of a wide range biologically active molecules for bone tissue regenerative purposes and/or treatment of bone diseases [15,39-45]. The structural and textural properties of mesoporous host matrices can be tailored depending on the guest molecule. Moreover, mesoporous silica walls are susceptible of undergoing chemical functionalization with different organic functions to achieve a better control over molecule loading and release performance [46].

The bioactive behavior, controlled delivery capability and resorbable nature of SMMs involve that once implanted, these bioceramics promote bone tissue formation and subsequently, they are degraded by the physiological fluids. These features make SMMs excellent candidates for the design of 3D scaffolds in bone tissue engineering. Tissue engineering techniques require the use of scaffolds, which served as 3D templates for the initial cell attachment and subsequent tissue formation and finally are degraded and substituted by new formed bone.

This chapter deals with the potential applications of SMMs for bone tissue regeneration. Firstly, the main aspects concerning the general properties and synthetic pathways are reviewed. Moreover, different aspects regarding biocompatibility of mesoporous silicas intended as biomaterials that must interact with biological systems are considered. The recent approaches carried out to improve the bioactive behavior of mesoporous materials on the basis of their chemical, textural and structural characteristics are also tackled. Special emphasis is given to the recent scientific and nanotechnological advances aimed at improving the performance of SMMs as local controlled delivery systems of biologically active molecules. Finally, the design and manufacture of porous scaffolds with 3D-dimensional interconnected hierarchical meso-macroporous structure are here described.

2. General Properties of Ordered Mesoporous Materials

SMMs were first reported in the early 1990s by Japanese researchers [47,48] and Mobil Oil Corporation scientists [49], who described for the first time the synthesis of KSW-n and M41S families of mesostructured materials. Mesoporous materials are a new generation of materials structurally unique, which exhibit order on the mesoscopic scale (2-50nm) and disorder on the atomic scale. The synthesis of mesoporous materials is based in the use of surfactants as mesostructure directing agents [50].

SMMs are characterized by regular arrays of uniform channels, whose dimensions can be tailored through the chemical nature of the surfactant, additives and synthesis conditions (pH, temperature) in the so-called *liquid crystal templating* (LCT) mechanism [51]. This process is based on the formation of liquid crystals in mixtures of polar solvents and surfactants with a non-polar tail group. However, deep investigations into the formation processes of SMMs led to postulate two different variations of the LCT mechanism (Figure 3). The first mechanism, known as *true liquid-crystal template* (TLCT) involves that the concentration of the surfactant is so high that under the existing conditions (temperature and pH) a lyotropic liquid-crystalline phase is formed without requiring the presence of the inorganic precursor.

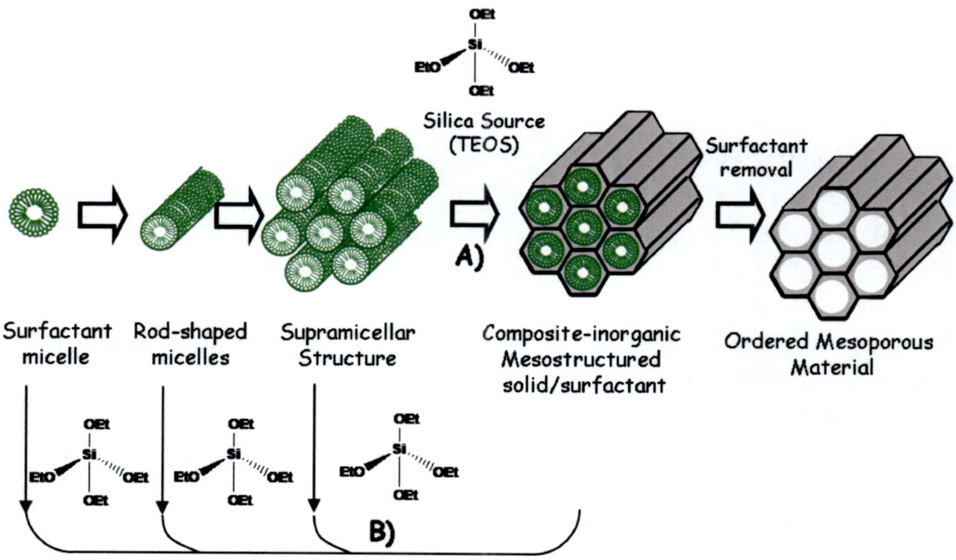

Figure 3. Schematic representation of A) true liquid-crystal template (TLCT) mechanism and B) cooperative liquid-crystal template (CLCT) mechanism used to describe the synthesis silica-based ordered mesoporous materials.

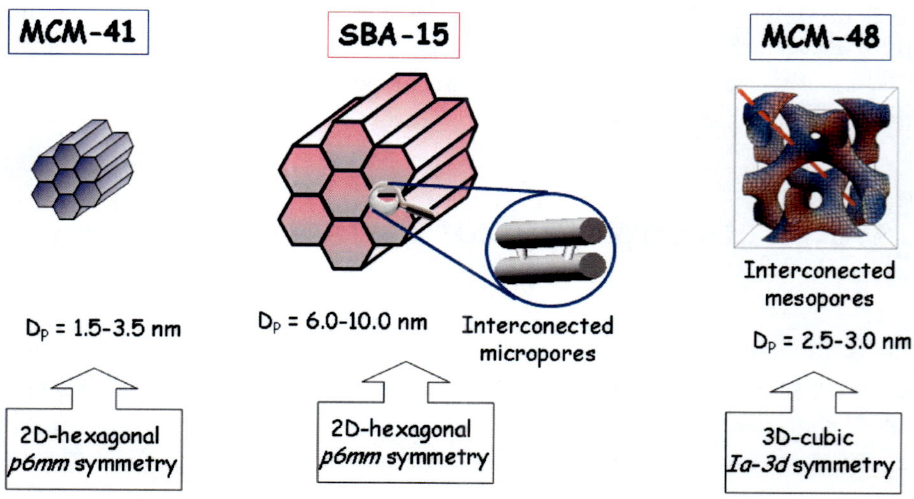

Figure 4. Models of different mesoporous structures, including their pore diameters (D_P) and symmetries.

TLCT mechanism assumes that the amount of surfactant dissolved in the aqueous solution is above the critical micellar concentration (*cmc*), which allows the surfactant molecules to cluster together forming micelles. These micelles are formed because the hydrophobic tails of the surfactant tend to congregate to minimize contact with water while their hydrophilic heads orientate to maximize the interaction with the aqueous medium. Once the lyotropic liquid-crystalline phase is formed, the silica source (normally tetraethyl- (TEOS) or tetramethylorthosilicate (TMOS)) is added, which condenses around the micelles.

The final mesostructure of the material will depend on the organization of the surfactant molecules into the micellar liquid crystals which are acting as templates for the assembly and subsequent condensation of inorganic precursors. The second proposed mechanism is the *cooperative liquid crystal template* (CLCT), which suggests that it is also possible that the lyotropic liquid-crystalline phase is formed even at lower concentrations of surfactant molecules (below the *cmc*), when there is a cooperative assembly of the surfactant and the already added silica precursor. Independently of the synthetic pathway followed, the last step in the synthesis of SMMs consists in the surfactant removal, by calcination or solvent extraction. The surfactant removal gives rise to a network of cavities within the silica framework that governs the physicochemical properties of the material.

Different mesoporous structures can be obtained depending on the synthesis procedure, being the most representative the MCM-n (Mobil Composition of Matter) series [49,51-55], SBA-n (Santa BArbara) series [56-58], MSU-n (Michigan State University) series [59], KIT-n (Korean Advanced Institute of Science and Technology) series [60], FSM-n (Folded Sheet Material) series [61], and AMS-n (Anionic surfactant templated Mesoporous Silica) series [62].

3. Biocompatibility of Silica-Based Mesoporous Materials

Bioceramics intended as bone implant in orthopedic surgery, as any biomaterial, must be in contact with physiological fluids. Consequently, they must fitful mandatory requirements such as long-term biocompatibility, which have been reported to depend on the site implantation, the shape and size of the material and also on its surface chemistry [63]. When a biomaterial is implanted into a living tissue, a series of reactions take place at the bone tissue-implant interface [12,64]. Firstly, there is an adsorption of certain proteins onto the biomaterial surface. Depending on the type of protein, this process is followed by the adhesion of small disk-shaped cells called "platelets". Such reactions originate an inflammatory response that leads to the encapsulation of the "foreign body", in which the biomaterial is isolated by a fibrous capsule [65]. Although encapsulation can be considered as a normal response and does not mean a non-biocompatible state, the collagen capsule could difficult an appropriate implant performance. When dealing with biomaterials acting as controlled delivery systems of biologically active agents, the collagen capsule would impede the diffusion of the released molecule into the surrounding tissue. Besides, the nutrient supply to the encapsulated cells would be disrupted by the presence of this fibrous capsule. Moreover, the activation of platelets leads to the formation of thrombi on the surface. Almost all biomaterials are known to cause surface-induced thrombosis that could lead to serious medical complications following thrombotic events. In this context, one major advantage of implant materials with controlled delivery capability is the possibility of confining different drugs to treat adverse inflammatory and encapsulation processes [66]. Among bioceramics, SMMs seem good candidates as biomaterials, because they can host a wide variety of biologically molecules able to treat bone inflammation or infection and/or molecules that promote bone tissue regeneration.

Albeit the biocompatibility and degradability with time of different silica materials have been described [31-33,67,68], few research works concerning the inherent cytotoxycity and biocompatibility of SMMs have been reported. *In vitro* cytotoxicity studies demonstrated that mesoporous silicas exhibited low toxicity at low concentrations [67,69-74] and that this toxicity increased at higher concentrations [72]. Such toxicity seems to be dependent on the particle size [59]. Recently, *in vitro* cytotoxicity studies of MCM-41 mesoporous material, MCM-41 functionalized with aminopropyl groups (MCM-41-AP) and mercaptopropyl groups (MCM-41-MP) and spherical silica nanoparticles (SiO_2) toward human neuroblastoma cells have been reported [76]. Since the particles studies were not soluble in aqueous media, authors introduced a new quantity to measure the cytotoxicity of these materials, Q_{50}, which is the number of particles required to inhibit normal cell growth by 50%. This study revealed that Q_{50} increased in the order: MCM-51 < MCM-41-MP < MCM-41-AP ≈ SiO_2. In view of these results, MCM-41 would be the most cytotoxic material studied. Although the chemical origins of the cytotoxic effect of these materials are not clear, the exposed surface area of the particle could be an important factor in cellular death. In this sense, the most toxic mesoporous silica materials were those with the largest surface areas. However, the chemical nature of the attached functional groups should not be overruled. Moreover, surface area may not be the basis for cytotoxicity since spherical silica nanoparticles, which exhibited relatively small surface area, displayed cytotoxicity similar to that of MCM-41-AP, which had higher surface area. All these findings suggest that cell death could also depend on other factors, such as size and shape.

In vivo studies have shown a low toxicity with small quantities of 1-2μm SBA [77] and MCF mesoporous particles [72]. In addition, mesoporous particles (~ 100 nm) fused with iron oxide amorphous silica particles exhibited low toxicity when intravenously administrated in mice [78]. Recently, *in vivo* studies using MCM-41, MCM-48 and mesocelullar silica-foams (MCF) mesoporous materials have been reported [79]. Following subcutaneous injection of mesoporous materials at the sciatic nerve in rats, a good biocompatibility on histology at all time points was observed. The applicability of these materials for intraperitoneal and intravenous use was evaluated by injection into mices. This study demonstrated that doses of 1 mg or less were well tolerated by animals. However mice injected with more than 5 mg of mesoporous material resulted in death. It seems that pulmonary embolism and/or thrombosis could be the cause of death. The role of silica in the etiology of this pathogenesis is still unclear. Although local tissue reaction of mesoporous silicas was benign, they caused somewhat systemic toxicity. Authors suggest that toxicity could be mitigated by modification of the materials, by means of surface adsorption of proteins, functional groups or polymers and so forth. However, these preliminary results evidence the need of performing *in vivo* test through the implantation of SMMs into living bone. The isolated cytotoxicity and biocompatibility assays reported up to date can not provide a clear vision of what will happen when implanted in bone. The effect of the bioactive response of SMMs together with their capability to host different therapeutic and/or osteogenic agents could lead to a synergic effect aimed at enhancing the biocompatibility of these materials. This is undoubtedly an added value when considering mesoporous silicas as bone implant materials, but much research effort is needed before being applied to the clinical practice.

4. Bioactivity of Silica-Based Ordered Mesoporous Materials

As previously-mentioned, one of the current challenges for the scientific community is the design of third generation ceramics able to stimulate bone regeneration. Sometimes, the synthesis of a third generation bioceramic consists in incorporating and additional value to a bioactive second generation bioceramic. The bioactive response of conventional sol-gel glasses depends on the presence of silanol groups (Si-OH) and porosity. Moreover, porosity has been revealed as key factor that modulates the kinetics of formation of the CHA layer [80-84]. Similarly, SMMs are expected to induce bioactive response because they exhibit a high density of silanol groups, which could act as nucleation sites for CHA. In addition, they present high surface areas, ordered pore networks and high pore volumes that could lead to enhanced kinetic of CHA formation.

Taking into consideration all these aspects, *in vitro* bioactive responses of the three well-known mesoporous materials MCM-41, MCM-48 and SBA-15 were evaluated [85,86]. An accepted method to try to evaluate the bone-bonding capability of bioceramics consists in performing *in vitro* bioactivity assays and test if a nanocrystalline CHA layer is formed onto the materials surface. These tests were carried out at 37 ºC by soaking disk-shaped pieces of material into a simulated body fluid (SBF), which is a solution with ionic composition similar to that of human plasma buffered at the physiological pH of 7.4 [87]. The changes induced in the surface of the SMMs are then monitored using different characterization techniques, such as Fourier transmission infrared spectroscopy (FTIR) and X-ray diffraction (XRD). Scanning electron (SEM) and transmission electron (TEM) microscopy together with energy dispersive using X-ray (EDX) and electron diffraction (ED) are also employed. In the case of bioactive materials, all these techniques allow to confirm the formation of a new layer, mainly consisting in CHA, into the materials surface. As expected, MCM-41, MCM-48 and SBA-15 mesoporous materials, which exhibit different pore diameter and diverse structural features, also presented different rate of formation of the CHA layer. Therefore, the obtained results evidenced that SBA-15 and MCM-48 were able to induce the formation of a nanocrystalline CHA layer onto their surfaces after 30 and 60 days of assay, respectively. However, no evidence of formation of such layer was observed onto the surface of MCM-41. The different bioactive behavior of these three SMM could be explained attending to their different concentration of silanol groups and their diverse textural and structural properties (Table 1). Therefore, the relatively small silanol density in MCM-41 (~ 2 mmol Si-OH·m^2) compared to that in SBA-15 and MCM-48 (~ 13 mmol Si-OH·m^2) could explain its non-bioactive response after 60 days of test. However, there is an important difference in the rate of formation of the CHA layer between SBA-15 and MCM-48, which exhibited similar silanol density. This fact could point to the relevance of the textural and structural features of these SMMs, which would also play a relevant role in the rate of formation of the CHA layer. In this sense, mesoporous matrices with large and accessible pore networks should favor the ionic diffusion through the mesoporous framework and consequently the formation of the CHA layer would be promoted. Certainly, SBA-15, with the greatest pore diameters (~ 9 nm) and 2D-hexagonal pore arrangement with interconnected microporosity, exhibited the fasted bioactive behavior (Table 1).

Table 1. Textural properties: Surface area (S_{BET}), mesopore diameter (D_p), total pore volume (V_p), micropore volume ($V_{\mu p}$). Structural characteristics, composition (% in mol) and time of bioactive response of different mesoporous materials

Matrix	S_{BET} (m^2/g)	D_p (nm)	Vp (cm^3/g)	Vμp (cm^3/g)	Structure	Composition (% in mol)	Bioactivity*
MCM-41	1157	3.6	0.98	–	2D-hexagonal (p6mm)	$SiO_2$100	>60 days
MCM-48	1166	3.6	1.05	–	3D-cubic (Ia-3d)	$SiO_2$100	60 days
SBA-15	787	8.8	1.05	0.061	2D-hexagonal (p6mm)	$SiO_2$100	30 days
P-MCM41	721	2.5	0.91	–	2D-hexagonal (p6mm)	$SiO_2$99-$P_2O_5$1	15 days
G-MCM41	1131	2.3	0.80	–	2D-hexagonal (p6mm)	$SiO_2$95.6-CaO4.0-$P_2O_5$0.4	1 day
MG-S58m	195 [95]	9.4	0.46 [0.35]	–	2D-hexagonal (p6mm) +wormlike	$SiO_2$58-CaO37-$P_2O_5$5	1 day [3 days]
MG-S75m	393 [117]	6.0	0.59 [0.21]	–	2D-hexagonal (p6mm) + orthorhombic (p2mm)	$SiO_2$75-CaO20-$P_2O_5$5	8 hours [3 days]
MG-S85m	427 [227]	5.7	0.61 [0.24]	–	3D-cubic (Ia-3d)	$SiO_2$85-CaO10-$P_2O_5$5	4 hours [3 days]

(*) Induction time for hydroxycarbonate apatite (HCA) layer formation onto the surface of materials determined by FTIR through the detection of the double-bands at (601-563 cm^{-1}). The values in brackets correspond to the textural values and bioactive responses obtained for conventional sol-gel glass with analogous composition [14,83,84].

MCM-48, which exhibited 3D-cubic pore arrangement and pore sizes close to 4 nm, exhibited a slower bioactive response than SBA-15. And finally, MCM-41, with 2D-hexagonal pore networks and pore diameter around 4 nm did not exhibit bioactive response after 60 days soaked into SBF solution.

All these findings evidence the textural and structural properties play an important role in the kinetics of formation of CHA layer onto the surfaces of SMMs. However, these are not enough conditions to achieve a satisfactory bioactive behavior, because the formation of the CHA layer is much slower than that of conventional sol-gel glasses (3 days) (Table 1). Consequently, the presence of elements such as calcium and/or phosphate is required to accelerate the formation of the CHA layer. The following sections overview the different chemical procedures developed up to date aimed at accelerating the bioactivity of SMMs. These methods include the incorporation of phosphorous into the silica matrix or doping with small amounts of bioactive glasses. Special attention is dedicated to describe the outstanding bioactive behaviors of the recently reported mesoporous bioactive glasses (MBGs).

4.1. Incorporation of Phosphorous into the Mesoporous Matrix

In vitro bioactivity assays carried out in bioactive sol-gel glasses revealed that the presence of phosphorous into the glass network highly affected the formation of the CHA layer [88]. This fact suggested the incorporation of small amounts of phosphorous (~ 1 %) into the MCM-41 silica network [89]. The structural and compositional characterization of this new material (P-MCM-41) using XRD, N_2 adsorption porosimetry, SEM-EDX and TEM-EDX techniques indicated that a 2D-hexagonal ordered mesoporous material with *p6mm* symmetry was obtained (Table 1). Moreover, it was also evidenced that the phosphorous content (~ 1% in weight) was heterogeneously distributed and it was mainly located in the outer rim of the particles and not in the inner core. The in vitro bioactivity tests showed that P-MCM-41 material was able to form an apatite-like layer on its surface after 15 days of assay. If we compare the time of bioactive response of P-MCM-41 to SBA-15 and MCM-48 materials, the incorporation of phosphorous into the silica network is a step forward towards the enhancement of the bioactive behavior of mesoporous materials and opens ups numerous alternatives in the field of SMMs for bone tissue regeneration applications.

4.2. Addition of Small Amounts of Bioactive Glasses

A widely employed strategy to promote bioactivity in different materials consists in preparing biphasic mixtures by incorporating another phase that acts as accelerator of the nucleation of apatite [90]. With this goal in mind, MCM-41 as the main phase (90% in weight) was mixed with a bioactive sol-gel glass in the system SiO_2-CaO-P_2O_5 (10% of weight) [85], giving rise to the denominated G-MCM-41. The *in vitro* bioactivity of this material revealed that the formation of the apatite layer started just only after 3 hours of assay, being completed in 1 day (Table 1). These results confirm that the addition of small amounts of bioactive glasses is an attractive strategy to induce bioactive behavior to SMMs materials.

4.3. Ordered Mesoporous Bioactive Glasses

By comparing the bioactive behavior of conventional sol-gel BGs with that of pure SMMs, it is evident that the bioactive response of ordered mesoporous silicas is not fully satisfactory. Only if small amounts of bioactive glasses are added to the SMMs the rate of formation of the CHA layer is accelerated. This fact inspired the idea of synthesizing sol-gel glasses with the textural and structural properties of mesoporous matrices. The research group of Prof. Zhao in 2004 demonstrated that the synthesis of highly ordered MBGs in the system SiO_2-CaO-P_2O_5 could be successfully carried out by using block copolymers as mesostructure directing agents [36]. The synthesis of these MBGs was performed by using the evaporation-induced self-assembly (EISA) method [91] in the presence of a non-ionic triblock copolymer as template (Pluronic® P123, $EO_{20}PO_{70}EO_{20}$). The enhanced textural properties of MBGs promoted by the template led to highly bioactive responses compared to conventional BGs [92-94]. Moreover, the textural and structural properties of MBGs can be tailored by modifying the CaO content of mesoporous glasses [37]. Usually, the CaO incorporation into multicomponent SiO_2-CaO-P_2O_5 systems is performed by using $Ca(NO_3).4H_2O$ as precursor. Moreover, tetraethylorthosilicate (TEOS) and triethylphosphate (TEP) are used as silicon and phosphorous precursors, respectively. By keeping a constant ratio between the network former precursors (TEOS and TEP) and the template (P123) and decreasing the CaO content different MBGs with diverse structural and textural properties were obtained. Figure 5 shows the structural characterization by TEM of different mesoporous glasses (MG-S58m, MG-S75m, MG-Si85m), in which an evolution from 2D-hexagonal to 3D-bicontinuous cubic structure was observed (Figure 5). Moreover, an increase in the textural properties was observed when decreasing the CaO content (Table 1) [37].

The *in vitro* assays into SBF revealed that MBGs exhibited faster bioactive responses than conventional BGs. In fact, whereas conventional BGs with analogous compositions exhibited bioactive response after 3 days of assay, the time of bioactive response ranges from 4 hours to 1 day in the case of MBGs (Table 1). It should be highlighted that in conventional SiO_2-CaO-P_2O_5 sol-gel glasses the kinetic of formation of the CHA layer is mainly governed by the CaO content, *i.e.* the higher the CaO the higher the rate of CHA formation. However, the governing factors that modulate bioactive behavior in MBGs are the pore structure and surface area. This fact was evidenced when MBG materials with the lowest CaO content (MG-S85m) but having 3D-bicontinuous cubic structure and the highest surface area values exhibited faster bioactive response than MBG materials with the highest CaO content (MG-S58m). FTIR and TEM-ED studies revealed that the formation of the nanocrystalline CHA layer took place after only 4 hours of assay in MG-S85s (Figures 6A and 6C).

In this case, the 3D pore system provided not only high surface area and porosity, but also favored the interchange of ions, increasing mass transport and diffusion processes, which resulted in the fastest CHA formation reported up to date in silica-based bioactive materials.

Moreover, the Ca^{2+} concentration and pH in SBF as a function of soaking time of MG-Si85m material did not experience significant changes, with values that were kept almost constant at around 100 ppm and 7.45, respectively (Figure 6.B). This is an interesting feature as bioceramic for bone tissue regeneration, because one of the main drawbacks of conventional BGs is their extremely high reactivity due to the initial burst effect, where the Ca^{2+} is quickly released to the surrounding medium. In this sense, MBGs with low CaO content could avoid the undesired cytotoxic effect that high local pH values could produce in living tissues.

Recently, a new fascinating property that derives from the textural and structural characteristics of MBGs has been reported. This is their biomimetic mechanism, where a sequential transition from amorphous calcium phosphate (ACP)–octacalcium phosphate (OCP)–CHA maturation, similar to the *in vivo* biomineralization process, has been observed for the first time [38].

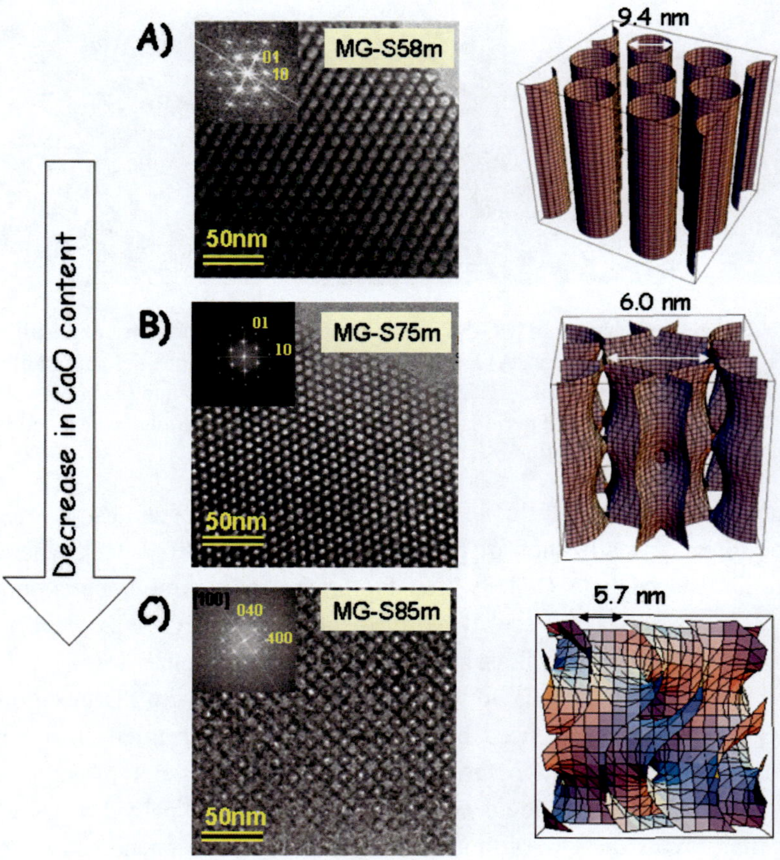

Figure 5. TEM images, their corresponding Fourier diffractograms and 3D structures of ordered mesoporous bioactive glasses with different CaO content. A) Correspond to the MG-S58m with the electron beam parallel to the pore-channel in 2D-hexagonal structure with *p6mm* space group; B) correspond to the sample MG-S75m with the electron beam parallel to the pore-channel in 2D-hexagonal structure with *p6mm* space group; and C) correspond to the [100] direction of 3D-bicontinuous cubic structure with *Ia-3d* space groups symmetry (sample MG-S85m).

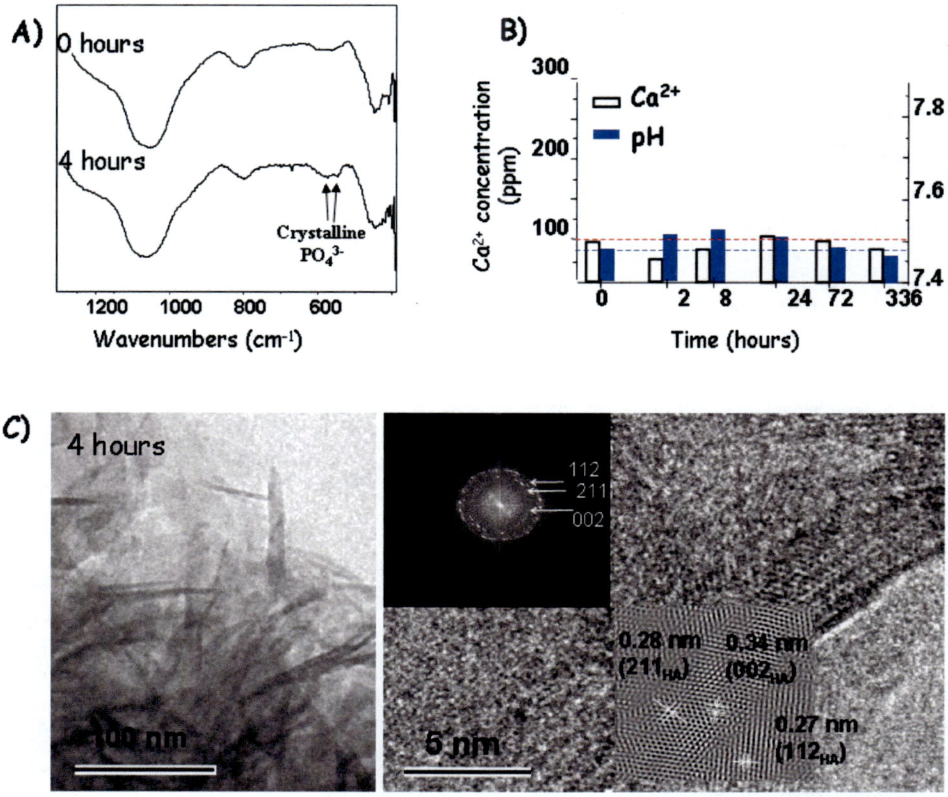

Figure 6. *In vitro* bioactive behavior of MG-S85 sample, with 3D-bicontinuous cubic structure and $85SiO_2$-10%CaO-5%P_2O_5 composition. A) FTIR spectra of material surface before and after 4 hours soaked into a simulate body fluid (SBF). B) Variation of calcium content and pH values of SBF after soaking the materials during different periods. C) High resolution TEM study corresponding to the surface of mesoporous glasses after 4 hours soaked into SBF solution.

The formation mechanism of the CHA layer into bioactive ceramics reported up to date consists in the direct crystallization of previously precipitated ACP [95], whereas previous formation of the intermediate OCP, which is formed in natural bone biomineralization process [96-98], does not take place. It worth mentioning that OCP is a metastable phase whose existence is limited to pH values in the crystallization system below 7.

Therefore, the biomimetic behavior of MG-S58m sample, with 2D-hexagonal structure and high CaO content was evidenced by TEM. This MBG permitted an intense Ca^{2+}–H^+ exchange as a consequence of the open channel array, the high textural parameters and the relatively high CaO content. This ionic exchange led to local acid pH values of 6.5 during the first stages, which favors the OCP formation (Figure 7.A). This phenomenon does not take place in the case of bioactive glasses, because the local pH is dept at pH 7.4 or even slightly increased from the beginning of the bioactive process, which would avoid the existence of OCP phase. This biomimetic behavior was monitored by TEM (Figure 7.B). After 1 hour soaked into the SBF, MG-S58m sample develops a large amount of newly formed ACP layer with a Ca/P ratio of 1.2. This event has been widely observed in any bioactive compounds, and corresponds to the step 4 of the bioactive process described by Hench [99].

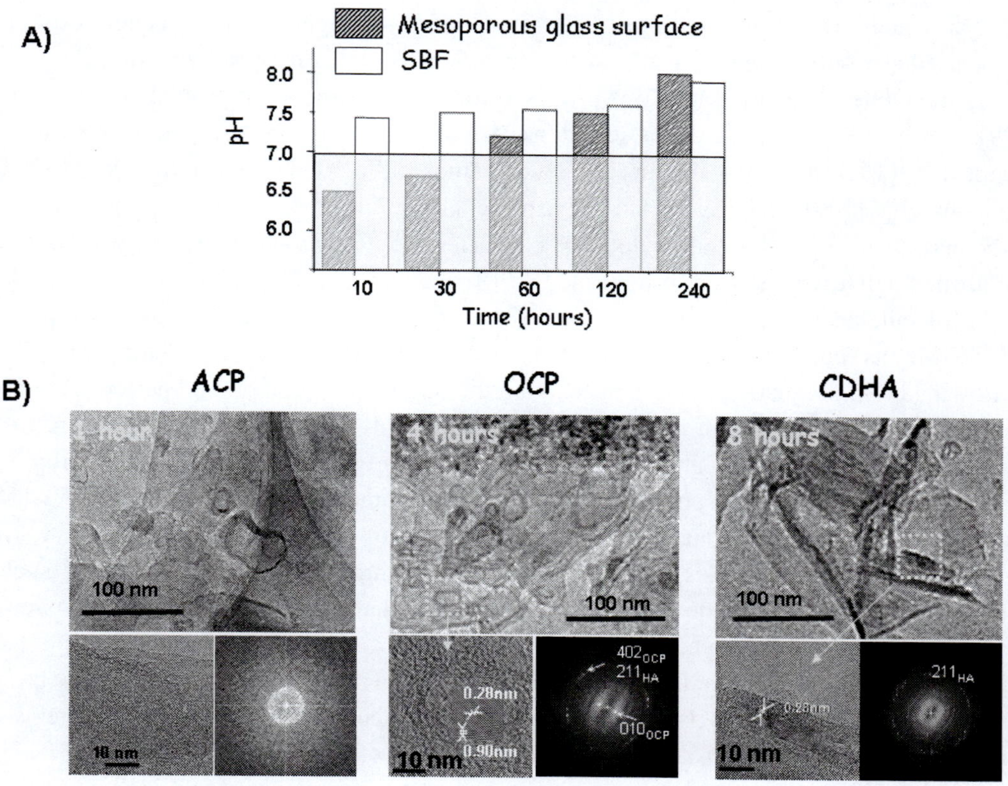

Figure 7. Bioactive in vitro study of MG-S58m mesoporous glass with a 2D-hexagonal structure and $58SiO_2$-37%CaO-5%P_2O_5 composition. A) Evolution of pH at the material surface as a function of time being soaked into a SBF solution. The pH range in which OCP phase is more stable is highlighted. B) High resolution TEM study of mesoporous glass surface after different soaking times into SBF. A sequential transition from ACP, OCP and CHA can be observed.

Up to date, the accepted mechanism involved the direct crystallization of CHA phase from the ACP. However, MBG revealed a unique phenomenon with the growing of nanocrystalline oval biphasic nuclei composed by OCP with a small fraction of HA after 4 hours in SBF, with a Ca/P ratio of 1.3. The transformation from oval OCP nuclei to needle-like nanocrystalline CHA is finally evident after 8 hours soaked into SBF.

All these results evidence the possibility of controlling the reactive properties of MBGs by tailoring their compositional, textural and structural properties. This new family of ordered mesoporous materials widens the range of possibilities for the use SMMs as a new generation of bioceramics with outstanding bone-bonding capability.

5. Mesoporous Materials as Local Controlled Delivery Systems

The local administration of therapeutic agents by host matrices presents advantages over conventional therapies, because it allows a better control over loading and controlled release of molecules, keeping constant plasma levels and reducing undesired side effect [100].

SMMs, which exhibit outstanding structural and textural properties, are excellent candidates to be used as reservoir matrices to host a wide variety of biologically active molecules.

Since 2001, when MCM-41 was proposed for the first time as controlled delivery system [39], several SMMs have been tested as delivery systems of different drugs, such as ibuprofen [101-104], gentamicin [105,106], amoxicillin [107], erythromycin [102,108], vancomycin [109], naproxen [110], aspirin [111], diflunisal [109], captopril [112], itraconazole [113] and alendronate [114,115]. Besides, SMMs have been also proposed as controlled delivery systems of proteins [116-118] and amino acids [119].

Molecule adsorption and *in vitro* delivery assays are indispensable steps in the research of SMMs as controlled delivery systems. Molecule adsorption is usually carried out following an impregnation method by soaking the SMMs for a determined period (commonly 24-48 hours) into a solution containing a given molecule with a high concentration. In this way, the loading solvent must be selected attending to the polarity of the drug [41]. Therefore, in the case of polar molecules, such as amoxicillin [107], gentamicin [106], captopril [112] and alendronate [114,115], the solvent used is water. On the contrary, when loading non-polar molecules, such as ibuprofen, is targeted non-polar solvents, such as hexane or pentane, are needed. There are also intermediated cases, such as erythromycin, in which acetonitrile is employed [108].

The choice of the loading conditions, such as pH and temperature, has to be also carefully carried out. This is especially important when the confinement of proteins and enzymes are aimed. For instance, the surface charges of the protein and the SMM, which depend on the pH of the loading solution, must be complementary to allow molecule adsorption. Moreover, the loading conditions should allow the preservation of the biological activity of proteins. Therefore, several research works have revealed that different proteins retained their functionality without being denatured inside the mesoporous silica frameworks [120-127]. In some cases the protein activity is not only retained after adsorption into SMM but also improved compared to proteins solved in aqueous solutions or covalently immobilized [120]. For instance, penicillin acylase exhibited an activity after adsorption into MCM-41 more than 5-fold greater than after being cross-linked to silylated MCM-41 using glutaraldehyde as cross-linking agent [128]. In addition, Deere *et al.* [129] reported that the peroxidative activity of the adsorbed cytochrome c onto different SMMs is higher than that of the aqueous protein.

In vitro delivery assays are performed by soaking the loaded SMM into SBF or 0.9% NaCl aqueous solution. Normally, temperature and pH are 37 °C and 7.4, respectively, to try to mimic physiological conditions. The amount of molecule released is monitored by spectroscopic techniques by employing high performance liquid chromatography (HPLC) or direct ultraviolet (UV) measurements.

These general aspects have to be considered when establishing the loading conditions, however the textural properties of the host SMMs are also key factors that govern the molecule loading and release processes. Therefore, the influence of pore diameter, surface area and pore volume on loading and release of biologically active molecules in SMMs are tackled and critically discussed in the following sections.

However, the organic modification or functionalization of the silica surface has been revealed as the keystone in the performance of SMMs as controlled delivery systems. The different functionalization approaches developed up to date and the chemical strategies reported so far to improve the performance of SMMs are also described within the next sections.

5.2. Influence of Textural Properties

Pore Diameter

The adsorption of molecules into SMMs is governed by size-selectivity criteria, *i.e.* the mesopore size determines the size of the guest molecule to be confined. Thus, if the size of the guest molecule is smaller than the pore diameter, the molecule could penetrate into the pore channel and accede to the internal surface area of the mesoporous matrix. On the contrary, if the pore opening is smaller than the molecule size, the molecule would adsorb only on the external surface of the material. Considering than the mesoporous diameter can be tailored between 1.5 nm and several tens of nanometers, SMMs are expected to host from small molecules to large-size molecules such as proteins.

Pore diameter is the limiting factor in molecule adsorption when the confinement of really large-size molecules is targeted. Deere *et al.* evaluated the adsorption of globular proteins of MCM-41 exhibiting different pore diameters ranging from 2 to 5 nm [120]. In general, proteins with hydrodynamic dimensions larger than the mesopore diameter were adsorbed on the outer surface of MCM-41. Moreover, adsorption assays of proteins exhibiting different pore diameters into a SBA-15-type matrix evidenced that only proteins with dimensions smaller than the mesopore diameter showed significant adsorption [130]. These assays evidenced that the SMM acts as a molecular sieve and that this size selectivity is rigorous.

Among the different existing proteins, it should be highlighted the case of serum albumins. Albumins are one of the major components in plasma proteins in humans. Albumin is usually composed of a single-chain of 582 amino acids with an average length of 10 nm and width of 6 nm [131-133]. One of the most remarkable properties of albumin is its ability to bind reversibly a wide variety of ligands. Moreover, albumins are also capable of binding different drugs than can be delivered to sites of pharmacological action. As a result, albumins could be used to store, protect, transport and deliver certain biologically active agents with special interest in bone regeneration technologies. However, when the confinement of albumins into SMMs is intended, large-mesopore matrices are needed. This fact led to the group of Prof. Vallet-Regí to use SBA-15 as host carrier and applying an improved method to increase the pore diameter of SBA-15. Thus, the increase in the mesopore diameter was achieved by increasing the time of hydrothermal treatment during the mesoporous synthesis, as previously reported [134,135]. Therefore, pore diameters ranging from 8.2 nm to 11.5 nm were obtained for SBA-15 materials submitted to hydrothermal treatment periods ranging from 1 to 7 days [117]. Moreover, loading assays of bovine serum albumin (BSA) were carried out, evidencing the dependence of BSA loading on SBA-15 diameter (Figure 8.A). Hence, the amount of BSA loaded was 151 mg/g, 234 mg/g, 242 mg/g and 270 mg/g for SBA-15 with mesopore size of 8.2 nm, 9.5 nm, 10.1 nm and 11.4 nm, respectively.

Furthermore, pore diameter has been demonstrated to strongly influence molecule release rate. Several MCM-41 matrices were synthesized by using several cationic surfactants with different chain lengths, which led to MCM-41 materials with different pore diameters ranging from 2.5 nm (employing short-chain surfactants) to 3.6 nm (employing long-chain surfactants) [136]. Ibuprofen release profiles revealed than the release kinetics is highly dependent on the pore diameter (Figure 8.B). Thus, the amount of drug released to the delivery medium diminished as the pore diameter decreased, evidencing that pore diameter acts as a release rate modulator.

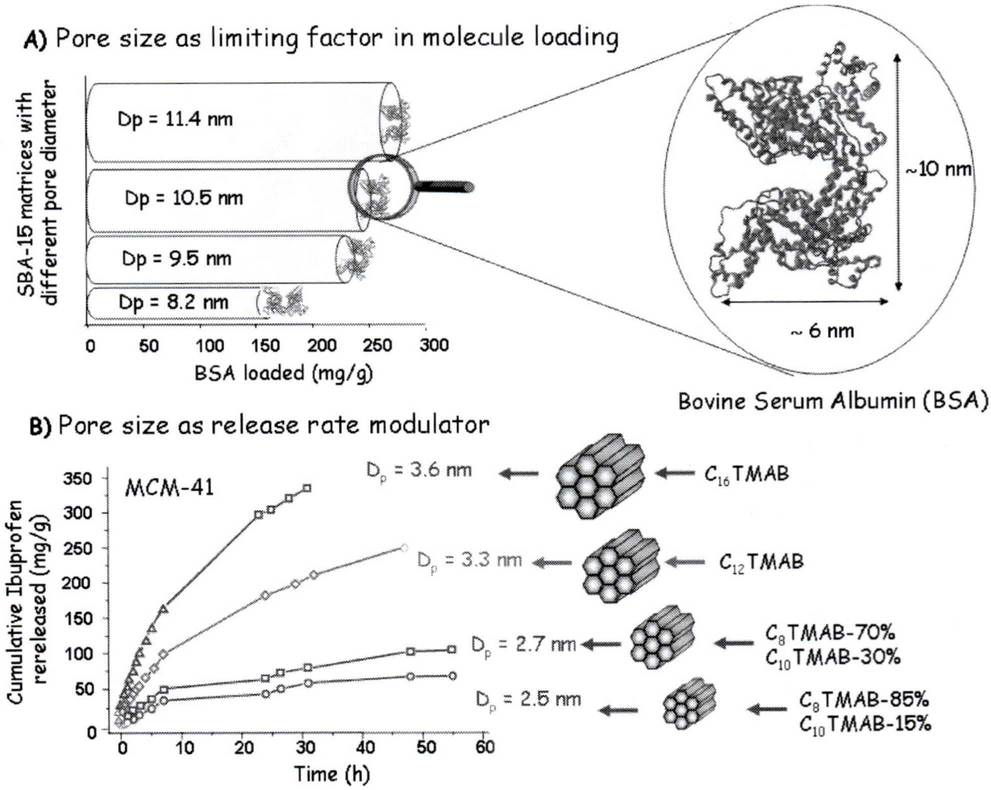

Figure 8. A) Influence of mesopore diameter in the loading of BSA into SBA-15 mesoporous matrices B) Ibuprofen release profiles from MCM-41 materials exhibiting different pore diameter. The surfactants used during the synthesis are indicated for each case. C_8TAB=trimethyloctylammonium bromide; C_{10}TAB=decyltrimethylammonium bromide, C_{12}TAB dodecyltrimethylammonium bromide; C_{16}TAB hexadecyltrimethylammonium bromide; C_{18}TAB octadecyltrimethylammonium bromide.

Surface Area

The adsorption of molecules into SMMs is a surface phenomenon that is mainly governed by the chemical interactions between silanol groups covering the silica surface and the functional groups of the guest molecule. The surface area of mesoporous matrices is the textural parameter that represents the available silica surface susceptible to interact with the guest molecule. Consequently, the surface area should determine the amount of molecules that can be confined into the silica matrix. It is expected that the higher the surface area the higher the amount of molecule loaded. This fact was confirmed when several MCM-41 matrices exhibiting different surface area values were employed as ibuprofen delivery systems [136]. Thus, MCM-41 mesoporous materials exhibiting surface areas of 768 m^2/g, 936 m^2/g, 1087 m^2/g and 1157 m^2/g loaded 110 mg/g, 190 mg/g, 230 mg/g and 340 mg/g of drug, respectively. This effect was also observed by Qu et al [112], who reported the captopril loading and release in several 2D-hexagonal structures (MCM-41_{12}, MCM-41_{16} and SBA-15) (Table 2).

Table 2. Captopril loading data from MCM-41 and SBA-15 mesoporous matrices exhibiting different surface areas. The surfactant employed for the synthesis of each material is also displayed. C_{16}TAB is hexadecyltrimethylammonium bromide, C12TAB is dodecyltrimethylammonium bromide and P123 is the polyoxyethylene-polyoxypropylene block copolymer (PEO_{20}-PPO_{70}-PEO_{20})

Material	Surfactant	Surface Area (m^2/g)	Amount of captopril loaded (mg/g)
MCM-41_{16}	C_{16}TAB	1211	339.9
MCM-41_{12}	C_{12}TAB	940	236.0
SBA-15	Pluronic ® P123	910	225.7

Again there was a direct dependence of the amount of captopril loaded on the surface area of the SMM, *i.e.* the highest surface areas promoted the greatest amounts of drug loaded. Moreover, MCM-41 and SBA-15 matrices, with surface areas of 1157 and 719 m^2/g, respectively, have been tested as alendronate delivery systems [114]. Alendronate is a potent bisphosphonate, which is orally administrated and is commonly used for osteoporosis treatments. The maximum loads of alendronate obtained were 139 mg/g and 83 mg/g for MCM-41 and SBA-15, respectively. Therefore, the surface area is tightly correlated with the maximum load of the SMM.

Pore Volume

The adsorption of molecules into SMMs takes place by *molecule-surface* interactions, and consequently, the amount of molecules loaded depends on the pore diameter as the size selective limiting factor, and also on the surface area. Recently, it has been reported that successive impregnations of MCM-41 ibuprofen solutions permit to achieve a complete pore filling leading to higher drug loading [137]. This fact was explained by the increase in the intermolecular ibuprofen interactions (Figure 9.A), as evidenced by solid-state nuclear magnetic resonance (NMR) spectroscopy studies [138]. In this case, the amount of ibuprofen adsorbed depended on the pre volume of the SMM, *i.e.* the larger the pore volume the greater the amount of drug loaded.

However, when the confinement of large-volume molecules, such as certain proteins, is targeted, the volume available to host the guest molecule could also be an important aspect influencing adsorption process. Recently, mesostructured cellular foams (MCFs) have been reported as host matrices of several enzymes and proteins [139,140]. The synthesis of MCFs was performed by using triblock copolymer surfactants and adding a swelling agent, commonly trimethylbenzene, into the structure directing template solution [141,142].

Recently, loading and release tests of BSA were performed into SBA-15 and MCF materials [118]. TEM and N_2 adsorption studies of SBA-15 revealed the presence of 2D-hexagonal pore networks with pore sizes of around 8 nm, being 1.1 cm^3/g the pore volume value (Figure 9.B). In the case of MCF, these studies evidenced the presence of spherical cells of around 28 nm with windows of around 18 nm, being the pore volume of 1.9 cm^3/g. The BSA loading assays revealed that the amount of BSA loaded was higher in MCF (240 mg/g) than in SBA-15 (150 mg/g). In this case, this difference could be ascribed to the difference in pore volume, *i.e.* the greater the pore volume, the higher the amount of BSA loaded. However, the contribution of other parameters, such as pore diameter, can not be overridden. The pore diameter of SBA-15 is just on the limit of the protein dimensions, which could make difficult the protein adsorption. On the contrary, the wide pore opening of MCF would facilitate BSA adsorption.

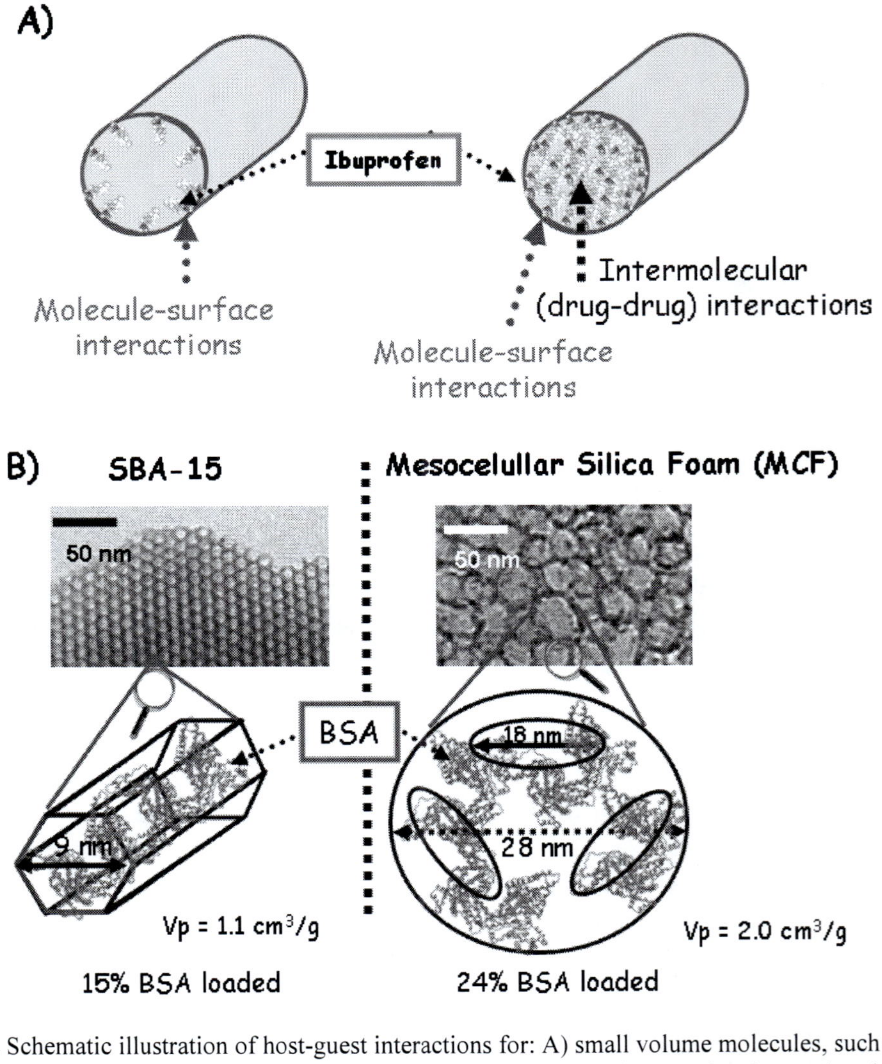

Figure 9. Schematic illustration of host-guest interactions for: A) small volume molecules, such as ibuprofen into the hexagonal mesopores of MCM-41; and B) large-volume molecules, such as bovine serum albumin (BSA) protein into SBA-15 and mesocelullar silica foam (MCF) matrices.

5.2. Organic Functionalization of Mesoporous Matrices

Functionalization using different organic groups has represented the real milestone in the development of SMMs as controlled delivery systems [2,46,143,144]. The surface of silica walls contains high density of silanol groups that can undergo organic modification by covalently grafting organic silanes ($(RO)_3SiR'$) [145].

In general, three different functionalization methods can be applied:

(i) *Co-condensation method*: also known as one-pot route, involves the addition of the organic group, commonly a silane containing reactive groups, such as chloride, methoxy or ethoxy groups, during the mesoporous synthesis and all the functionalization process is performed in one step. When using the co-condensation method, the organic groups are linked to the outer and to the inner part of the silica walls. Consequently, the functionalization degree can not exceed 40% mol to avoid loosening of mesoporous structure.

(ii) *Post-synthesis method*: the organic modification process is performed under anhydrous conditions once the free-surfactant SMM has been already obtained. Although the post-synthesis grafting leads to heterogeneous distributions of the functional groups, they result in well defined structured controlled by the silica matrix. In addition, this method ensures that the organic groups are located in the outer surface of mesopore walls, leading to higher functionalization degrees [101].

(iii) *Selective functionalization*: this is an improved post-synthesis functionalization method that involves the selective surface modification of the external surface and the pores. Starting from the free-surfactant SMM and a chemical agent exhibiting low-reactivity, only the more accessible external surface is functionalized. The subsequent treatment with more reactive agents leads to the functionalization inside the pores [146]. Recently, another alternative consists in starting from the mesoporous matrix containing the surfactant inside the pores. After linking a functional group at the external surface, the surfactant is removed and the inner side of the pores further functionalized.

The choice of the functionalization method depends on the molecule to be hosted and subsequently released. For example, MCM-41 functionalized with amine-groups following co-condensation and post-synthesis methods was used as host matrix for ibuprofen [101]. These studies demonstrated that the decrease in the textural properties (pore diameter, surface area and pore volume) of SMMs was more noticeable in MCM-41 functionalized by post-synthesis method. In addition, ibuprofen release tests revealed that the drug delivery rate from MCM-41 functionalized by post-synthesis was smaller than that of MCM-41 functionalized using co-condensation route. This could be explained considering that aminopropyl groups are placed in the outer surface of the silica matrix, yielding higher functionalization degree susceptible of interacting with ibuprofen and inducing higher drug retention. The existence of host-guest ionic interactions between amino groups from functionalized matrix and carboxylic group of ibuprofen was confirmed by ^{1}H NMR spectroscopy [147]. More recently, Song *et al.* [116] reported organic modification of SBA-

15 using aminopropyl groups and following the two functionalization routes previously described, *i.e.* co-condensation and post-synthesis. In this case, ibuprofen and BSA were chosen as model molecules and loading and release test were carried out. The results showed that functionalization with aminopropyl groups using post-synthesis method led to a decrease in the release rate of ibuprofen compared to SBA-15 modified by the co-condensation route, in agreement with the results previously reported for MCM-41. On the contrary, the BSA release rate was smaller from SBA-15 functionalized by co-condensation than that from SBA-15 functionalized by post-synthesis. This could be explained by the balance of electrostatic interaction and hydrophilic interaction between BSA and the functionalized SBA-15 matrix that would be more favorable in matrices synthesized by one-pot synthesis.

The nature of the host-guest chemical interaction can be tailored by an appropriate choice of the organic groups depending on the targeted molecule and its application. Two main approaches have been widely reported. The first strategy concerns the use of different organic groups able to induce attracting interactions with the functional groups of the guest molecule. The influence of the matrix-molecule chemical interaction on the adsorption and release of molecules was investigated by organically modifying MCM-41 with several organic functional groups (chloropropyl, phenyl, benzyl, mercaptopropyl, cyanopropyl and butyl) and using the post-synthesis method [148]. Ibuprofen was chosen as model drug and adsorption and delivery assays were performed. As a consequence of the different interaction of carboxylic group of ibuprofen with the tested organic functions, diverse load and release behaviors were observed. Therefore, MCM-41 functionalized with polar groups loaded higher amounts of ibuprofen than MCM-41 functionalized with non-polar groups. Moreover, ibuprofen release rate was smaller from matrices modified with mercapto or amino groups because such functions induced strong attracting electrostatic interactions with the carboxylic acid. The second strategy involves the use of hydrophobic species to functionalize the mesoporous silica walls. The main relevant aspects concerning both strategies are described in the next sections, being mainly focused in the functionalization using amino groups and the functionalization with hydrophobic groups.

Functionalization with Amine Groups

The strategy of organically modifying SMMs with amino groups has been extensively reported. MCM-41 and SBA-15 materials functionalized with aminopropyl groups using the post-synthesis method have been tested as alendronate controlled delivery systems [114]. The results evidenced that the amount of drug loaded into these amino-modified matrices (MCM-41-NH_2 and SBA-15-NH_2) was almost 3-fold greater than that on unmodified matrices (Table 3). Comparing both mesoporous matrices, MCM-41-NH_2 loaded more alendronate (366.1 mg/g) than unmodified MCM-41 (139.2 mg/g). Analogously, SBA-15-NH_2 (233.0 mg/g) matrix adsorbed higher alendronate amounts than unmodified SBA-15 (82.8 mg/g). Regarding alendronate release behavior, amino functionalization of these SMM resulted in slower release kinetics compared to unmodified materials. Thus the percentage of alendronate released after 24 hours of assay was 28% and 58% from the total drug loaded for MCM-41-NH_2 and unmodified MCM-41, respectively.

The same trend was observed for SBA-15-NH_2 and unmodified SBA-15, which released 11% and 56% of the total alendronate loaded, respectively, after 24 hours.

Table 3. Alendronate (AL) release data from MCM-41 and SBA-15 before and after amine functionalization

Material	AL loading (mg/g)	% AL released after 24 h	AL total delivery time (h)
MCM-41	139.2	58	72
MCM-41-NH_2	366.1	28	264[a]
SBA-15	82.8	56	264
SBA-15-NH_2	223.0	11	264[b]

[a] Incomplete delivery (76%), [b] incomplete delivery (69%).

Recently, SBA-15 materials organically modified with aminopropyl groups and different functionalization degrees have been reported as good candidates to modulate alendronate dosage [115]. The organic modification was carried out through the post-synthesis method but improved by adding a catalyst during the functionalization process. A linear dependence of the amount of alendronate loaded on the functionalization degree was observed. Moreover, this gradual functionalization allowed to achieve a better control over drug release, *i.e.* the higher the functionalization degree the smaller the total amount of alendronate released to the delivery medium. This would allow the modulation of drug dosage. These results are of great interest for bone implant technologies, because due to the high potency of bisphosphonates, only small local doses are needed.

In addition, amino-functionalization of SMMs permits to control the release behavior of proteins such as BSA [116,117]. SBA-15 materials with different pore diameters synthesized using different hydrothermal treatments were functionalized by post-synthesis route [117]. As previously commented organic functionalization always leads to a decrease of pore diameter. In the case of BSA loading, this protein is just on the limit of SBA-15 mesopore dimensions, and consequently, after amino functionalization, the amount of BSA incorporated decreased compared to unmodified matrices. However, the attracting interactions taking place between amine groups of functionalized matrices and amide groups of BSA notably affected the protein release kinetics. In this sense, the initial burst effect observed in BSA release from unmodified matrices (~90%) was reduced almost three times (~30%) after amino functionalization. In addition, the release of protein from all SBA-15-NH_2 mesoporous materials was incomplete, whereas the total amount of loaded BSA was released after 192 hours from unmodified matrices.

Furthermore, amino-functionalization of large-pore and large-volume MCF materials has been also probed to increase the affinity towards BSA molecule [118] (Figure 10). The results revealed that the amount of BSA loaded was higher in MCF-NH_2 than in unmodified MCF. This fact can be easily explained because despite of the reduction of pore diameter as a consequence of functionalization, the pore size of MCF-NH_2 (~ 16nm) is still big enough to allow the BSA incorporation. Again, amino functionalization exerts a noticeable effect in BSA release profiles. The initial burst effect of unmodified MCF (~60%) was drastically reduced in MCF-NH_2 (~10%).

All these findings demonstrate that amino functionalization of SMMs is a satisfactory strategy for the design of controlled delivery systems of many biologically active molecules exhibiting organic groups which are capable of undergoing attracting interactions with amino functions.

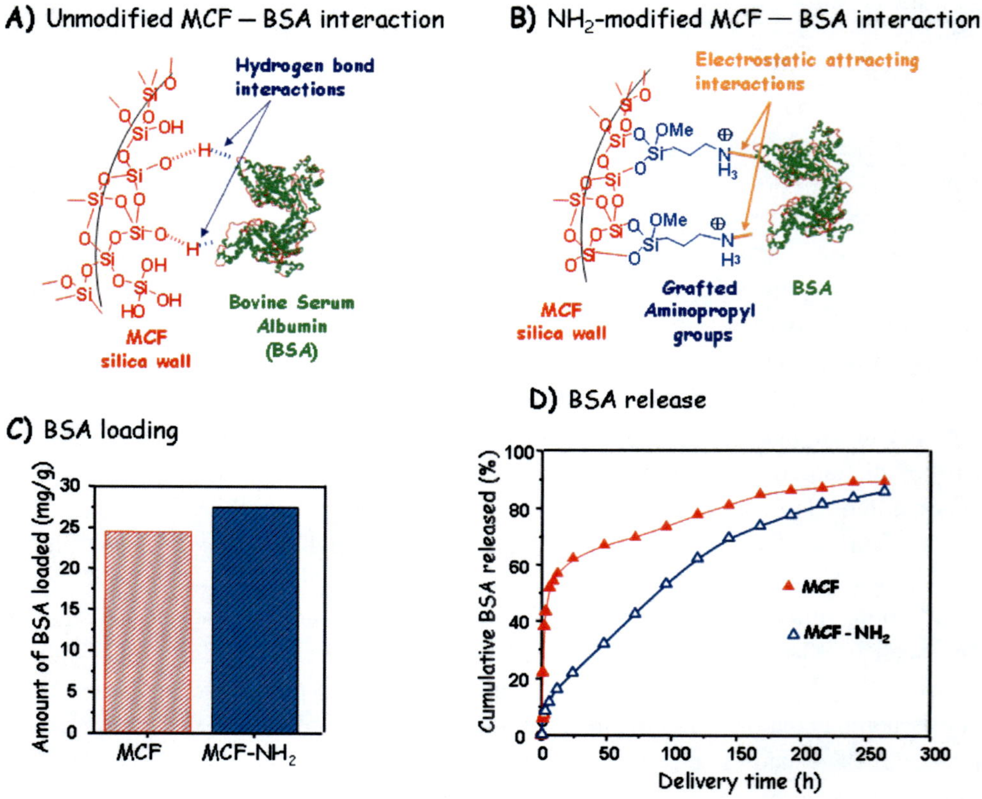

Figure 10. Schematic representation of mesoporous matrix-bovine serum albumin (BSA) host-guest interactions for: A) pure mesoporous mesocellular silica foam (MCF); and B) aminopropyl-functionalized MCF (MCF-NH_2). C) BSA loading and D) BSA release profiles are also displayed.

Functionalization with Hydrophobic Groups

The functionalization of SMMs with hydrophobic groups is an alternative approach commonly used to control the loading and release of certain molecules. For instance, the functionalization of SBA-15 with different alkyl chains, octyl (C_8) and octadecyl (C_{18}) has been carried out and controlled delivery tests of erythromycin, a hydrophobic antibiotic, have been reported [108].

Albeit the diminution in the textural properties due to the functionalization led to a decrease in the amount of erythromycin loaded (130 mg/g and 180 mg/g for SBA-15-C_8 and SBA-15-C_{18}, respectively) compared to unmodified SBA-15 (340 mg/g), there was a remarkable decrease in the delivery rate. This fact was attributed to the decrease of the wettability of the functionalized surfaces, which made difficult the penetration of the aqueous release medium inside the mesopores and induced slower drug delivery kinetics.

Moreover, SBA-15 materials functionalized using hydrophobic groups have been proposed as controlled delivery systems of *L*-tryptophan (*L*-Trp) [119], a hydrophobic amino acid present in the 3D structure of many peptides, proteins and growth factors of interest in bone tissue regeneration technologies [149,150]. *L*-Trp exhibits a hydrophobic aromatic indol ring that makes necessary to modify the SBA-15 matrix, which contains high density of silanol groups. In fact, unmodified SBA-15 loaded less than 5 mg/g of *L*-Trp, probably due to the extremely different chemical nature of hydrophobic amino acid and hydrophilic SBA-15. With the aim of increasing host-guest interactions, SBA-15 was functionalized using quaternary amines with different alkyl lengths (~$C_3N^+Me_3$ and ~$C_3N^+Me_2C_{18}$) (Figure 11). The main forces that governed amino acid adsorption in SBA-15 functionalized with short alkyl chains (~$C_3N^+Me_3$) were coulombic attracting interactions between deprotonated carboxylic groups of amino acid (-COO^-) and protonated quaternary amines (-N^+R_4) covering the mesoporous surface (Figure 11.A). In this case the amount of *L*-Trp loaded into SBA-15-$C_3N^+Me_3$ matrix raised up to 43 mg/g.

When using long hydrocarbon chains (~$C_3N^+Me_2C_{18}$) two-thirds of the silica surface was functionalized. This high functionalization degree using hydrophobic chains induced strong interactions between mesoporous surface and indol group of *L*-Trp (Figure 11.B), leading to *L*-Trp loading amounts of 82 mg/g for SBA-15-$C_3N^+Me_2C_{18}$.

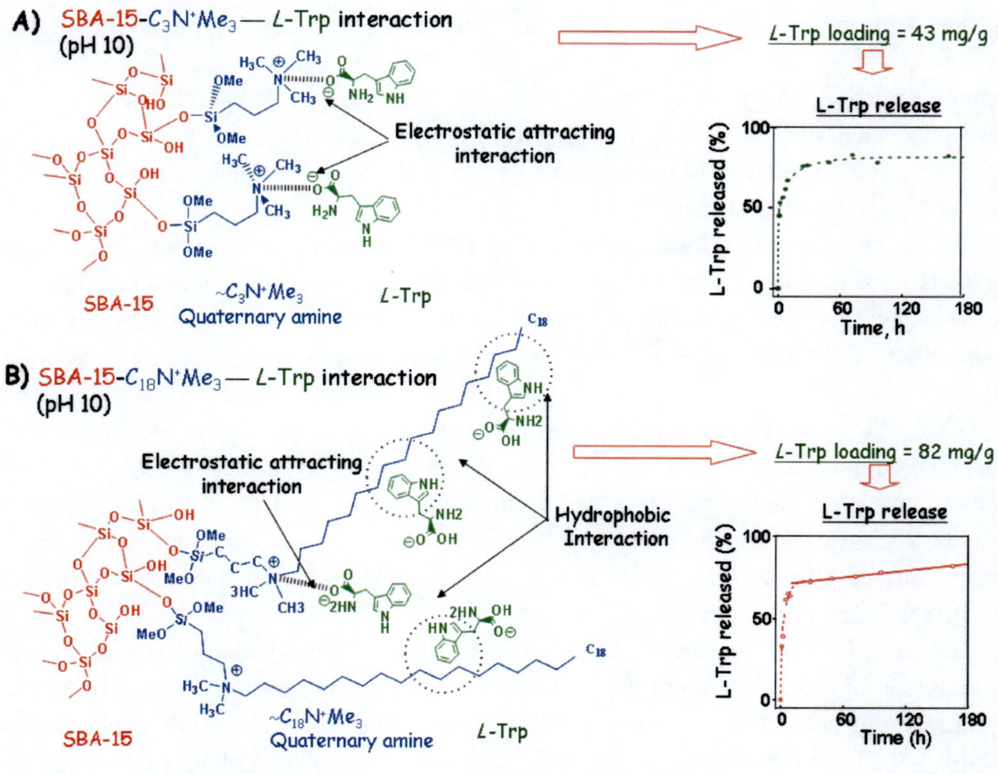

Figure 11. Molecular model of interaction between *L*-Trp and SBA-15 functionalized with A) short-chain quaternary amines (~$C_3N^+Me_3$) and B) long-chain quaternary amines (~$C_{18}N^+Me_3$). *L*-Trp loads and the corresponding *L*-Trp release profiles are also displayed for each case.

The *L*-Trp release patterns from both functionalized matrices (Figure 11) display an initial burst effect and the rest of amino acid is released in a sustained manner, following first-order and zero-order or linear kinetics from SBA-15-$C_3N^+Me_3$ and SBA-15-$C_3N^+Me_2C_{18}$ matrices, respectively.

6. Hierarchical Meso-Macroporous Scaffolds for Bone Tissue Engineering

In recent years, hierarchically porous scaffolds of multiple length scales have received great attention in bone tissue engineering. Hierarchically materials containing both interconnected meso-macroporous structures combine the outstanding properties of ordered mesoporous materials with the advantages of macroporous structures [151-154]. The presence of ordered pore networks allows the incorporation of osteogenic agents, such as certain drugs, growth factors, proteins, peptides, etc., to promote new bone formation (Figure 12). In addition, 3D-interconnected macroporosity allow bone cell penetration, adherence, growth and proliferation leading to bone tissue in-growth and eventually vascularization on implantation [155,156]. The combination of meso and macroporosity will result in an enhancement of the mass transport whereas maintaining the surface area on the meso-scale. Much effort is being carried out by the scientific community to develop hierarchically meso-macroporous materials with improved features [157]. The synthesis of these materials is commonly carried out by using surfactants as mesostructures directing agents and large-size substances, such as colloidal crystals [158,159], polymer foams [160], biocelluloses [161], emulsions [162], vesicles [163], inorganic salts [164] and ice crystals [165] to the direct creation of macroporous structures.

Due to the outstanding bioactive behavior of MBGs, these materials have been recently employed as raw materials for the design of hierarchically structured scaffolds. Therefore, Yun *et al.* reported the synthesis of ordered giant-, macro and 3D MBG scaffolds using a combination of sol-gel, double polymers templating and rapid prototyping (RP) techniques [94].

The resulting scaffold exhibited three lengths of porosity: mesopores (~5 nm) obtained by using a triblock copolymer template ($EO_{100}PO_{65}EO_{100}$, (F127)), macropores (~10-30 nm) produced by using methyl cellulose and giant-sized pores (~300-1000 μm) created by RP methods [29,166]. The *in vitro* bioactivity test revealed that a CHA layer was formed onto the material surface after 24 hours in soaked in SBF, evidencing the outstanding *in vitro* bone-forming capability of these scaffolds.

Moreover, Li *et al.* prepared hierarchically MBGs scaffolds by using P123 surfactant as soft template for the formation of the mesostructure and polyurethane (PUF) as positive hard template for macroporous structures [167]. The resulting materials exhibited hierarchical porosity with interconnected macropores of 200-400 or 500-700 μm in size and uniform mesopores of 3.68 nm. *In vitro* bioactivity test showed that this MBG scaffolds induced the formation of a CHA layer on their surface after 4 hours in SBF, and the crystallization of such layer was completed after 4 hours.

Other authors have also reported the employment of P123 and PUF to synthesize hierarchically structured 3D MBGs scaffolds with four different chemical compositions and *in vitro* bioactivity and cell adherence test were performed [168].

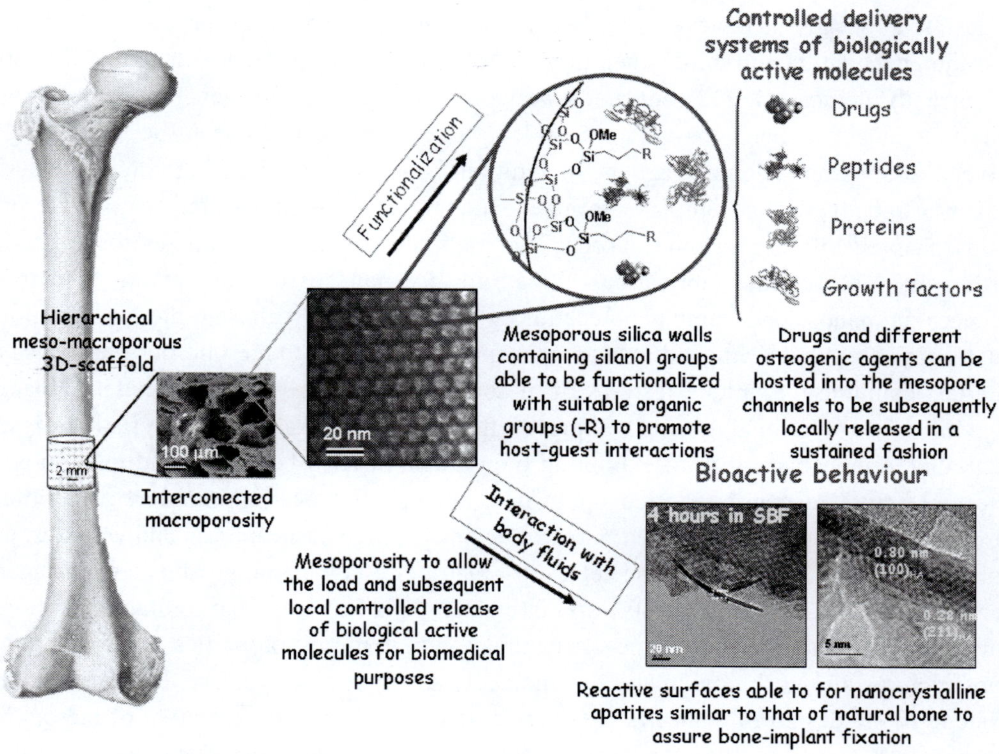

Figure 12. Schematic illustration of functional scaffold with hierarchically meso and macroporosity based in mesoporous silica and its corresponding functionality.

Different characterization techniques indicated that these scaffolds presented similar mesostructural and textural properties with interconnected macroporous networks (pore diameters of 200-400 µm) and mesopores of 4.9 nm in size. Bioactivity assays evidenced that the introduction of Ca and P into the network facilitated the formation of CHA layer on the materials surfaces. Cell cultures for 1, 3 and 7 days indicated that primary human bone-derived cells were able to attach and spread to different degrees on the different scaffold tested.

These authors indicate that the potential reason for the difference in supporting cell growth and differentiation exhibited by the different scaffolds could be relative to the CHA layer on the surface of scaffold, which has been reported to affect cell activity [169,170]. Moreover, the release of Ca and Si ions may be contributing to the modulation of cellular attachment [171]. However, further cell proliferation and differentiation assays are needed to determine the nature of cell interaction with the scaffolds.

Conclusion

This chapter describes the current scientific trends in the design of bioceramics for bone tissue regeneration. Bioactive ceramics able to develop bone-bonding apatite phases onto their surfaces when in contact with physiological fluids have been widely employed during the last four decades. However, the recent scientific challenge goes beyond just ensuring bone-implant fixation and third generation bioceramics able to stimulate new bone formation are currently demanded. This concept involves the design of third generation bioceramics exhibiting bioactive behavior with the added value of being capable to act as controlled delivery systems of osteogenic agents. In addition, bone tissue engineering allows the design of 3D scaffolds that act as templates for new bone in-growth. As it was demonstrated through in this chapter, silica based mesoporous materials are excellent candidates to be used as starting materials for the fabrication of scaffolds for bone tissue engineering. The recent advances in nanoscience and nanotechnology have allowed tailoring the compositional, structural and textural features of mesoporous matrices, leading to mesoporous glasses. These materials combine the unique features of mesoporous matrices with the excellent bioactive behavior of conventional glasses. Some of the more remarkable characteristics of such materials are their capability of exhibiting biomimetic *in vitro* behaviors and exhibiting the fastest bioactive response reported up to date among all bioceramics. Moreover, ordered mesoporous materials, with ordered pore arrangements, high surface areas and volumes, pore diameters in the 2-50 nm range, can act as host matrices of a wide range of osteogenic agents, such as certain drugs, growth factors, proteins, peptides, etc. that promote new bone formation. The tailoring of the structural and textural properties of mesoporous nanostructures allows the modulation of molecule adsorption and release. However, the real keystone in the design of controlled delivery systems is the functionalization of mesoporous materials with appropriated organic groups able to promote host-guest interactions.

This double scope, bioactivity and controlled delivery capability opens up novel insights in the use of mesoporous materials as starting materials for the manufacture of 3D scaffolds for bone tissue engineering. This is an emerging research field and the joint effort of chemists, physicists, biologists, engineers and physicians is needed to design and fabricate suitable 3D hierarchical meso-macro structures that fulfill the criteria for and ideal scaffold for both bone tissue engineering and *in situ* bone regeneration.

References

[1] Vallet-Regí, M. Ceramics for medical applications. Perspective Article. *J. Chem. Soc. Dalton Trans.* 2001, 97-108.

[2] Vallet-Regí, M. Revisiting ceramics for medical applications. Perspective Article. *J. Chem. Soc. Dalton Trans.* 2006, 5211-5220.

[3] Hulbert, SF. The use of alumina and zirconia in surgical implants. In Hench LL, Wilson J editors. An introduction to bioceramics. Singapore: World Scientific; 1993; 25-40.

[4] Muster, D; Demri, TJ; Hage-Ali, M. Physicochemical characterization of surface and interface on biomaterials and coatings. In Wise DL, Trantolo DJ, Altobelli DE, Yaszemski MJ, Gresser JD, Schwart ER editors. *Encyclopedic handbook of biomaterials and bioengineering. Part A. Materials.* New York: Marcel Dekker; 1995; 785-812.

[5] Hench, L; Splinter, RJ; Greenlee, TK; Allen, WC. Bonding mechanisms at the interface of ceramic prosthetic materials. *J. Biomed. Mater. Res.* 1971, 5, 117-141.

[6] Hench, LL. The story of Bioglass ®. *J. Mater. Sci: Mater Med.* 2006, 17, 967-978.
[7] Kokubo, T. Bioactive glass-ceramics: properties and applications. *Biomaterials*. 1991, 12, 155-163.
[8] Hench, LL. Bioceramics: From concept to clinic. *J. Am. Ceram. Soc.* 1991, 74, 1487-1570.
[9] Vallet-Regí, M. Bone repair and regeneration possibilities. *Mat.-wiss. u. Werkstofftech*. 2006, 37, 478-484.
[10] Kasemo, B. Biological Surface Science. *Surf. Sci.* 2002, 500, 656-677.
[11] Castner, DG; Ratner, BD. Biomedical surface science: Foundations to frontiers. *Surf. Sci.* 2002, 500, 28-60.
[12] Tirrell, M; Kokkoli, E; Biesalsk, M. The role of surface science in bioengineered materials, *Surf. Sci.* 2002, 500, 61-83.
[13] Vallet-Regí, M; Romero, AM; Ragel, V.; Legeros, RZ. XRD, SEM-EDS and FTIR studies of in vitro growth of an apatite-like layer on sol-gel glasses. *J. Biomed. Mater. Res*. 1999, 44, 416-421.
[14] Vallet-Regí, M; Ragel, CV; Salinas, AJ. Glasses with medical applications. *Eur. J. Inor. Chem*. 2003, 6, 1029-1042.
[15] Vallet-Regí, M. Ordered mesoporous materials in the context of drug delivery systems and bone tissue engineering, *Chem. Eur. J.* 2006. 12, 5934-5943.
[16] del Real, RP; Arcos, D; Vallet-Regí, M. Implantable magnetic glass-ceramic based on (Fe, Ca) SiO_3 solid solutions. *Chem. Mater*. 2002, 14, 64-70.
[17] Ruiz, E; Serrano, MC; Arcos, D; Vallet-Regí, M. Glass-glass ceramic thermoseeds for hyperthermic treatment of bone tumours. *J. Biomed. Mater. Res*. 2006, 79A, 533-543.
[18] Vallet-Regí M; Arcos D. Nanostructured hybrid material for bone tissue regeneration *Current Nanosci.* 2006, 2, 179-189.
[19] Colilla, M; Salinas, AJ; Vallet-Regí, M. Amino-polysiloxane hybrid materials for bone Reconstruction. *Chem. Mater*. 2006, 18, 5676-5683.
[20] Manzano, M; Arcos, D; Rodríguez-Delgado, M; Ruíz, E; Gil, FJ; Vallet-Regí, M. Bioactive star gels. *Chem Mater*. 2006, 18, 5696-5703.
[21] Hench, LL; Polak, JM. Third-generation biomedical materials. *Science*. 2002, 295, 1014-1017.
[22] Hollister, SJ. Porous scaffold design for tissue engineering. *Nat. Mater.* 2005, 5, 518-524.
[23] LeGeros, RZ. Calcium Phosphates in Oral Biology and Medicine. In Myers HM, editor. *Monographs in Oral Science*. Basel: Karger Press, 1991, vol. 15, 108-129.
[24] Glimcher, MJ. The nature of the mineral phase in bone: Biological and clinical implications. In: Avioli LV, Krane SM, editors. *Metabolic bone disease and clinically related disorders*. San Diego: Academic Press; 1998, 23-50.
[25] Vallet-Regí, M; González-Calbet, J. Calcium phosphates as substitution of bone tissues. *Prog. Solid State Chem.* 2004, 32, 1-31.
[26] Dorozhkin, SV. Calcium orthophosphates, *J. Mater. Sci.* 2007, 42, 1061-1095, 2007.
[27] Rho, JY; Uhn-Spearing, LK; Zioupos, P. Mechanical properties and the hierarchical structure of bone. *Med. Eng. Phys.* 1998, 20, 92-102.

[28] Frieβ, W; Warner, J. Biomedical Applications. In: Schüth F, Sing KSW, Weitkamp J. *Handook of Porous Solids. Vol. 5*, Weinheim (Federal Republic of Germany): Wiley-VCH; 2002; 2923-2970.

[29] Xie, B; Parkhill, RL; Warren, WL; Smay, JE. Direct writing of three-dimensional polymer scaffolds using colloidal gels. *Adv. Funct. Mater.* 2006, 16, 1685-1693.

[30] Vallet-Regí, M. Bioceramics: where do we come from and which are the future expectations. *Key Eng. Mater.* 2008, 377, 1-18.

[31] Kortesuo, P; Ahola, M; Karlsson, S; Kangasniemi, I; Yli-Urpo, A; Kiesvaara, J. Silica xerogel as an implantable carrier for controlled drug delivery-evaluation of drug distribution and tissue effects after implantation. *Biomaterials*. 2000, 21, 193-198.

[32] Chia, S; Urano, J; Tamanoi, F; Dunn, B; Zink, JI. Patterned hexagonal arrays of living cells in sol-gel silica films. *J. Am. Chem. Soc.* 2000, 122, 6488-6489.

[33] Radin, S; El-Bassyouni, G; Vresilovic, EJ; Schepers, E; Ducheyne, P. In vivo tissue response to resorbable silica xerogels as controlled-release materials. *Biomaterials*. 2005, 26, 1043-1052.

[34] Vogt, JC; Brandes, G; Krüger, I; Behrens, P; Nolte, I; Lenarz, T; Stieve, M. A comparison of different nanostructured biomaterials in subcutaneous tissue. *J. Mater. Sci.: Mater. Med.* 2008, 19, 2629-2636.

[35] Vallet-Regí, M; Ruiz-González, L; Izquierdo-Barba, I; González-Calbet, JM. Revisiting silica based ordered mesoporous materials: medical applications. *J Mater Chem*, 2006, 16, 26-31.

[36] Yan, XX; Yu, CZ; Zhou, XF; Tang, JW; Zhao, DY. Highly ordered mesoporous bioactive glasses with superior in vitro bone-forming bioactivities, *Angew. Chem. Int. Ed.* 2004, 43, 5980-5984.

[37] López-Noriega, A; Arcos, D; Izquierdo-Barba, I; Sakamoto, Y; Terasaki, O; Vallet-Regí. Ordered mesoporous bioactive glasses for bone tissue regeneration. M. *Chem. Mater.* 2006, 18, 3137-3144.

[38] Izquierdo-Barba, I; Arcos, D; Sakamoto, Y; Terasaki, O; López-Noriega, A; Vallet-Regí, M. High-Performance Mesoporous Bioceramics Mimicking Bone Mineralization. *Chem. Mater.* 2008, 20, 3191-3198.

[39] Vallet-Regí, M; Rámila, A; del Real, RP; Pérez-Pariente J. A new property of MCM-41: Drug delivery system. *Chem. Mater.* 2001, 13, 308-311.

[40] Vallet-Regí, M; Balas, F; Colilla, C; Manzano, M. Bioceramics and pharmaceuticals: A remarkable synergy. *Solid State Sci.* 2007, 768-776.

[41] Vallet-Regí, M; Balas, F; Colilla, M; Manzano, M. Drug confinement and delivery in ceramic implants. *Drug Metab. Lett.* 2007, 1, 37-40.

[42] Vallet-Regí, M; Arcos, D. Mesoporous materials for biomedical applications, In: Pannone PJ, editor. Trends in biomaterials research, New York: Nova Science Publishers; 2007; 109-142.

[43] Izquierdo-Barba, I; Manzano, M; Colilla, M; Vallet-Regí, M. Silica-Based ordered mesoporous materials for biomedical applications, *Key Eng. Mater.* 2008, 377, 133-150.

[44] Vallet-Regí, M; Colilla, M; Izquierdo-Barba, I. Bioactive mesoporous silicas as controlled delivery systems: application in bone tissue regeneration. *J. Biomed Nanotechnol.* 2008, 4, 1-15.

[45] Colilla, M; Izquierdo-Barba, I; Vallet-Regí, M. novel biomaterials for drug delivery, *Expert. Opin. Ther. Patents*, 2008, 18, 639-656.

[46] Vallet-Regí, M; Balas, F; Arcos, D. Mesoporous materials for drug delivery. *Angew. Chem. Int. Ed.* 2007, 46, 7548-58.

[47] Yanagisawa, T; Shimizu, T; Kuroda, K; Kato, C. The preparation of alkyltrimethylammonium-kanemite complexes and their conversion to microporous materials. *Bull. Chem. Soc. Jpn.* 1990, 63, 988-992.

[48] Inagaki, S; Fukushima, Y; Kuroda, K. Synthesis of highly ordered mesoporous materials from a layered polysilicate. *Chem. Comm.* 1993, 8, 680-682.

[49] Kresge, CT; Leonowicz, ME; Roth, WJ; Vartuli, JC; Beck, JS. Ordered mesoporous molecular sieves synthesised by a liquid-crystal template mechanism. *Nature*. 1992, 359, 710-712.

[50] Ying, JY; Mehnert, CP; Wong, MS. Synthesis and applications of supramolecular-templated mesoporous materials. *Angew. Chem. Int. Ed.* 1999, 38, 56-77.

[51] Beck, JS; Vartuli, JC; Roth, WJ; Leonowicz, ME; Kresge, CT; Schmitt, KD; Chu, CTW; Olson, DH; Sheppard, EW; McCullen, SB; Higgins, JB; Schlenker, JL. A new family of mesoporous molecular-sieves prepared with liquid-crystal templates. *J. Am. Chem. Soc.* 1992, 114, 10834-10843.

[52] Firouzi, A; Atef, F; Oertli, AG; Stucky, GD; Chmelka, BF. Alkaline lyotropic silicate-surfactant liquid crystals. *J. Am. Chem. Soc*. 1997, 119, 3596-3610.

[53] Zhang, J; Luz, Z; Goldfarb, D. EPR studies of the formation mechanism of the mesoporous material MCM-41 and MCM-50. *J. Phys. Chem. B*. 1997, 101, 7087-7094.

[54] Kruk, M; Jaroniec, M; Sakamoto, Y; Terasaki, O; Ryoo, R; Ko, CH. Determination of pore size and pore wall structure of MCM-41 by using nitrogen adsorption, transmission electron microscopy, and X-ray diffraction. *J. Phys. Chem. B*. 2001, 104, 292-301.

[55] Kaneda, M; Tsubakiyama, T; Carlsson, A; Sakamoto, Y; Ohsuna, T; Terasaki, O; Joo, SH; Ryoo, R. Structural study of mesoporous MCM-48 and carbon networks synthesised in the spaces of MCM-48 by electron crystallography. *J. Phys. Chem. B*. 2002, 106, 1256-1266.

[56] Zhao, DY; Feng, JL; Huo, QS; Melosh, N; Fredrickson, GH; Chmelka, BF; Stucky, GD. Triblock copolymer syntheses of mesoporous silica with periodic 50 to 300 angstrom pores. *Science*. 1998, 279, 548-552.

[57] Ravikovitch, PI; Neimark, AV. Experimental confirmation of different mechanisms of evaporation of ink-bottle type pores: equilibrium, pore blocking, and cavitation. *Langmuir*. 2002, 18, 9830-9837.

[58] Ravikovitch, PI; Neimark, AV. Density functional theory of adsorption in spherical cavities and pore size characterisation of templated nanoporous silicas with cubic and three-dimensional hexagonal structures. *Langmuir*. 2002, 18, 1550-1560.

[59] Bagshaw, SA; Prouzet, E; Pinnavaia, TJ. Templating of mesoporous molecular-sieves by non-ionic polyethylene oxide surfactants. *Science*. 1995, 269:1242-1244.

[60] Ryoo, R; Kim, JM; Ko, CH; Shin, CH. Disordered molecular sieve with branched mesoporous channel network. *J. Phys. Chem. B*. 1996, 100, 17718-17721.

[61] Inagaki, S; Koiwai, A; Suzuki, N; Fukushima, Y; Kuroda, K. Syntheses of highly ordered mesoporous materials, FSM-16, derived from kanemite. *Bull. Chem. Soc. Jpn.* 1996, 69, 1449-1457.

[62] Che, S; García-Bennett, AE; Yokoi, T; Sakamoto, K; Kunieda, H; Terasaki, O; Tatsumi, T. Mesoporous silica of novel structures with periodic modulations synthesised by anionic surfactant templating route. *Nat. Mater.* 2003, 2, 801-805.

[63] Park, H; Park, K. Biocompatibility issues of implantable drug delivery systems. *Pharm. Res.* 1996, 13, 1770-1776.

[64] Anderson, JM. Biomaterials-an introduction to materials in medicine. In: Ratner BD, Hoffman AS, Schoen FJ, Lemons JE, editors. *Biomaterials*. New York: Academic Press; 1996, 165-205.

[65] Anderson, JM. Biological responses to materials, *Annu. Rev. Mater. Res.* 2001, 31, 81-110.

[66] Tang, L; Eaton, JW; Inflammatory responses to biomaterials, *Am. J. Clin. Pathol.* 1995, 103, 466-471.

[67] Roy, I; Ohulchanskyy, TY; Pudavar, HE; Bergey, EJ; Oseroff, AR; Morgan, J; Dougherty, TJ; Prasad, PN. Ceramic-based nanoparticles entrapping water-insoluble photosensitizing anticancer drugs: A novel drug-carrier system for photodynamic therapy, *J. Am. Chem. Soc.* 2003, 125, 7860-7865.

[68] Barbé, C; Bartlett, J; Kong, L; Finnie, K; Lin, HQ; Larkin, M; Calleja, S; Bush, A; Calleja, G. Silica Particles: A Novel Drug-Delivery System. *Adv. Mater.* 16, 1959-1966, 2004.

[69] Son, YH; Park, M; Bin Choy, Y; Choi, HR; Kim, DS; Park, KC; Choy, JH. One-pot synthetic route to polymer-silica assembled capsule encased with nonionic drug molecule, *Chem. Commun.* 2007, 2799-2801.

[70] Lu, J; Liong, M; Zink, JI; Tamanoi, F. Mesoporous silica nanoparticles as a delivery system for hydrophobic anticancer drugs. *Small*. 2007, 3, 1341-1346.

[71] Radu, DR; Lai, CY; Jeftinija, K; Rowe, EW; Jeftinija, S; Lin, VS-Y. A polyamidoamine dendrimer-capped mesoporous silica nanosphere-based gene transfection reagent. *J. Am. Chem. Soc.* 2004, 126, 13216-13217.

[72] Blumen,, SR; Cheng, K; Ramos-Nino, ME; Taatjes, DJ; Weiss, DJ; Landry, CC; Mossman, BT. Unique uptake of acid-prepared mesoporous spheres by lung epithelial and mesothelioma cells. *Am. J. Respir. Cell. Mol.* 2007, 36, 333-342.

[73] Trewyn, BG; Nieweg, JA; Zhao, Y; Lin, VS-Y. Biocompatible mesoporous silica nanoparticles with different morphologies for animal cell membrane, penetration. *Chem. Eng. J.* 2008, 137, 23-29.

[74] Chung, TH; Wu, SH; Yao, M; Lu, CW; Lin YS; Hung, Y; Mou, CY; Chen, YC; Huang, DM. The effect of surface charge on the uptake and biological function of mesoporous silica nanoparticles 3T3-L1 cells and human mesenchymal stem cells. *Biomaterials*. 2008, 28, 2959-2966.

[75] Vallhov, H; Gabrielsson, S; Stromme, M; Scheynius, A; García-Bennett, AE; Mesoporous silica particles induce size dependent effects on human dendritic cells. *Nano Lett.* 2007, 7, 3576-3582.

[76] Di Pasqua, AJ; Sharma, KK; Shi, YL; Toms, BB; Ouellette, W; Dabrowiak, JC; Asefa, T. Cytotoxicity of mesoporous silica nanomaterials, *J. Inorg. Biochem.* 2008, 102, 1416-1423.

[77] Lopez, T; Basaldella, EI; Ojeda, ML; Manjarrez, J; Alexander-Katz, R. Encapsulation of valproic acid and sodic phenytoin in ordered mesoporous SiO_2 solids for the treatment of temporal lobe epilepsy. *Opt. Mater.* 2006, 9, 75-81.

[78] Wu, SH; Lin, YS; Hung, Y; Chou, YH; Hsu, YH; Chang C; Mou, CY. Multifunctional mesoporous silica nanoparticles for intracellular labelling and animal magnetic resonance imaging studies. *Chembiochem*. 2008, 9, 53-57.

[79] Hudson, SP; Padera, RF; Langer, R; Kohane, DS. The biocompatibility of mesoporous silicates, *Biomaterials*. 2008, 29, 4045-4055.

[80] Li, P; Ohtsuki, C; Kokubo, T; Nakanishi, K; Soga, N; Nakamura, T; Yamamuro, T. Apatite formation induced by silica-gel in a simulated body-fluid. *J. Am. Ceram. Soc.* 1992, 75, 2094-2097.

[81] Pereira, MM; Clark, AE; Hench, LL. Effect of texture on the rate of hydroxyapatite formation on gel-silica surface. J. *Am. Ceram. Soc.* 1995, 78, 2463-2468.

[82] Pereira, MM; Clark, AE; Hench, LL. Mechanisms of hydroxyapatite formation on porous gel-silica substrates. *J. Sol–Gel Sci. Technol.* 1996, 7, 59-68.

[83] Vallet-Regí, M; Arcos, D; Pérez-Pariente, Evolution of porosity during in vitro hydroxycarbonate apatite growth in sol-gel glasses, *J. Biomed. Mater. Res.* 2000, 51, 23-28.

[84] Balas, F; Arcos, D; Pérez-Pariente, J; Vallet-Regí, M. Textural properties of $SiO_2{\cdot}CaO{\cdot}P_2O_5$ glasses prepared by the sol-gel method. *J. Mater. Res.* 2001, 16, 1345-1348.

[85] Horcajada, P; Rámila, A; Boulahya, K; González-Calbet, J; Vallet-Regí, M. Bioactivity in ordered mesoporous materials. *Solid State Sci.* 2004, 6, 1295-1300.

[86] Izquierdo-Barba, I; Ruiz-González, L; Doadrio, JC; González-Calbet, JM; Vallet-Regí, M. Tissue regeneration: a new property of mesoporous materials. *Solid State Sci.* 2005, 7, 983-989.

[87] Kokubo, T; Kushitani, H; Sakka, S; Kitsugi, T; Yamamuro, T. Solutions able to reproduce *in vivo* surface-structure changes in bioactive glass-ceramic A-W3. *J. Biomed. Mater. Res.* 1990, 24, 721-734.

[88] Vallet-Regí, M; Izquierdo-Barba, I; Salinas, AJ. Influence of P_2O_5 on crystallinity of apatite formed *in vitro* on surface of bioactive glasses. *J. Biomed. Mater. Res.* 1999, 46, 560-565.

[89] Vallet-Regí, M; Izquierdo-Barba, I; Rámila, A; Pérez-Pariente, J; Babonneau, F; González-Calbet JM. Phosphorus-doped MCM-41 as bioactive material. *Solid State. Sci.*, 2005, 7, 233-237.

[90] Vallet-Regí, M; Rámila, A; Padilla, S; Muñoz, B. Bioactive glasses as accelerators of apatite bioactivity. *J. Biomed. Mater. Res.* 2003, 66, 580-585.

[91] Brinker, CJ; Lu, YF ; Sellinger, A ; Fan, HY. Evaporation-induced self-assembly: nanostructures made easy. *Adv. Mate*r. 1999, 11, 579-585.

[92] Yan, XX; Den, HX; Huang, XH; Lu, GQ; Qiao, SZ; Zhao, DY; Yu, CZ. Mesoporous bioactive glasses. I. Synthesis and structural characterization. *J. Non-Cryst. Solids*. 2005, 351, 3209-3217.

[93] Yan, XX; Huang, XH; Yu, CZ; Deng, HX; Wang, Y; Zhang, ZD; Qiao, SZ; Lu, CQ; Zhao, DY. The *in-vitro* bioactivity of mesoporous bioactive glasses. *Biomaterials*. 2006, 27, 3396-3403.

[94] Yun, HS; Kim, Se; Hyeon, YT. Highly ordered mesoporous bioactive glasses with *Im-3m* symmetry. *Mater. Lett.* 2007, 61, 4569-4572.

[95] Hench, LL; Wilson, J. Surface-active biomaterials. *Science*. 1984, 226, 630-636.

[96] Brown, WE; Eidelman, N; Tomazic, B. "Octacalcium phosphate as a precursor in biomineral formation. *Adv. Dent Res*. 1987, 1, 306-313.

[97] Bodier-Houlle, P; Steuer, P; Voegel, JC; Cuisinier, FJG. First experimental evidence for human dentine crystal formation involving conversion of octacalcium phosphate to hydroxyapatite. *Acta Crystallogr*. 1998, 54, 1377-1381.

[98] Nancollas, GH; Tomazic, B. Growth of calcium-phosphate on hydroxyapatite crystals - effect of supersaturation and ionic medium. *J. Phys. Chem*. 1974, 78, 2218-2225.

[99] Hench, LL; Andersson, O. Bioactive Glasses. In: Hench LL, Wilson J, editors. *An introduction to Bioceramics*. Singapore: World Scientific, 1993, 41-62.

[100] Langer, R. Drug delivery: Drugs on Target. *Science*. 2001, 293, 58-59.

[101] Muñoz, B; Rámila, A; Pérez-Pariente, J; Díaz, I; Vallet-Regí, M. MCM-41 organic modification as drug delivery rate regulator. *Chem. Mater.* 2003, 15, 500-503.

[102] Izquierdo-Barba, I; Martínez, A; Doadrio, AL; Pérez-Pariente, J; Vallet-Regí, M. Release evaluation of drugs from ordered three-dimensional silica structures. *Eur. J. Pharm. Sci.* 2005, 26, 365-373.

[103] Manzano, M; Aina, V; Areán, CO; Balas, F; Cauda, V; Colilla, M; Delgado, MR; Vallet-Regí, M. Studies on MCM-41 mesoporous silica for drug delivery: Effect of particle morphology and amine functionalization. *Chem. Eng. J.* 2008, 137, 31-37.

[104] Cauda, V; Fiorilli, S; Onida, B; Verné, E; Vitale-Brovarone, C; Viterbo, D; Croce, G; Milanesio, M; Garrone, E. SBA-15 ordered mesoporous silica inside a bioactive glass-ceramic scaffold for local drug delivery, *J. Mater. Sci.: Mater. Med.* 2008, 19, 3303-3310.

[105] Xue, JM; Shi, M. 2004. PLGA/mesoporous silica hybrid structure for controlled drug release. *J. Control. Release*. 2004, 98, 209-217.

[106] Doadrio, AL; Sousa, EMB; Doadrio, JC; Pérez-Pariente, J; Izquierdo-Barba, I; Vallet-Regí, M. Mesoporous SBA-15 HPLC evaluation for controlled gentamicin drug delivery. *J Control Release*. 2004, 97, 125-132.

[107] Vallet-Regí, M; Doadrio, JC; Doadrio, AL; Izquierdo-Barba, I; Pérez-Pariente, J. Hexagonal ordered mesoporous material as a matrix for the controlled release of amoxicillin. *Solid State Ionics*. 2004,172, 435-439.

[108] Doadrio, JC; Sousa, EMB; Izquierdo-Barba, I; Pérez-Pariente, J; Vallet-Regí, M. Functionalization of mesoporous materials with long alkyl chains as a strategy for controlling drug delivery pattern. *J. Mater. Chem.* 2006, 16, 462-467.

[109] Yang, Q; Wang, SH; Fan, PW; Wang, LF; Di, Y; Lin, KF; Xiao, FS. pH-responsive carrier system based on carboxylic acid modified mesoporous silica and polyelectrolyte for drug delivery. *Chem. Mater*. 2005, 17, 5999-6003.

[110] Cavallaro, G; Pierro, P; Palumbo, FS; Testa, F; Pasqua, L; Aiello, R. Drug delivery devices based on mesoporous silicate. *Drug Delivery*. 2004, 11, 41-46.

[111] Zeng, W; Qian, XF; Zhang, YB; Yin, J; Zhu, ZK. Organic modified mesoporous MCM-41 through solvothermal process as drug delivery system. *Mater. Res. Bull.* 2005, 40, 766-772.

[112] Qu, FY; Zhu, GS; Huang, SY; Li, SG; Sun, JY; Zhang, DL; Qiu, SL. Controlled release of captopril by regulating the pore size and morphology of ordered mesoporous silica. *Microporous Mesoporous Mater.* 2006, 92, 1-9.

[113] Mellaerts, R; Mols, R; Jammaer, JAG; Aerts, CA; Annaert, P; Van Humbeeck, J; Van den Mooter, G; Augustijns, P; Martens, JA. Increasing the oral bioavailability of the poorly water soluble drug itraconazole with ordered mesoporous silica. *Eur. J. Pharm. Biopharm.* 2008, 69, 223-230.

[114] Balas, F; Manzano, M; Horcajada, P; Vallet-Regí, M. Confinement and controlled release of bisphosphonates on ordered mesoporous silica-based materials. *J. Am. Chem. Soc.* 2006, 128, 8116-8117.

[115] Nieto, A; Balas, F; Colilla, M; Manzano, M; Vallet-Regí, M. Functionalization degree of SBA-15 as key factor to modulate sodium alendronate dosage. *Microporous Mesoporous Mater.* 2008, 116, 4-13.

[116] Song, S-W; Hidajat, K; Kawi, S. Functionalized SBA-15 materials as carriers for controlled drug delivery: Influence of surface properties on matrix-drug interactions. *Langmuir*. 2005, 21, 9568-9575.

[117] Vallet-Regí, M; Balas, F; Colilla, M; Manzano, M. Bone-regenerative bioceramic implants with drug and protein controlled delivery capability. *Prog Solid State Chem*, 2008, 36, 163-191.

[118] Colilla, M; Manzano, M; Vallet-Regí, M. Recent advances in ceramic implants as drug delivery systems for biomedical applications, *Int. J. Nanomed.* 2008, 3, 403-414.

[119] Balas, F; Manzano, M; Colilla, M; Vallet-Regí, M. *L*-Trp adsorption into silica mesoporous materials to promote bone formation. *Acta Biomater.* 2008, 4, 514-522.

[120] Deere, J; Magner, E; Wall, JG; Hodnett, BK. Mechanistic and structural features of protein adsorption onto mesoporous silicates. *J. Phys. Chem. B*. 2002, 106, 7340-7347.

[121] Cheng, YY; Lin, SH; Chang, HC; Su, MC. Probing adsorption, orientation and conformational changes of cytochrome c on fused silica surfaces with the soret band. *J. Phys. Chem. A*. 2003, 107, 10687-10694.

[122] Lei, J; Fan, J; Yu, C; Zhang, LY; Jiang, SY; Tu, B; Zhao, DY. Immobilization of enzymes in mesoporous materials: controlling the entrance to nanospace. *Microporous Mesoporous Mater.* 2004, 73:121-128.

[123] Vinu, A; Murugesan, V; Tangermann, O; Hartmann, M. Adsorption of cytochrome c on mesoporous molecular sieves: Influence of pH, pore diameter, and aluminium incorporation. *Chem. Mater*. 2004, 16, 3056-3065.

[124] Hartmann M. Ordered mesoporous materials for bioadsorption and biocatalysis. *Chem. Mater.* 2005, 17:4577-93.

[125] Katiyar, A; Ji, L; Smirniotis, PG; Pinto, NG. Adsorption of bovine serum albumin and lysozyme on siliceous MCM-41. *Microporous Mesoporous Mater.* 2005, 80, 311-320.
[126] Lee, CH; Mou, CY; Ke, SC; Lin, TS. Effect of spin configuration on the reactivity of cytochrome c immobilized in mesoporous silica. *Mol. Phys.* 2006, 104, 1635-1641.
[127] Slowing, II; Trewyn, BG; Lin, VS-Y. Mesoporous silica nanoparticles for intracellular delivery of membrane-impermeable proteins. *J. Am. Chem. Soc.* 2007, 129, 8845-8849.
[128] He, J.; Li, X.; Evans, D. G.; Duan, X.; Li, C. A new support for the immobilization of penicillin acylase. *J. Mol. Catal. B: Enz.* 2000, 11, 45-53.
[129] Deere, J; Magner, E; Wall, JG; Hodnett, BK. Adsorption and activity of cytochrome c on mesoporous silicates, *Chem. Commun.* 2001, 465-466.
[130] Yiu, HHP; Wright, PA. Enzymes supported on ordered mesoporous solids: a special case of an inorganic-organic hybrid. *J. Mater. Chem.* 2005, 15, 3690-3700.
[131] Peters, T. All about albumin: biochemistry, genetics and medical applications, SanDiego: Academic Press; 1996.
[132] Sugio, S; Kashima, A; Mochizuki, S; Noda, M; Kobayashi, K. Crystal structure of human serum albumin at 2.5 angstrom resolution. *Protein Eng.* 1999, 12, 439-446.
[133] Research Collaboratory for Structural Bioinformatics (RCSB). 2008. Protein Data Bank. Accessed 22 September 2008. URL: http://www.pdb.org.
[134] Kruk, M; Jaroniec, M Sayari, A. New approach to evaluate pore size distributions and surface areas for hydrophobic mesoporous solids. *J. Phys. Chem. B.* 1999, 103, 4590-4598.
[135] El-Safty, SA; Hanaoka, T; Mizukami, F. Ddesign of highly stable, ordered cage mesostructured monoliths with controllable pore geometries and sizes. *Chem. Mater.* 2005, 17, 3137-3145.
[136] Horcajada, P; Rámila, A; Pérez-Pariente, J; Vallet-Regí, M. Influence of pore size of MCM-41 matrices on drug delivery rate. *Microporous Mesoporous Mater.* 2004, 68, 105-109.
[137] Charnay, C; Begu, S; Tourné-Péteilh, C; Nicole, L; Lerner, D; Devoisselle, JM. Inclusion of ibuprofen in mesoporous templated silica: Drug loading and release property. *Eur. J. Pharm. Biopharm.* 2004, 57, 533-540.
[138] Azaïs, T; Tourné-Péteilh, C; Aussenac, F; Baccile, N; Coelho, C; Devoisselle, JM; Babonneau, F. Solid-state NMR study of ibuprofen confined in MCM-41 material. *Chem. Mater.* 2006, 18, 6382-6390.
[139] Han, YJ; Stucky, GD; Butler, A. Mesoporous silicate sequestration and release of proteins. *J. Amer. Chem. Soc.* 1999, 121, 9897-9898.
[140] Zhang, X; Guan, RF; Wu, DQ; Chan, KY. Preparation of amino-functionalized mesostructured cellular foams and application as hosts for large biomolecules. *J. Mater. Sci.: Mater. Med.* 2007, 18, 877-882.
[141] Schmidt-Winkel, P; Lukens, WW; Zhao, DY; Yang, P; Chmelka, BF; Stucky, GD. Mesocellular siliceous foams with uniformly sized cells and windows. *J. Amer. Chem. Soc.* 1999, 121, 254-255.
[142] Schmidt-Winkel, P; Lukens, WW; Yang, P; Margolese, DI; Lettow, JS; Ying, JY; Stucky, GD. Microemulsion templating of siliceous mesostructured cellular foams with well-defined ultralarge mesopores. *Chem. Mater.* 2000, 12, 686-696.

[143] Lin, VS-Y; Lay, C-Y; Huang, J; Song, S-A; Xu, S. Molecular recognition inside of multifunctionalized mesoporous silicas: Toward selective fluorescence detection of dopamine and glucosamine. *J. Am. Chem. Soc.* 2001, 123, 11510-11511.

[144] Mal, NK; Fujiwara, M; Tanaka, Y. Photocontrolled reversible release of guest molecules from coumarin-modified mesoporous silica. *Nature*. 2003, 421, 350-353.

[145] Hoffmann, F; Cornelius, M; Morell, J; Froba, M. Silica-based mesoporous organic-inorganic hybrid materials, *Angew. Chem. Int. Ed.* 2006, 45, 3216-3251.

[146] de Juan, F; Ruiz-Hitzky, E. Selective functionalization of mesoporous silica. *Adv. Mater.* 2000, 12, 430-432

[147] Babonneau, F; Camus, L; Steunou, N; Rámila, A; Vallet-Regí, M. Encapsulation of ibuprofen in mesoporous silica: Solid state NMR characterization. *Mater. Res. Soc.* 2003, 775, 3261-3266.

[148] Horcajada, P; Rámila, A; Férey, G. Vallet-Regí, M. Influence of superficial organic modification Of MCM-41 matrices on drug delivery rate. *Solid State Sci.* 2006, 8, 1243-1249.

[149] Suva, LJ; Winslow, GA; Wettenhall, R; Hammonds, RG; Moseley, JM; Diefenbachjagger, H. A parathyroid hormone-related protein implicated in malignant hypercalcemia: cloning and expression. *Science*. 1987, 237, 893-896.

[150] Valin, A; García-Ocaña, A; DeMiguel, F; Sarasa, JL; Esbrit, P. Antiproliferative effect of the C-terminal fragments of parathyroid hormone-related protein, PTHrP-(107-111) and (107-139), on osteoblastic osteosarcoma cells. *J. Cell. Physiol.* 1997, 160, 209-215.

[151] Cabañas, MV; Peña, J; Román, J; Vallet-Regí, M. Room temperature synthesis of agarose/sol-gel glass pieces with tailored interconnected porosity. *J. Biomed. Mater. Res.* 2006, 78A, 508-514.

[152] Padilla, S; Sánchez-Salcedo, S; Vallet-Regí, M. Bioactive glass as precursor of designed-architecture scaffolds for tissue engineering. *J. Biomed. Mater. Res.* 2007, 81A, 224-232.

[153] Román, J; Cabañas, MV; Peña, J; Doadrio, JC; Vallet-Regí, M. An optimized beta-tricalcium phosphate and agarose scaffold fabrication technique. *J. Biomed. Mater. Res.* 2008, 99-107.

[154] Sánchez-Salcedo, S; Werner, J; Vallet-Regí, M. Hierarchical pore structure of Calcium phosphate scaffolds by a combination of gel-casting and multiple tape-casting methods. *Acta Biomater.* 2008, 4, 913-922.

[155] Jones, JR; Lee PD, Hench LL. Hierarchical porous materials for tissue engineering. *Phil. Trans. R. Soc. A*. 2006, 364, 263-281.

[156] Rekow, D; Van Thompson, P. and Ricci, J.L. Influence of scaffold meso-scale features on bone tissue response, *J. Mater. Sci*. 2006, 41, 5113-5121.

[157] Yuan, ZY; Su, BL. Insights into hierarchically meso-macroporous structured materials. *J. Mater. Chem.* 2006, 16, 663-677.

[158] Yang, PD; Deng, T; Zhao, DY; Feng, PY; Pine, D; Chmelka, BF; Whitesides, GM; Stucky, GD. Hierarchically ordered oxides. *Science*. 2006, 282, 2244-2246.

[159] Lebeau, B; Fowler, CE; Mann, S; Farcet, C; Charleux, B; Sanchez, C. Synthesis of hierarchically ordered dye-functionalised mesoporous silica with macroporous architecture by dual templating. *J. Mater. Chem.* 2000, 10, 2105-2108.

[160] Maekawa, H; Esquena, J; Bishop, S; Solans, C; Chmelka, BF. Meso/macroporous Inorganic oxide monoliths from polymer foams. *Adv. Mater.* 2003, 15, 591-596.

[161] Wang, LQ; Shin, Y; Samuels, WD; Exarhos, GJ; Moudrakovski, IL; Terskikh, VV; Ripmeester, JA. Magnetic resonance studies of hierarchically ordered replicas of wood cellular structures prepared by surfactant-mediated mineralization. *J. Phys.Chem. B.* 2003, 107, 13793-13802.

[162] Zhang, H.F; Hardy, GC; Rosseinsky, MJ; Cooper, AI. Uniform emulsion-Templated silica beads with high pore volume and hierarchical porosity. *Adv. Mater.* 2003, 15, 78-81.

[163] Antonelli, DM. Synthesis of macro-mesoporous niobium oxide molecular sieves by a ligand-assisted vesicle templating strategy. *Microporous Mesoporous Mater.* 1999, 33, 209-214.

[164] Zhao, DY; Yang, PD; Chmelka, BF; Stucky, GD. Multiphase assembly of Mesoporous-macroporous membranes. *Chem. Mater.* 1999, 11, 1174-1178.

[165] Nishihara, H; Mukai, SR; Yamashita, D; Tamon, H. Ordered macroporous silica by ice templating. *Chem. Mater.* 2005, 17, 683-689.

[166] Yeong, WY; Chua, CK. Rapid prototyping in tissue engineering: challenges and potential, *Trends Biotechnol.* 2004, 22, 643-652.

[167] Li, X; Wang, X, Chen, H; Jiang, P; Dong, X; Shi, J. Hierarchically poprous bioactive glass scaffolds synthesized with a PUF and P123 cotemplated approach. *Chem. Mater.* 2007, 19, 4322-4326.

[168] Zhu, Y; Wu, C; Ramaswamy, Y; Kockrick, E; Simon, P; Kaskel, S; Zreiqat, H. Preparation, characterization and in vitro bioactivity of mesoporous bioactive glasses (MBGs) scaffolds for bonte tissue engineering. *Microporous Mesoporous Mater.* 2008, 112, 494-503.

[169] Wu, CT; Chang, J; Zhai, WY; Ni, SY. A novel bioactive porous bredigite ($Ca_7MgSi_4O_{16}$) scaffold with biomimetic apatite layer for bone tissue engineering. *J. Mater. Sci.: Mater. Med.* 2007, 18, 857-864.

[170] Olmo, N; Martín, AI; Salinas, AJ; Turnay, J; Vallet-Regí, M; Lizarbe, MA. Bioactive sol-gel glasses with and without a hydroxycarbonate apatite layer as substrates for osteoblast cell adhesion and proliferation. *Biomaterials*. 2003, 24, 3383-3393.

[171] Valerio, P; Pereira, MM; Goes, AM; Leite, MF. The effect of ionic products from bioactive glass dissolution on osteoblast proliferation and collagen production. *Biomaterials*. 2004, 25, 2941-2948.

In: Bioceramics: Properties, Preparations and Applications ISBN: 978-1-60741-056-0
Editors: W. Kossler, J. Fuchs, pp. 201-221

Chapter IV

Two New Routes to Form Porous Bioceramic Beads

Chih-Kuang Wang**[*1], **Wen-Cheng Chen**[2], **Chun-Cheng Hung**[2], **Yin-Chih Fu**[3] and **Mei-Ling Ho**[4]

[1]Faculty of Medicinal and Applied Chemistry,
Kaohsiung Medical University, Kaohsiung 807, Taiwan
[2]Faculty of Dentistry, Kaohsiung Medical University,
Kaohsiung 807, Taiwan
[3]Department of Orthopaedic Surgery,
Kaohsiung Medical University Hospital, Kaohsiung 807, Taiwan
[4]Department of Physiology, Kaohsiung Medical University,
Kaohsiung 807, Taiwan

Abstract

Granulate systems for the delivery and application of drugs are claimed to have enhanced bioavailability, predictable therapeutic response, greater efficacy and safety, and controlled and prolonged drug release time. Therefore, the development of granulate systems of calcium phosphate-based drugs (e.g. antibiotics, antimicrobial agents, growth factors, etc.) with controlled drug release kinetics have increasingly become an important area of research, in view of the prevalent rates of infection in bone and dental surgery. Further, porous calcium phosphate ceramics are also expected to play important roles in treating bone problems with the emerging tissue engineering approach, as it involves loading proper cells into porous ceramics (scaffolds) and implanting the cell-loaded scaffolds into a host body for achieving bone tissue regeneration. Porous spherical HAp granules of 50-2000 μm diameter have been produced by the dispersion of well-mixed HAp/polymer slurry in a dispersion medium for example. Several studies have reported the development of HAp granulates by various techniques with irregular or spherical geometry. Various studies have been conducted using different polymers (such as gelatin, collagen, chitosan, etc.) as matrices for the preparation of HAp microbeads and

[*] Corresponding author: e-mail: ckwang@kmu.edu.tw, Tel: +886-7-312-1101 ext.2677, Fax: +886-7-312-5339

researchers have recently reported that HAp microspheres were prepared by using oil-in-water emulsions and solvent evaporation technique. We herein will report the preparation and characterization of porous calcium phosphate beads from two kinds of new strategy route. One is that porous bead prepared by alginate-interacting Ca ions mechanism on addition of a pore-forming PE powder by sintering process, another one is by water-in-oil emulsions in higher temperature and fast condensation shaping technique.

Keywords: bioceramic, hydroxyapatite, porous bead, fabrication.

Introduction

Various calcium phosphate materials have been proposed as candidates for artificial bones. From the perspective of biocompatibility, hydroxyapatite ($Ca_{10}(PO_4)_6(OH)_2$, HAp) seems to be the most suitable ceramic material for hard tissue replacement implants [1-3]. Additionally, β-tricalcium phosphate (β-TCP) is another highly bioactive-implantable material. While being exposed to bodily fluids and undergoing a biointegration process involving biodissolution/biodegradation, apatite crystals are precipitated and the eventual formation of new bone occurs on the implant site [4-6]. Some scholars [7-9] have recently attempted to develop biphasic calcium phosphate (BCP) comprising HAp and β-TCP as well. Although the synthetic pathways of these calcium phosphates are the most commonly discussed, the wet method typically involves distribution of a small particle size with a high surface area. Of precipitation-based wet methods, the reactions of orthophosphoric acid (H_3PO_4) with calcium hydroxide ($Ca(OH)_2$) are among the most popular procedures employed. This is a more convenient approach and suitable for the applications to obtain pure HAp, TCP, and biphase comprising HAp and β-TCP, because water is the only by-product [10]. In any case, HAp has attracted a great deal of attention because of its high affinity with biopolymers such as proteins and enzymes [11].

Granulate systems for the delivery and application of drugs are claimed to have enhanced bioavailability, predictable therapeutic response, greater efficacy and safety, and controlled and prolonged drug release time [12-18]. Therefore, the development of granulate systems of calcium phosphate-based drugs (e.g. antibiotics, antimicrobial agents, growth factors, etc.) with controlled drug release kinetics have increasingly become an important area of research, in view of the prevalent rates of infection in bone and dental surgery [14-16].

Several studies have reported the development of HAp granulates by various techniques with irregular or spherical geometry [12-15,17]. Further, porous calcium phosphate ceramics are also expected to play important roles in treating bone problems with the emerging tissue engineering approach, as it involves loading proper cells into porous ceramics (scaffolds) and implanting the cell-loaded scaffolds into a host body for achieving bone tissue regeneration. Summery of the literatures review [15,17-21], a procedure for synthetic of porous spherical HAp granules has been conducted using different polymers (such as gelatin, collagen, chitosan, etc.) as matrices for the preparation of HAp microbeads. For examples, Paul at al. (1999) had porous spherical HAp granules of 200-1000 μm diameter using the synthetic procedures of well-mixed HAp/chitosan slurry in a dispersion medium, the latter being a mixture of heavy and light liquid paraffins [15]. Another procedure for synthetic of porous spherical HAp granules by using oil-in-water emulsions and solvent evaporation technique has been used in the literatures. For example, the porous spherical HAp granules of 50-2000 μm diameter have been produced by the dispersion of well-mixed HAp/polymer slurry in aqueous solution of gelatin and vegetable oil as a dispersion medium [14-16,22].

The first aim of this work was to synthesize and characterize properties of calcium phosphate powders. These precipitations of single phase or biphasic particles have been further examined to reveal the relationships among pH value, Ca/P ratio and especially the amount of glycerol added. The reason for the addition of the glycerol in this work was to increase the solubility of $Ca(OH)_2$ [23]. The second aim was to develop and prepare porous HAp beads by an alginate-interacting Ca ions mechanism on addition of a pore-forming PE powder by sintering process and by using novel water-in-oil emulsions in higher temperature and fast condensation shaping technique. In the present study, we herein report the preparation and characterization of porous beads of definite size with sphere morphology and porosity, by optimizing the quantities of HAp solid powders added and stirring speed, without the modification of other experimental and preparative parameters. Our initial cytotoxic analyses on such calcium phosphates beads demonstrated their potential use for specific applications such as bone filler and drug delivery systems.

Materials and Methods

Synthesis of Calcium Phosphate Powders

The synthesis of HAp has been interpreted in details in our previous study [24,25]. Briefly, Calcium phosphates were synthesized by aqueous precipitation using $Ca(OH)_2$ (Showa, Japan) and H_3PO_4 (Showa, Japan) as the reagents. In the preparation of $Ca(OH)_2$ suspension, the powders were added to the distilled water with a volume percentage of glycerol and stirred using a propeller-like stirrer for 0.5 h.

During the synthesizing procedures, 0.5 M H_3PO_4 aqueous and 0.5 M $Ca(OH)_2$ suspension in distilled water were used. The H_3PO_4 aqueous was slowly added to the $Ca(OH)_2$ suspension at a rate of 30-40 ml/min until the Ca/P molar ratio reached the required value (e.g. 1.5, 1.67 and 2.0). The reaction mixtures were vigorously stirred during the precipitation process, which proceeded at 37 °C. Beginning the reaction period, 1 M tris-(hydroxymethyl) aminomethane (Tedia, USA) and hydrogen chloride solution (0.45 M HCl) (Showa, Japan) were used to adjust the pH value.

The resulting gelatinous precipitate was allowed to react for 24 h, washed three times in distilled water, and then lyophilized for 48 h. The as-synthesized powders were heated from 600 °C to 800°C or 1300 °C for 2 h to examine apatite thermal stability and phase variation at elevated temperatures.

Preparation of Porous Beads by Process (I)

Due to the crosslinking between the carboxylate anions of glucuronate units in alginate and the calcium ions, and biocompatibility alginate gel has also been investigated as a drug delivery device [26]. This study of porous calcium phosphate beads was made by an alginate-interacting Ca ions mechanism on addition of a pore-forming PE powder by sintering process. Aqueous solution of 4% sodium alginate (Lancaster Corp.) was prepared at 50 °C, as a dispersion media. Impart porosity to the ceramic body; the polyethylene (PE) was burned out during firing, leaving free space in the resulting body. The calcination of calcium phosphate powders and near 150 μm size PE (Goodfellow Cambridge Limited, UHMW) powders were added to the sodium alginate solution. The amount of calcium phosphate powder was 3 g in 25 ml of alginate solution, and the PE powder possessed 55% of calcium phosphates. To improve the even dispersion of PE powders existing in the slurry, 1% polyvinyl chloride (PVA) was permitted as an additive. After that, the mixture slurry was squeezed out into small spherical drops by a #18 syringe needle, and then dispersed in 500 ml of 1.5% $CaCl_2$ aqueous solution in a reaction flask by stirring with a Teflon paddle stirrer at 300 rpm. The stirring resulted in bead formation due to the alginate interacting with Ca^{2+} ions. These composite beads were washed in distilled water, and then dried at 50 °C in air for 12 h. They were heated initially at 600 °C for 30 min to burn-off any polymer next. Finally, they were heated at 1250 °C for 120 min in an air furnace to sinter the beads. Briefly the route diagram of the porous calcium phosphates beads prepared by alginate-interacting Ca ions mechanism on addition of a pore-forming PE powder by sintering process was showed in figure 1.

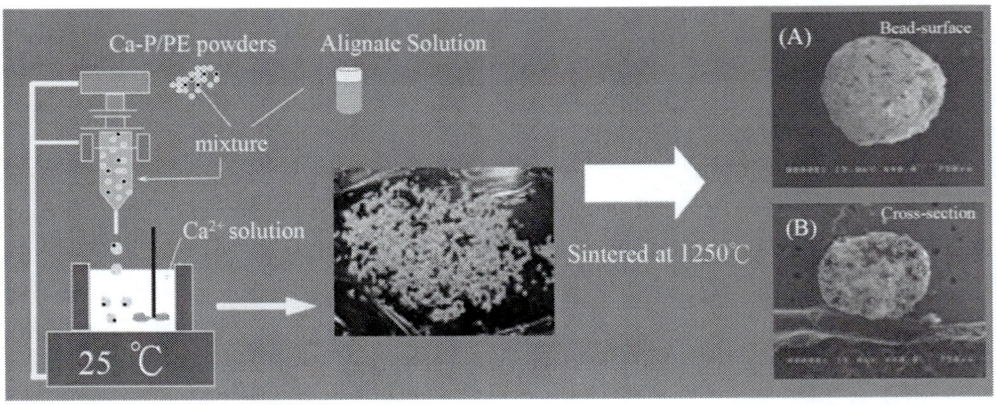

Figure 1. Route diagram of porous hydroxyapatite beads prepared by alginate-interacting Ca ions mechanism on addition of a pore-forming PE powder by sintering process.

Preparation of Porous Beads by Process (II)

Initially, an oil phase with 160 ml olive oil and co-surfactant (1.125% w/v) was prepared by using a magnetic stirrer in a one-liter beaker. The hydrophilic-lipophilic-balance (HLB) value of co-surfactant at 5 was achieved by mixing span80 (Sorbitan monooleate, Showa, Japan) and Brij35 (POE (10) lauryl ether, Acros, USA) with appropriate ratios as calculated.

A solution of 6 wt% agar (Scharlau Microbiology, Spain) in 32 ml water at 80 °C was prepared, and HAp powders (11.76 and 13.23 wt%, respectively) were added into the beaker after calcination at 800 °C, then mixed evenly with homogenizer afterwards. The emulsion of water-in-oil (w/o) was made by pouring the water phase into the oil phase by mixing vigorously at high speed under high temperature. The w/o emulsion was stirred at two different revolutions (ranging from 800~870 and 900~1100 rpm, respectively) with Hot Plates/Stirrers (Corning PC420, USA) at 90±5 °C, and continued for 20 min. The reaction temperature was then reduced to quickly stabilize the particle shape by using a large volume of chilled (4 °C) distilled water. These composite beads were washed with chilled distilled water again, and lyophilized for 48 hr. Next, they were heated initially at 600 °C for 30 min to burn-off any polymer present, and then sintered at 1250 °C for 120 min in an air furnace. The effect of HAp powder quantities and stirring speed on the particle shape, size ranking, porosity analysis and XRD were then evaluated. Briefly the route diagram of porous hydroxyapatite beads prepared by emulsion in higher temperature and fast condensation shaping technique was showed in figure 2. Besides, the different processes of method (II) with their respective processing parameters employed were showed in Table 1.

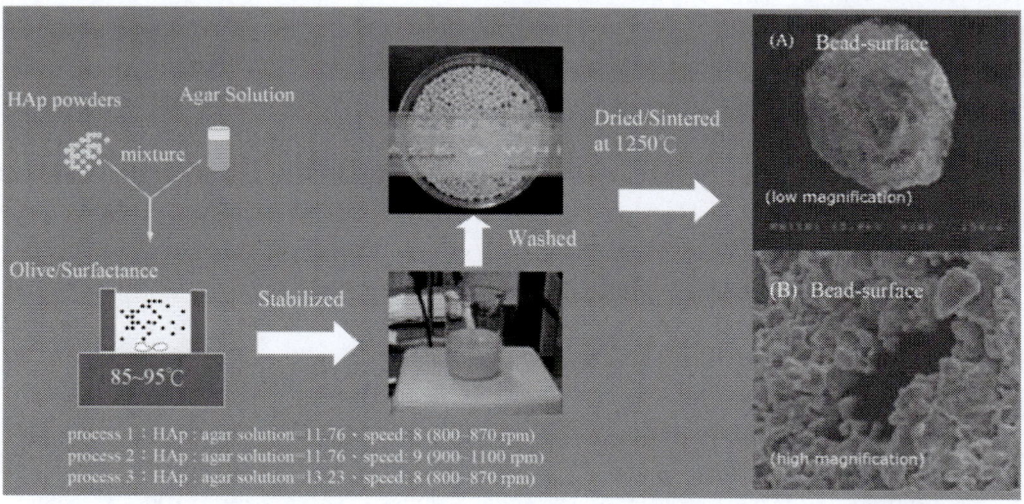

Figure 2. Route diagram of porous hydroxyapatite beads prepared by emulsion in higher temperature and fast condensation shaping technique.

Characterization of Powders

An X-ray diffractometer (Rigaku D-max IIIV, Japan), at 30 kV and 20 mA with a scanning speed of 4°/min, was adopted to identify the phases of various powders. The phase weight percentage was calculated using a standard calibration curve. In brief, a number of control samples were made from the pure materials over a composition range that overlaps the expected range in the target. Diffraction patterns were then prepared for each control sample, and the intensity ratio was calculated based upon two unobscured peaks from each phase. The relative intensity ratio (RIR) of HAp:β-TCP was estimated using the intensity peaks of peaks (211) and (0210) of HAp and β-TCP, respectively, according to the formula

$RIR = I_{\beta\text{-}TCP} / (I_{HAp} + I_{\beta\text{-}TCP})$ [19,27,28]. An FTIR spectrometer (JASCO Corp. FT/IR-410, Japan) was adopted to characterize various functional groups - most importantly, hydroxyl and phosphate groups [29,30]. During the FTIR analysis in the transmittance absorption mode, the heated treatment samples were ground to powder, and mixed with KBr in a weight ratio of 1:100. The analysis was performed over the 400 to 4000 cm^{-1} range.

Characterization of Porous Beads

HAp beads were then sifted and categorized according to the particle size distribution as determined by the use of three different kinds of mesh (200 μm-500 μm, 500 μm-800 μm, and 800 μm-1300 μm) in a utensil. Porosity analysis was carried out using an Archimedes' Principle [31]. This method requires initial measurement of the dry mass of the scaffold followed by pre-wetting with ethanol under negative pressure to saturate the scaffold with water. The scaffold is then removed from water and weighed to determine its wet mass. Subsequently, the scaffold is totally immersed in water and its submerged mass is then recorded. Percent porosity can then be expressed as: $\%\text{Porosity} = (M_{\text{wet}} - M_{\text{dry}})/(M_{\text{wet}} - M_{\text{submerged}}) \times 100\%$. In addition, the volume of the pore size on process (I) samples that lower than 10 μm was valuated by mercury porosimetry (Quantachrome PoreMaster 60, Germany). Morphological investigation of HAp porous beads with different processing was carried out after sintering, using a scanning electron microscope (SEM) (S-4200, Hitachi, Japan). The Ca/P ratios of the synthesized powders were determined using an energy dispersive spectrometer (EDS) (Noran, USA) and an the inductively coupled plasma - optical emission spectrometer (ICP-OES) (Perkin-Elmer, OPTIMA-2000, USA).

Toxic Evaluation on Cell Culture

The mice mesenchymal stem cell-line (D1) was used in toxic evaluation. Cells were cultivated in Dulbecco's modified Eagle's medium (DMEM) containing 10% fetal calf serum (FCS), 0.01% ascorbic acid, nonessential amino acids and 100 U per ml penicillin/streptomycin (Gibco-BRL, USA) at 37 °C in a humidified incubator containing 5% CO_2. The culture medium was replenished every two days and for subculture, the cell monolayers were rinsed with phosphate-buffered saline (PBS) and detached by incubating them with 0.25% Trypsin-EDTA for 5 min at 37 °C. Changes in the cell viability of the D1 cells were quantitatively assessed with 3-(4, 5-dimethylthiazol-2-yl)-diphenyl tetrazolium bromide (MTT) (Sigma, USA) at 24 h culture periods. The MTT assay is a rapid colorimetric method to determine viable cell numbers, which is based on mitochondrial conversion of MTT to MTT formazan.

For the evaluation of the cytotoxicity in direct contact with cells, a concentration of 2,000 cells per well was seeded on a 96-well cell culture plate and cultured at 37 °C in a humidified incubator containing 5% CO_2. After cells reached confluence, the porous beads (previously sterilized by exposure under ultra violet overnight) were placed onto each well and cultured at 37 °C in a humidified incubator containing 5% CO_2. Culture plates without porous beads were used as controls. After 20 h of cultivation, 10 μl of MTT solution (5 mg per ml in PBS) was added to each well and incubated for another 4 h (at 37 °C) for MTT formazan formation. Purple formazan on each well was extracted with 200 μl dimethyl sulfoxide (DMSO). The optical density (OD) of produced MTT formazan in the solution was measured with an ELISA reader (SLT, Crailheim, Germany) at a wavelength of 570 nm, with readings of wells containing solely DMSO as blanks. Data were collected and averaged from the six to eight different wells per experimental condition. Finally, the *t*-test statistical analysis was used to evaluate the statistical significance of the cell toxicity data.

Results and Discussions

Preparation of Porous Beads by Process (I)

Characterization of Calcium Phosphate Powders (I) - Phase Structure Analysis

Figure 3(a) presents the X-ray powder diffraction patterns from the pH value of 7.4 with the Ca to P ratio of 1.67 raw material. The reaction temperature of 37 °C was chosen because it was very near to the body temperature. The precipitated calcium phosphates give a similar poorly crystallized apatite structure (JCPDS file number 9-432) as shown in the as-synthesized pattern of figure 3(a). As in the figure 3(a) 800 °C pattern, the slight β-TCP phase coexisted in the main HAp phase by calcination at 800 °C. This is probably because the precipitates are formed as CDHA, so that it is considered to decompose partly by calcination into β-TCP, [29,32] a stable phase. The β-tricalcium phosphate (JCPDS file number 9-169) is another type of highly bioactive implantable material, exposed to the body's fluids, the β-TCP underwent a biointegration process involving biodissolution/biodegradation, then apatite crystal will be precipitated, and the final bone formation onto the implant surface [2,32]. Besides, upon heating to 800 °C, the powder showed a substantial increase in peak height, and an associated drop in peak width, which corresponded to an increase in crystallinity. Consequently, the (102), (210) and (202) of the apatite diffractograms appeared around 28°, 29° and 34° [29]. The phase weight percentage was calculated by using the standard calibration curve and the relative intensity ratio (RIR) of the HAp:β-TCP was estimated using the intensity peaks of peaks (211) and (217) of HAp and β-TCP respectively, using the formula, $RIR=I_{\beta\text{-TCP}} / (I_{HAp}+I_{\beta\text{-TCP}})$. Figure 3(a) depicts the HAp/β-TCP was close to 92/8 after 800 °C heat treatment.

Figure 3(b) presents the X-ray powder diffraction patterns from the pH value of 6.4 with the Ca to P ratio of 1.5 raw material. The XRD patterns of the as-synthesized calcium phosphates gave a very poor crystalline structure as well, but the structure almost appeared to be the β-TCP phase when the heating temperature reached 800 °C. The phase weight percentage calculation result showed the HAp/β-TCP was close to 10/90 after 800 °C heat treatment. Several studies have explained that the CDHA would transfer to β-TCP without the second phase of CaO at high temperature, but the stoichiometric HAp phase exhibited phase transformation to β-TCP with the second phase of CaO at high temperatures [2,32-34].

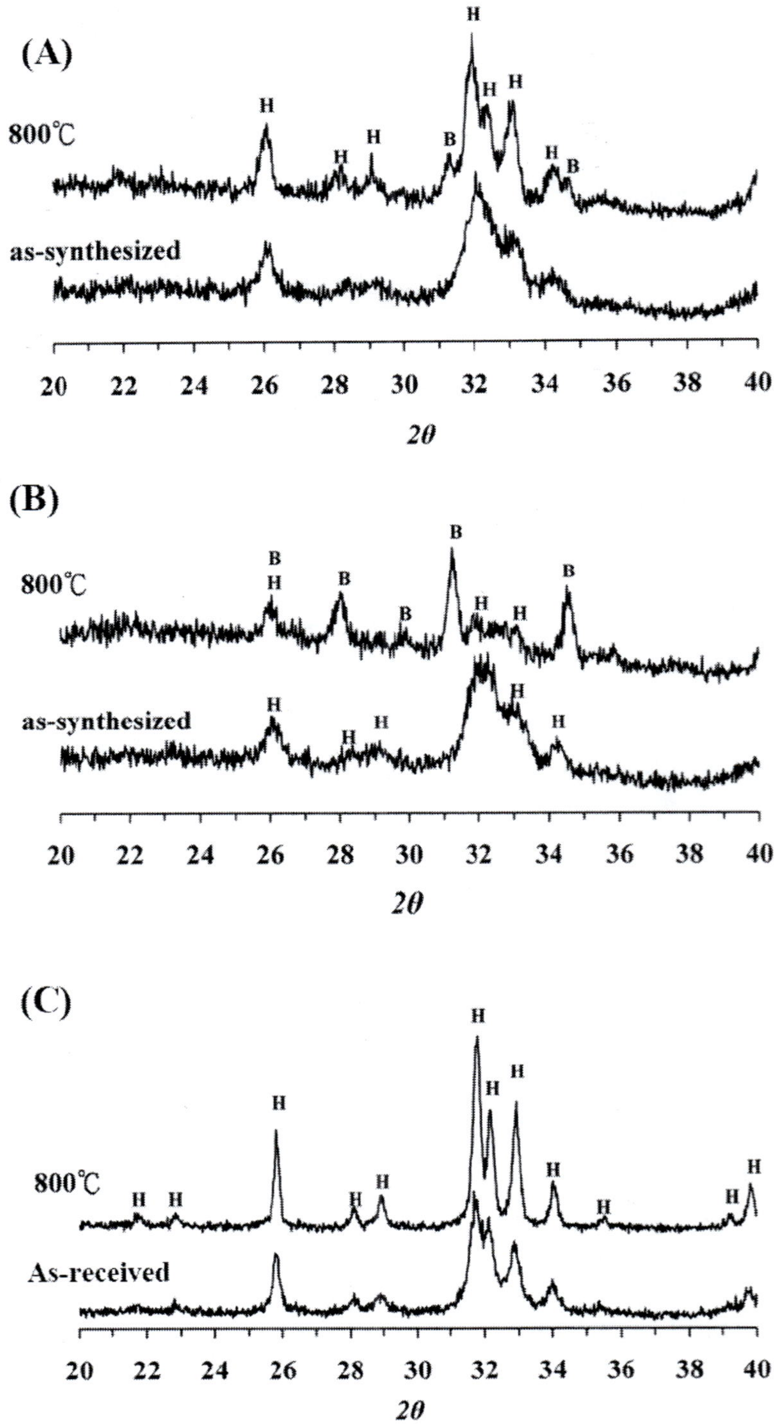

Figure 3. XRD patterns of as-synthesized/as-received powders and heat treated at 800 °C. Synthesis conditions were pH value of 7.4 and Ca/P ratio of 1.67 (A) and pH value of 6.4 and Ca/P ratio of 1.5 (B). As-received powder of Alfa Aesar® HAp (A Jahnson Matthey Company) was (C). (H: apatite, B: β-TCP).

Other researches have described the mechanisms of the solid state transformation of a CDHA into BCP at elevated temperatures as being an alternative route to obtain BCP materials [35,36]. However, the figure 3(c) of XRD was showed as a single-phase HAp after 800 °C heated treatment from commercial HAp powder (Alfa Aesar®) and it showed a substantial increase in peak height, and an associated drop in peak width, which corresponded to an increase in crystallinity still. The results showed this commercial HAp powder had excellent thermal stability. Generally, the as-synthesized calcium phosphate product with Ca to P ratios distant from 1.67 was known to be less thermally stable [37].

Characterization of Calcium Phosphate Powders (I) - Functional Group Analysis

Figure 4 presents the FTIR spectral patterns of 800 °C heat treated samples from β-TCP rich phase (the pH value of 6.4 with the Ca to P ratio of 1.5) raw material (A) and HAp rich phase (the pH value of 7.4 with the Ca to P ratio of 1.67) raw material (B). They were found to correspond with the XRD pattern of figure 3(b) and figure 3(a), respectively. The characteristic OH group absorption bands of 640 cm^{-1} and the bands at 1092 cm^{-1}, 1044 cm^{-1}, 1036 cm^{-1}, 960 cm^{-1}, 573 cm^{-1}, and 475 cm^{-1} were assigned to the vibration in the phosphate group of the HAp [38,39]. Additionally, the vibration in the phosphate group absorption bands of β-TCP was at 1120 cm^{-1}, 1042 cm^{-1}, 971 cm^{-1}, 948 cm^{-1}, 604 cm^{-1} and 433 cm^{-1}, respectively [5,37].

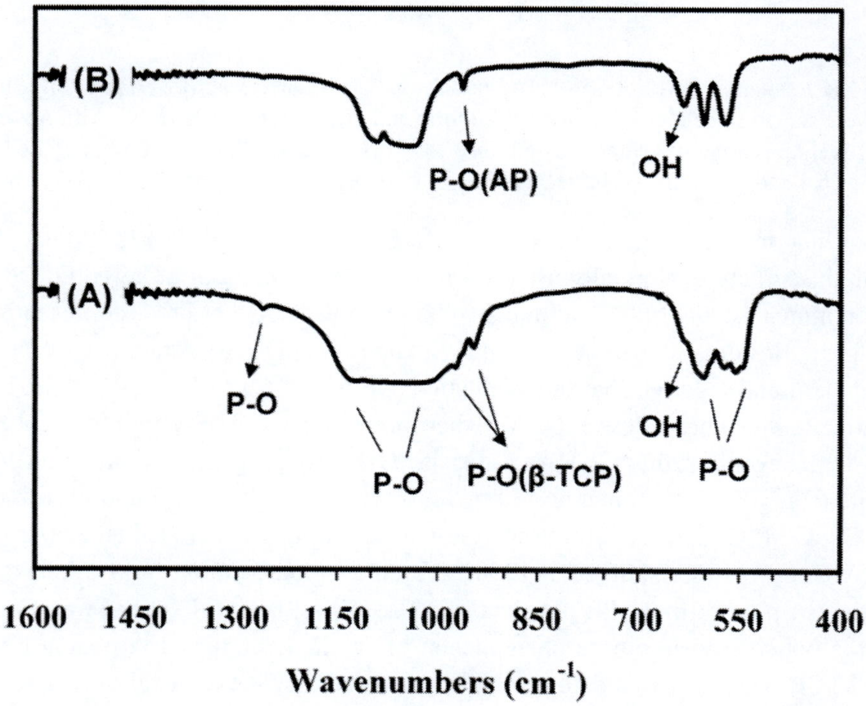

Figure 4. FTIR spectra of as-synthesized powder heat treated at 800 °C. Synthesis conditions were pH value of 7.4 and Ca/P ratio of 1.67 (A) and pH value of 6.4 and Ca/P ratio of 1.5 (B).

Characterization of Porous Beads (I) - Phase Structure Analysis

Figure 5 shows the X-ray powder diffraction patterns at 1250 °C sintered porous beads from three kinds of powders were made in the above mentioned. The patterns all demonstrated neither to be HAp peaks nor β-TCP peaks.

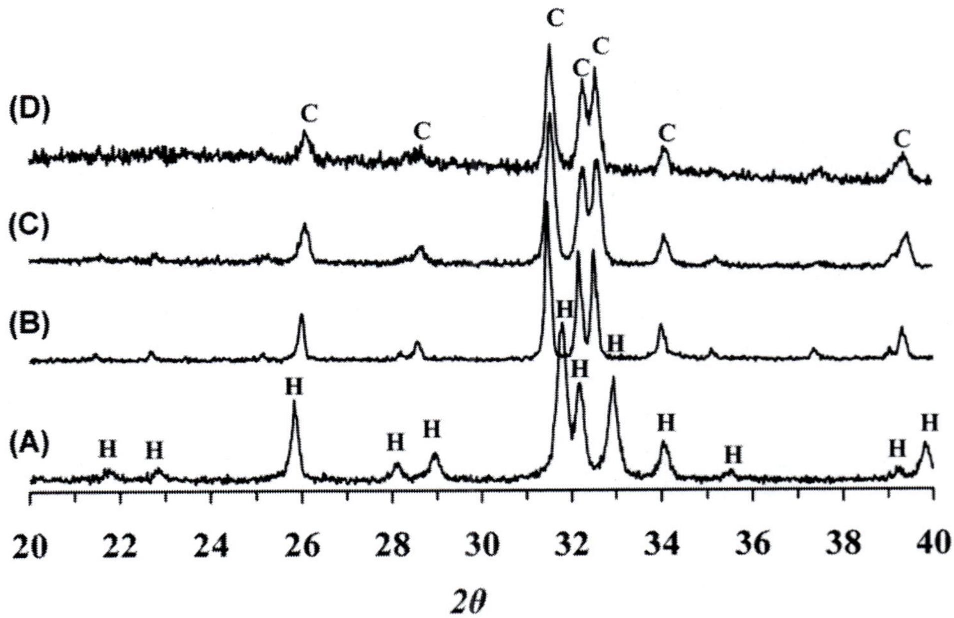

Figure 5. XRD patterns of Alfa Aesar® HAp powder at 800 °C heat treatment (A) and three kinds powder were shown since they were made bead form and then sintered at 1250 °C. Alfa Aesar® HAp powder (B). HAp powder of synthesis conditions were pH value of 7.4 and Ca/P ratio of 1.67 (C) and pH value of 6.4 and Ca/P ratio of 1.5 (H: apatite, C: CDHA) (D).

According to the JCPDS file number 46-0905, the $Ca_9(HPO_4)(PO_4)_5OH$ phase was correct in this structure. Normally, BCP is produced by sintering of a $Ca_9(HPO_4)(PO_4)_5OH$ at the temperatures 1000-1200 °C although the mechanism of this process presently remains unclear [36]. Besides, de Groot et al. [2] studied the high-temperature characteristics of synthetic HAp and reported that the synthetic HAp with a Ca to P ratio near 1.67 was only stable at the temperature below 1200 °C, when sintered in a dry or wet air atmosphere. It was claimed that beyond 1200 °C, HAp loses its OH^- groups gradually and transforms into oxyapatite ($Ca_{10}(PO_4)_6O$). When heated to 1450 °C, oxyapatite was found to heat dissociate into β-TCP, $Ca_2P_2O_7$ and $Ca_4P_2O_9$. Regardless of the starting materials being HAp, β-TCP or biphase, when they were sintered at 1250 °C by the alginate-interacting Ca ions mechanism on addition of pore-forming PE powders, the $Ca_9(HPO_4)(PO_4)_5OH$ phase was formed only. This is the opposite view on the phenomenon of calcium-deficient HAp being divided into HAp and TCP. Then, it was a defective structure created by the removal of a mole CaO from the stoichiometric HAp [40,41]. However, in this study, we provided calcium ions from $CaCl_2$ aqueous for the alginate-interacting Ca ions mechanism, so it may have formed HAp with Ca-rich residual first, then CDHA appeared by elevating the temperature to 1250 °C and removing CaO. Finally, CDHA loses its HPO_4 group gradually and transforms into nonstoichiometry CDHA beyond 1250 °C. From this chemical point of view, the following relation of (1), (2), and (3) may exist in TCP, CDHA and HAp:

$$3Ca_3(PO_4)_2 + Ca^{2+} + 2OH^- \leftrightarrow Ca_{10}(PO_4)_6(OH)_2 \quad (1)$$

$$Ca_{10}(PO_4)_6(OH)_2 \leftrightarrow Ca_9(HPO_4)(PO_4)_5OH + CaO \quad (2)$$

$$Ca_9(HPO_4)(PO_4)_5OH \leftrightarrow Ca_{9-x}(HPO_4)_x(PO_4)_{5-x}(OH)_{1-x}\ (0\leq x\leq 1) \quad (3)$$

Characterization of Porous Beads (I) - Porosity and Pore Volume Analysis

The most important novel porous bead method used in this study to produce macro- and micro- porous calcium phosphate bioceramic parts, were shown to be successful in the achievement of total porosity values over the range of 62.5±3.7% from HAp rich phase raw material and 55.7±5.3% from β-TCP rich phase raw material (Table 2).

The main control of the porosity values in the final, sintered CDHA samples were found to be attained by essentially changing the amounts of PE, concentrations of agar solution, and the raw materials phase used in the processing of the slurries, which yielded the green beads. Owing to the density of theory of hyroxyapatite (3.156 g/cm^3) higher than the density of theory of β-TCP (3.07 g/cm^3) [29], while adding with the same 55 vol% PE, the PE amount within HAp rich phase which being added can be more than β-TCP rich phase. However, it can obtain the more porosity at raw material of HAp phase rich than at raw material of β-TCP phase rich.

Table 1. Different processes of method (II) with their respective processing parameters employed

Process no.	HAp : agar solution (weight ratio)	Speed of stir
1	11.76	800~870 rpm
2	11.76	900~1100 rpm
3	13.23	800~870 rpm
4	13.23	900~1100 rpm

Table 2. Porosity of beads were obtained by method (I)

Raw Materials	Synthesis conditions were pH value of 7.4 and Ca/P ratio of 1.67 (HAp rich phase)	Synthesis conditions were pH value of 6.4 and Ca/P ratio of 1.5 (β-TCP rich phase)
Porosity of porous beads	62.5±3.7%	55.7±5.3%

In addition, the lower than 10 μm micopore part in our CDHA bioceramics produced with 20.3 vol.% from HAp rich phase raw material and 12.5% vol.% from β-TCP rich phase raw material. Because the concentration of agar was the same condition in this research, so the difference of micropores mainly comes from the amount of PE and raw material structure differently. Whatever, it assumed that the higher porosity presented by these materials can provide diffusion pathways and ample room for drug adsorption and drug delivery.

Characterization of Porous Beads (I)- Surface and Cross Section Morphology

A view of a porous bead is shown in figure 6(a) from HAp rich phase raw material. The bead shape appeared as a porous sphere, and their sizes were between 0.9 mm and 1.1 mm in diameter. There were some larger pores from 60 µm to 120 µm on the surface, which were made by PE powder residual. The cross-section of the porous bead as shown in figure 6(b), showed well-dispersed pores when a little PVA surfactant was used. However, the pore size within the inner part of the beads was similar to the appearance of the pores on the surface. The porous bead was made from the raw material of β-TCP rich phase, as shown in figure 7(a) and (b). The porous characteristics were similar between the HAp raw material and the β-TCP rich phase raw material.

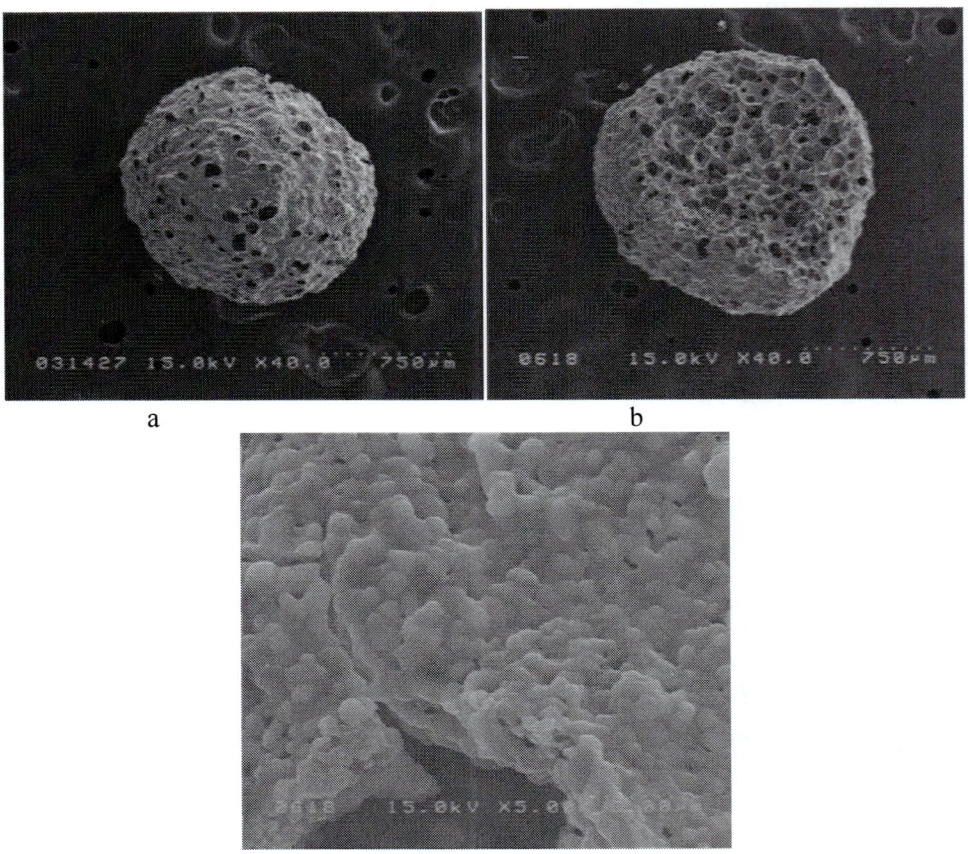

Figure 6. SEM photographs of porous calcium phosphate bead, which raw powder synthesized at pH value of 7.4 and Ca/P ratio of 1.67. surface (×40) (A); cross-section (×40) (B); surface (×5000) (C).

As SEM shows in figure 6(c) from HAp raw material, there were irregular micropores lower than 10 µm and crevices were observed; these were considered to be the densification process hindered at the sintering stage, since the alginate sodium and PE burnt off. The grain sizes of the surface and within the bead were 0.2 μm to 1.2 μm. Besides, this grain surface appeared smooth. Similar observations were shown in figure 7(c) from β-TCP raw material.

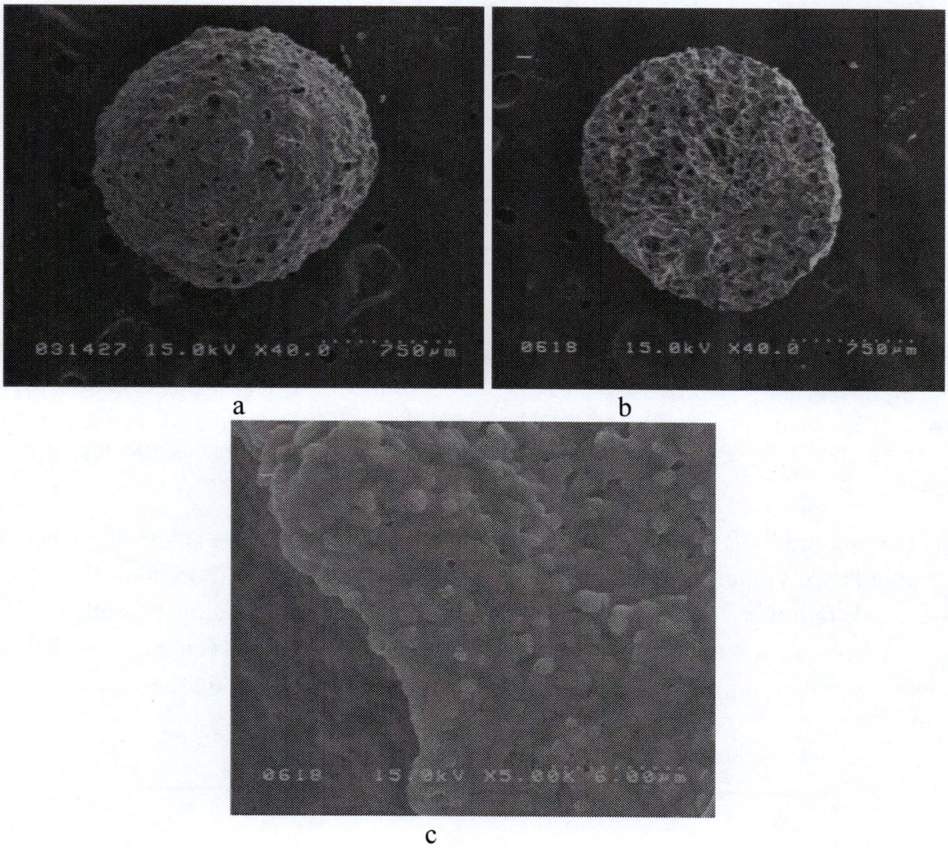

Figure 7. SEM photographs of porous calcium phosphate bead, which raw powder synthesized at pH value of 6.4 and Ca/P ratio of 1.5. surface (×40) (A); cross-section (×40) (B); surface (×5000) (C).

Preparation of Porous Beads by Process (II)

Characterization of Calcium Phosphate Powders (II) - Phase Structure Analysis

Figure 8 presents the XRD patterns of as-synthesized samples which were synthesized at a Ca/P ratio of 2.0, a pH value of 10 and 10-vol% glycerol in aqueous $Ca(OH)_2$. It was presented as a single-phase HAp at 1300 °C. The apatite synthesized under such reaction conditions exhibited good thermal stability. From the evolution of the Ca/P ratio of figure 8 sample showed as-synthesized HAp was presented 1.78 and 1.68, as determined from EDS and ICP-OES, respectively. The little but consistently higher Ca/P ratio of the as-received powders determined by EDS were slightly but consistently the higher, found in the as-received powder suggests that the electron beam bombarded the to samples, causing a little highly-volatile phosphorus to escape from calcium phosphates.

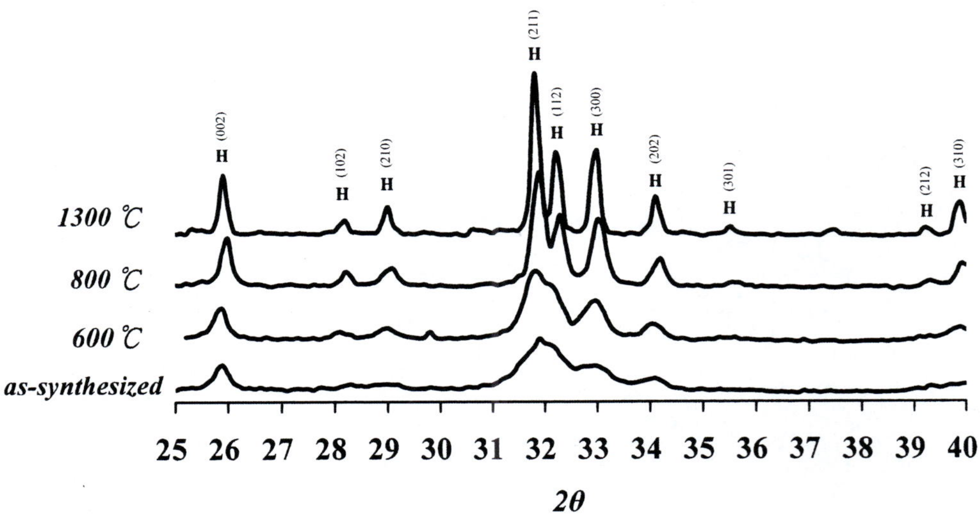

Figure 8. XRD patterns of as-synthesized and heat-treated samples at a synthesis Ca/P ratio of 2.0 with a pH value of 10.0 and 10-vol% glycerol in aqueous $Ca(OH)_2$. (ACP: amorphous calcium phosphates, H: apatite, B: β-TCP).

Therefore, the Ca/P ratio was close to the theoretical value of the HAp, which is regarded as the pure HAp. Therefore, the addition of 10-vol% glycerol would not alter the stability of apatite at all, following heat treatment at 1300 °C in this study. Obviously, both a higher pH value (ex. between 8.4 and 10) and a critical Ca/P ration (ex. between 1.67 and 2.0) during synthesis were two important factors that greatly exhibit influence on the stability of apatite at 1300 °C.

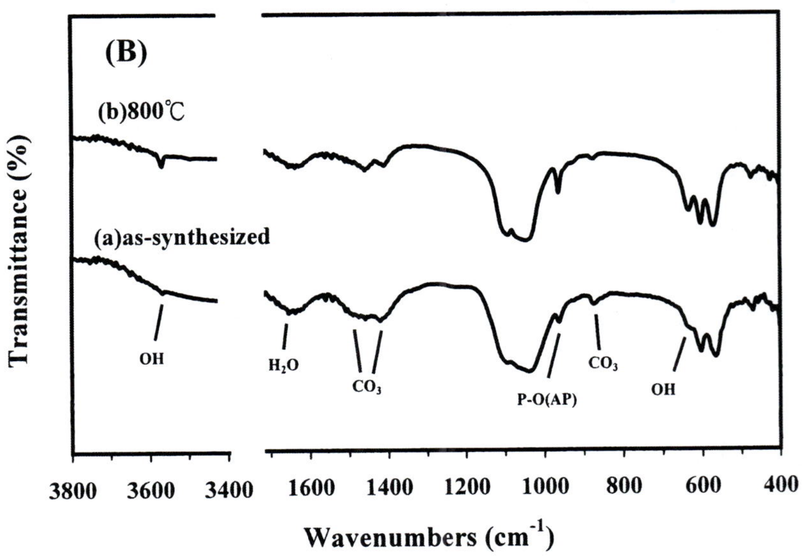

Figure 9. FTIR patterns of as-synthesized and heat-treated samples at a synthesis Ca/P ratio of 2.0 with a pH value of 10.0 and 10-vol% glycerol in aqueous $Ca(OH)_2$.

Characterization of Calcium Phosphate Powders (II)- Functional Group Analysis

Figure 9 presents the FTIR spectral patterns of the as-synthesized (a) and 800 °C heat-treated (b) samples which were precipitated at a pH of 10, a Ca/P ratio of 1.67, and 10-vol% of glycerol. This precipitation was consistent with the XRD patterns of pure HAp, as presented in figure 8. The characteristic hydroxyl group absorption bands from HAp were at 3575 cm^{-1} and 640 cm^{-1} respectively. The other bands at 1092 cm^{-1}, 1044 cm^{-1}, 1036 cm^{-1}, 960 cm^{-1}, 573 cm^{-1} and 475 cm^{-1} were assigned to the vibrations in the PO_4^{3-} group of the HAp. The pure HAp structure appears to have stable OH and C-O bands at 800 °C. The overall apatite structure of HAp remained undisturbed at 800 °C, as indicated by the aforementioned XRD results (figure 8). Based on the above XRD and FTIR data, the synthesis temperature of 37 °C with a Ca/P ratio of 2.0, a pH value of 10 and a 10-vol% of glycerol, will achieve the formation of thermally stable apatite phase.

Characterization of Porous Beads (II) - Shrinkage Observation and Particle Size Distribution

It has been well-documented by various researchers that different experimental parameters of the emulsion process will have influence on porous bead properties after sintering (such as shrinkage ratio of porous beads, particle size distribution and porosity, etc.). These above-mentioned experimental parameters include concentration of agar gel, temperature of hydroxyapatite calcination, solid to water ratio in aqueous $Ca(OH)_2$ solution, stirring speed in the emulsion, water phase to oil phase ratio, emulsion temperature, and surfactant types, etc. However, according to the author's experience (for example, emulsions were unable to promote the formation of spherical bodies from raw materials when stirring speed was less than 600 rpm). Furthermore, data from scientific literature also indicated that the low-hydrophile-lipophile-balance (HLB) is dominantly hydrophobic and is added to the oil phase) [42]. Our approach in current study established a novel emulsion system where the quantities of HAp solid powder added and stirring speed were two crucial parameters considered. In Table 1, the parameters of four processes are shown and compared.

In Process 4, the tendency to form rodlike granules was mainly due to the high solid-to-liquid ratio (13.23) and high stirring speed (900-1100 rpm). In other words, when the viscosity of HAp/agar slurry was too high, samples were easily transformed into the short-rodlike shape by strong shear force. Morphologically, samples tended to wrap gas into their interiors and become suspended, resulting in the failure of formation of emulsified spheres. Sound spherical granules were achieved by all other three processes. Process 2, with higher stirring speed and lower solid-to-liquid weight ratio (11.76), was found that gas could sometimes easily be wrapped inside to cause a suspension state at higher stirring speed, whereas spheres with higher shrinkage rate could be obtained once agar had shrunk and gas was extracted during the lyophilizing process. It is clear that residual pores and barrier (ex. agar) will cause lower densification at the sintering stage [43]. Additionally, lower stirring speed and lyophilization treatments tended to yield higher shrinkage rates after sintering and resulted in the production of high-density spheres.

Figure 10 demonstrates that the particle distribution range between 200~1300 μm in diameter for three processes. The distributions of weight percentage of spheres with different diameters were similar between Processes 1 and 3, with the majority (~78%) being within the 800~1300 μm in size range whereas 19% of the spheres were within the 500~800 μm size range. Only a small percentage of spheres were within the 200~500 μm size range. However, in Process 2, almost 59 % of spheres were within the 500~800 μm size range. This is likely due to the fact that higher stirring speed and lower emulsion viscosity make it easier to create smaller spheres with more even sizes. In support of this, Pradeesh et al. [22] have explained the breaking down of larger droplets into smaller droplets in the dispersed phase with increased stirring speed.

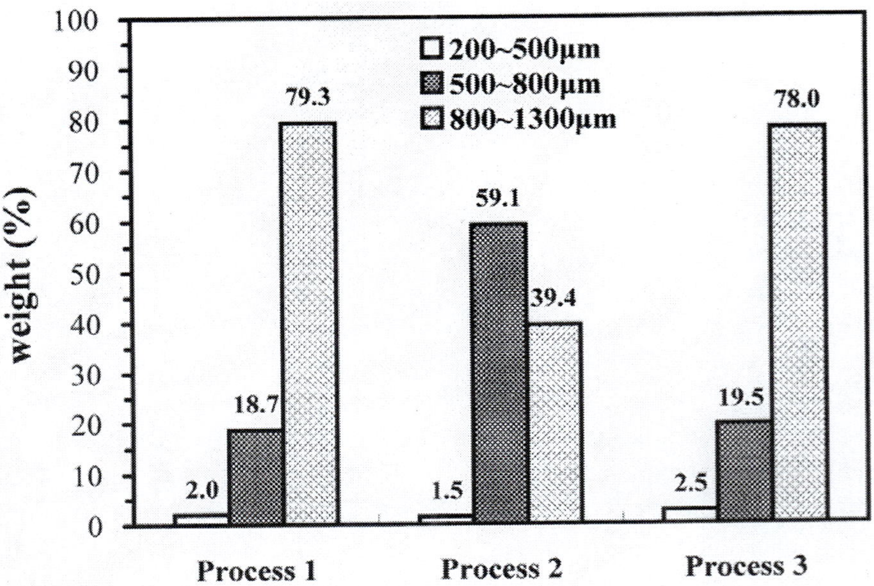

Figure 10. The weight ratios of size distribution of porous beads were measured for different processes. Raw materials were synthesized at a Ca/P ratio of 2.0 with a pH value of 10 and 10-vol% glycerol in aqueous $Ca(OH)_2$.

Characterization of Porous Beads (II)-Surface Morphology and Porosity

As per the SEM photographs of porous beads shown in figure 11 (A, B) from Process 1, there were irregular smaller pores (smaller than 3 μm) and crevices than those shown in figure 11 (C, D) (smaller than 15 μm) from Process 2 observed. Moreover, the grain structure of surface of spheres obtained from Process 1 appeared closer to that obtained from Process 2. These were considered to result from the densification process hindering the sintering stage, due to pore residue and agar burn-off. Besides, the grain sizes of the surface were about 0.5 to 3 μm in these two processes. Additionally, spheres obtained from Process 1 exhibited better strength for density, when the porous beads were being crushed and examined bare-handed, than those from Process 2.

Table 3 shows the results of porosity analyses on beads from Processes 1 and 3 were ~57.4±2.2% porosity and ~58.6±3.7% porosity respectively; whereas the result for Process 2 was ~61.4±3.1% porosity, indicating both Processes 1 and 3 achieved higher degrees of densification after sintering. On the other hand, the lower degree of densification by Process 2 was mainly due to more pore residues remaining after completion of the process.

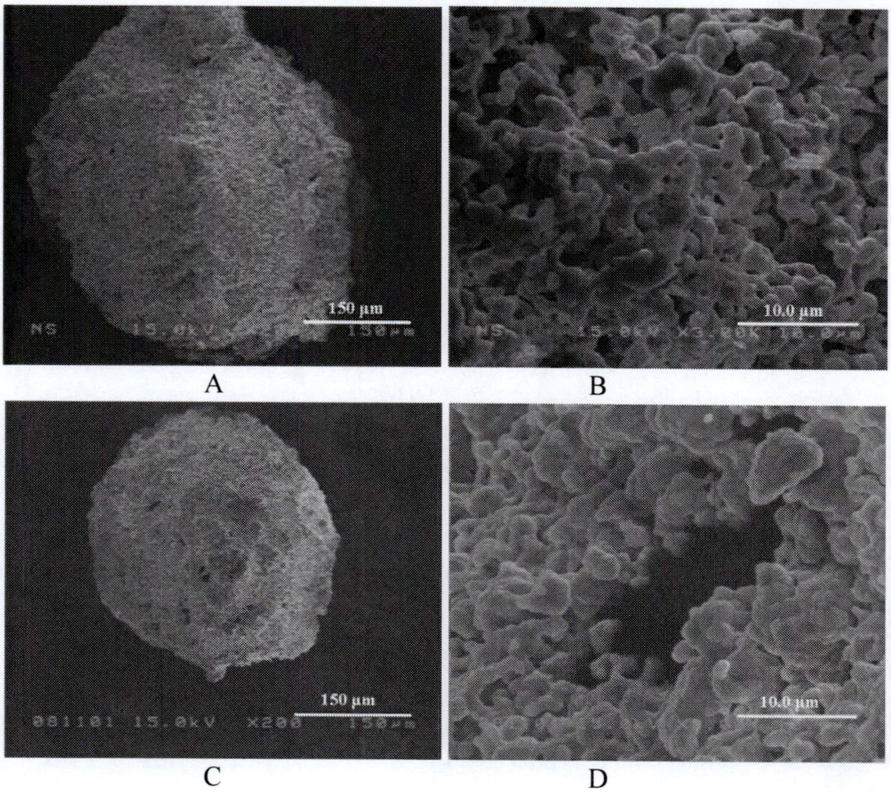

Figure 11. SEM photographs of porous bead sintered at 1250 °C (A and B from Process 1, C and D from Process 2, respectively), with raw materials synthesized at a Ca/P ratio of 2.0 with a pH value of 10 and 10-vol% glycerol in aqueous $Ca(OH)_2$.

Table 3. Porosity of beads were obtained by different processes of method (II)

	Process 1	Process 2	Process 3
Porosity of porous beads	57.4%±2.2	61.4±3.1%	58.6%±3.7

Furthermore, the higher degree of porosity with adequate mechanical pressures could enhance the adhesion of cells and flowing of liquid nutrients through the materials, which are basic and essential requirements for any biomaterial aimed at being used as a supporting scaffold of cell/tissue cultures or controlled drug-releasing vectors.

Characterization of Porous Beads (II) - Phase Structure Analysis

Figure 12 presents the X-ray powder diffraction patterns of porous beads sintered at 1250 °C from all process. It is clear that the HAp peaks are still present. Besides, Zhou et al. [34] studied the high-temperature characteristics of synthetic HAp and reported that the synthetic

HAp with a Ca/P ratio near 1.67 was stable only below 1200 °C, when being sintered either in a dry or wet air atmosphere.

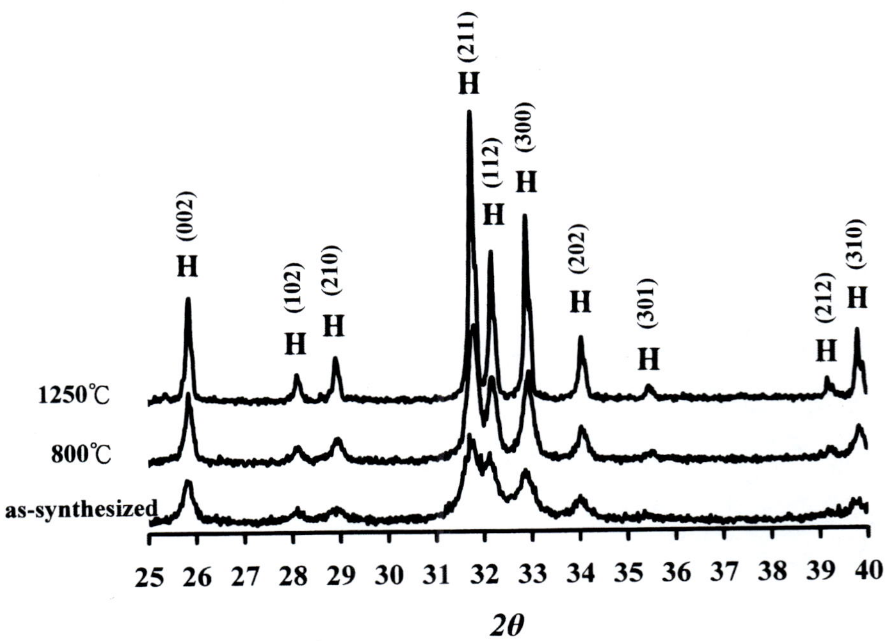

Figure 12. The XRD patterns of as-synthesized apatite powder, heat-treated at 800 °C, and porous bead sintered at 1250 °C. Raw materials were synthesized at a Ca/P ratio of 2.0 with a pH value of 10 and 10-vol% glycerol in aqueous Ca(OH)2.(H: apatite).

It was claimed that HAp loses its OH^- groups gradually and transforms into oxyapatite ($Ca_{10}(PO_4)_6O$) when the reaction temperature was elevated beyond 1200 °C. When being heated to 1450 °C, oxyapatite was found to dissociate into β-TCP, $Ca_2P_2O_7$ and $Ca_4P_2O_9$. However, the XRD patterns showed no significant difference between hydroxyapatite and oxyapatite.

Cell Toxicity Evaluation

Cytotoxicity testing includes numerous methods, both qualitative and quantitative. In this study, we used an indirect test in which the metabolic activity (conversion of MTT to MTT formazan) indicated the degree of cytotoxicity.

Table 4. Evaluation of cell toxicity of beads obtained from two methods by MTT assays

	Control	HAp rich phase of method (I)	Process (1, 2, 3) of method (II)
MEAN (O.D.)	0.506	0.501	0.508
SD	0.053	0.025	0.0253
t-TEST	0.500	0.452	0.467

The effects of porous bead samples (from Processes 1-3) and control group on the viability of mice mesenchymal stem cell-line (D1) were measured with MTT test. As results shown in Table 4, MTT activity values of the both of porous beads were found the MTT-absorbing value of cell activation on porous beads can still maintain a good quantity, and the *t*-test results show P value to be significantly greater than 0.05 as well. Therefore, we believe that HAp porous beads obtained in this study should not be toxic to cells.

Conclusion

The data introduce that β-TCP rich, CDHA rich and pure HAp can be obtained at the beginning of the synthesis by controlling various factors such as the pH value, the Ca/P ratio, the heat-treated temperature and the addition of some glycerol. Additionally, the presence of glycerol unaffected the stability of the apatite phase of spheres when being heat-treated from 800 °C to 1300°C. The thermal stability of hydroxyapatite phase was obtained to 1300 °C, while synthesis was done at the pH value of 10.0 with a Ca/P ratio of 2.0 and a synthesis temperature of 37 °C and 10-vol% glycerol in aqueous $Ca(OH)_2$.

In this report we introduce two new routes to form porous bioceramic beads, one is that porous bead prepared by alginate-interacting Ca ions mechanism on addition of a pore-forming PE powder by sintering process, another one is by water-in-oil emulsions in higher temperature and fast condensation shaping technique. Experimental results of the former were showed that, regardless of the raw materials being HAp rich, TCP rich or pure HAp, when they were sintered at 1250 °C by the alginate-interacting Ca ions mechanism on addition of a pore-forming polyethylene (PE) powder, the $Ca_9(HPO_4)(PO_4)_5OH$ phase (CDHA) was formed only. Porous beads of various calcium phosphates with different sizes (0.9-1.1 mm) and pore size groups (60-120 μm and lower than 10 μm) appeared. Besides, the novel water-in-oil system for the preparation of HAp beads, our data indicated that can succeed in forming porous bead. Besides, differences in stirring speeds and solid-to-liquid ratios could largely influence the size, morphology, and porosity of the beads made. The inclusions of agar, olive, and surfactants (e.g. span80, Brij35) still maintain the apatite phase structure of porous HAp beads sintered at 1250 °C during the preparation process. Our assays of such porous calcium phosphates beads on cell cytotoxicity also indicated their incapability of inducing toxicity to D1 cells, which evidently enhance their potential future application as a carrier for therapeutic delivery potential and bone formaton of filler.

Acknowledgements

The authors gratefully acknowledge the support for this research by the Ministry of Economic Affairs and National Science Council in Taiwan under the grant numbers 94-EC-17-A-17-S1-041 and NSC92-2218-E-037-001, respectively.

References

[1] L.L. Hench, Bioceramics, *J. Am. Ceram. Soc.* 81 (1998) 1705.

[2] K. de Groot, C.P.A.T. Klein, J.G.C. Wolke, H.J.M.A. dB, in: T. Yamamoto, L.L. Hench, J. Wilson (Ed.), CRC *Handbook of Bioactive Ceramics Volume II Calcium Phosphate and Hydroxylapatite Ceramics*, CRC press, Boca Raton, Florida, 1990, p.3.

[3] C.P.A.T. Klein, A.A. Driessen, K. de Groot, A. van den Hooff, *J. Biomed. Mater. Res.* 17 (1983) 769.

[4] G. Daculsi, O. Laboux, O. Malard, P. Weiss, *J. Mater. Sci. Mater. Med.* 14 (2003) 195.

[5] M. Jarcho, R.L. Salsbury, M.B. Thomas, R.H. Doremus, *J. Mater. Sci. Mater. Med.* 14 (1979) 142.

[6] F.H. Lin, C.J. Liao, K.S. Chen, J.S. Sun, *Biomaterials* 19 (1998) 1101.

[7] N. Kivrat, A.C. Tas, *J. Am. Ceram. Soc.* 81 (1998) 2245.

[8] L.C. Whelan, M.P. Morgan, G.M. McCarthy, *Front Biosci* 10 (2005) 530.

[9] R.Z. LeGeros, S. Lin, R. Rohanizadeh, D. Mijares, J.P. LeGeros, *J. Mater. Sci. Mater. Med.* 14 (2003) 201.

[10] S.W.K. Kweh, K.A. Khor, P. Cheang, *J. Mater. Pro. Tech.* 89-90 (1999) 373.

[11] K. Kandori, A. Fudo, T. Ishikawa, *Colloids Surf. B: Biointerf.* 24 (2002) 145.

[12] K. Ioku, G. Kawachi, M. Toda, S. Sasaki, H. Fujimori, S. Goto, in: N.M. Nakahara, M. Ueno, K. Yasuoka, K. IAPWS Watanabe (Ed.), *Proceedings of the 14th International Conference on the Properties of Water and Steam*, Kyoto, Japan, 2005, p.259.

[13] V.S. Komlev, S.M. Barinov, E. Girardin, S. Oscarsson, A. Rosengren, F. Rustichelli, *Sci. Tech. Adv. Mater.* 4 (2003) 503.

[14] V.S. Komleva, S.M. Barinova, E.V. Koplikb, *Biomaterials* 23 (2002) 3449.

[15] W. Paul, S.T. Sharma, *J. Mat. Sci. Mat. Med.* 10 (1999) 383.

[16] T.S. Pradeesh, M.C. Sunny, H.K. Varma, P. Ramesh, *Bull. Mater. Sci.* 28 (2005) 383.

[17] T. Matsumoto, M. Okazaki, M. Inoue, S. Yamaguchi, T. Kusunose, T. Toyonaga, *Biomaterials* 25 (2004) 3807.

[18] M. Sivakumar, P.K. Rao, *Biomaterials*, 23 (2002) 3175.

[19] W.C. Chen, C.P. Ju, J.C. Wang, C.C. Hung, J.H. *Chern Lin, Dent. Mater.* (2008) March, accepted.

[20] Y.J. Wang, F.H. Lin, J.S. Sun, Y.C. Huang , S.C. Chueh, F.Y. Hsu, *Artif. Org.* 27 (2003) 162.

[21] T.J. Wu, H.H. Huang, C.W. Lan, H. C. Lin, F.Y. Hsu, Y.J. Wang, *Biomaterials* 25 (2004) 651.

[22] T.S. Pradeesh, M.C. Sunny, H.K. Varma, P. Ramesh, *Bull. Mater. Sci.* 28 (2005) 383.

[23] M.H. Kish, M. Nouri, *J. Appl. Polym. Sci.* 72 (1999) 631.

[24] B.H. Chen, K.I Chen, M.L. Ho, H.N. Chen, C.K. Wang, *Mater. Chem. Phy.* (2008) June, accepted.

[25] Y.C. Fu, M.L. Ho, S.C. Wu, H.S. Hsieh, C.K. Wang, *Mater. Sci. Eng.* C 28 (2008) 1149.

[26] Kikuchi, M. Kawabuchi, S. Sugihara, Y. Sakurai, Okano T., *J. Control. Release* 47 (1997) 21.

[27] E.C. Victoria, F.D. Gnanam, Trends Biomater. *Artif. Organs* 16 (2002) 12.

[28] Y.E. Greish, P.W. Brown, *J. Biomed. Mater. Res. Part B: Appl. Biomater*. 67B (2003) 632.

[29] C.K. Wang, C.P. Ju, J.H. Chern Lin, *Mater. Chem. Phy*. 53 (1998) 138.

[30] C.K. Wang, J.H. Chern Lin, C.P. Ju, H.C. Ong, R.P.H. Chang, *Biomaterials,* 18 (1997) 1331.

[31] T.M.G. Chu, D.G. Orton, S.J. Hollister, S.E. Feinberg, J.W. Halloran, *Biomaterials* 23 (2002) 1283.

[32] C.P.A.T. Klein, A.A. Driessen, K. de Groot, A. Van den Hooff, *J. Biomed. Mater. Res*. 17 (1983) 769.

[33] M.H. Santos, M. de Oliveira, L.P. de Freitas Souza, H.S. Mansur, W.L. Vasconcelos, *Mater. Res.* 7 (2004) 625.

[34] J. Zhou, X.D. Zhang, J. Chen, S. Zeng, K. de Groot, *J. Mater. Sci. Mater. Med.* 4 (1993) 83.

[35] J.M. Bouler, R.Z. LeGeros, G. Daculsi, *J. Biomed. Mater. Res*. 51 (2000) 680.

[36] S.V. Dorozhkin, E.I. Dorozhkina, *Chem. Mater*. 14 (2002) 4267.

[37] C. Cameron, B.N. Besim, Internat. *Ceram. Monogra*. 1 (1994) 79.

[38] M. Jarcho, R.L. Salsbury, M.B. Thomas, R.H. Doremus, *J. Mater. Sci. Mater. Med.* 14 (1979) 142.

[39] O.U. José F de, S. Lidia Á de, C.P. Carlos A. de, A. Paula F. de, M.R. Alexandre, A.S. Glória, *Mater. Res*. 8 (2005) 1439.

[40] M.T. Fulmer, R.I. Martin, P.W. Brown, *J. Mater. Sci. Mater. Med.* 3 (1992) 299.

[41] L. Yubao, C.P.A.T. Klein, J. de Wijn, S. Van de Meer, K. de Groot, *J. Mater. Sci. Mater. Med.* 5 (1994) 263.

[42] A.T. Florence, D. Whitehill, in: D.O. Shah (Ed.), *Macro- and Microemulsions: Theory and Applications. ACS Symposium Series 272*, Washington, DC, 1985, p.359.

[43] W.D. Kingery, B. Francois, in: G.C. Kuczynski, N.A. Hooton, G.F. Gibbon (Eds), *Sintering and Related Phenomena*, Gondon Breach, New York, 1967, p.471.

In: Bioceramics: Properties, Preparations and Applications ISBN: 978-1-60741-056-0
Editors: W. Kossler, J. Fuchs, pp. 223-234

Chapter V

Application of the Sol-Gel Process in the Preparation of Bioceramics

Katalin Sinkó and Anikó Meiszterics
Institute of Chemistry, L. Eötvös University, Pázmány st 1/a.,
H-1117, Budapest, Hungary

Abstract

The $CaO - SiO_2$ or $CaO - SiO_2 - P_2O_5$ ceramic materials can be applied for biomedical applications due to the bioactive character. The essential condition for bioactive glasses or ceramics to bond to living bone is the formation of a bone-like apatite layer on their surfaces. The bioceramic materials can be synthesized by two methods: by classic melt-quenching process starting from inorganic powders ⌈*e.g.* $CaCO_3$, SiO_2, P_2O_5⌋ and by sol-gel technique starting from metal alkoxides ⌈ *e.g.* $Si(OR)_4$⌋ or inorganic salts ⌈$Ca(NO_3)_2$⌋.

One of the most important advantages of the sol-gel technique is the low energy requirement, much lower than that of conventional powder or melting technologies; <1000 °C in contrast to 1500-2000 °C. In addition, the sol–gel processing allows one to produce gel glasses with compositions lying within the liquid–liquid immiscibility dome of several silicate systems.

For example as with many multicomponent glasses, only a certain range of $CaO - SiO_2$ compositions can be melting derived. According to some published results, the bioactivity of the sol-gel derived glass-ceramics is unambiguously better than that of ceramics prepared by quenching of melts. The increase in bioactivity can be explained by the great differences in the textural properties of the materials synthesized by different techniques. The crystallinity and porosity out of the texture parameters influence strongly the bioactivity. The structure of a higher porosity obtained by sol-gel method can more fit the porous bone tissues than the compact one. The amount and position of crystalline particles (*e.g.* carbonates) can be much easier controlled via sol-gel than melting processes.

Introduction

The bioactive glass-ceramics and composites have been successfully used for the repair, reconstruction, and replacement of diseased or damaged parts of the body, especially bone or tooth. The most bioactive glasses and ceramics have been based on a silicate network due to the slight and slow solubility of silicates in human body fluid. Hereby these bioactive materials can be used as long-term implants. The bioactivity can be attributed to the bone bonding behaviour. On the surface of bioactive materials, a biologically active carbonate hydroxyapatite layer forms that provides the bonding interface with living tissues. SiO_2 seems very important for the bioactive behaviour of the glass [1]. First a silica hydrogel layer evolves that allows subsequent crystallisation of the apatite-like phase [2]. This hydrated silica is responsible for the hydroxyapatite nucleation. The silicate glasses or ceramics are generally amorphous solid materials with crystallisation nuclei. A disordered structure resulted by network modifiers (*e. g.* Ca^{2+} ion) is needed for the high bioreactivity in an aqueous environment of the glasses. The alkaline or earth alkaline ions (*e. g.* Na^{+} or Ca^{2+} ions) on the surface can be replaced by H^{+} ion to produce silanol (Si-OH) groups. The silanol group on the surface of the biomaterial is reported to be essential for the formation of hydroxyapatite. The silanol group provides favourable sites for hydroxyapatite nucleation [3-9].

The first bioactive glass studied was Bioglass® 45S5, introduced by Hench in 1971, which still remains the most used in clinical applications and the most promising one [10]. Bioglass® 45S5 is produced by fusion, and its specific composition is 45% SiO_2, 24.5% CaO, 24.5% Na_2O, 6% P_2O_5. The calcium phosphates (*e. g.* apatite) have been of remarkable interest to biologists, mineralogists, inorganic and industrial chemists. Calcium phosphate biomaterials have many clinical applications in the repair of bone defects, bone augmentation and coatings for metal implants. The most used calcium phosphate in implant production is hydroxyapatite as being the materials most similar to the mineral component of the bones. The hydroxyapatite exhibits valuable properties; biomaterial, biocompatibility, bioactivity, osteoconductivity, *etc.*, but its mechanical properties are poor [11]. Considering the required mechanical strength and bioactivity of bioceramics, many authors focus the synthesis of calcium silicate(-phosphate) materials [12-15]. The considerable number of authors, who study the bioactivity, concentrates on the apatite nucleation upon the role of the silanol groups existing on the silicate glass surfaces [9, 16, 17].

Melting and sol–gel are two well known methods for producing glasses or ceramics. The melt-quenching technique has some disadvantages: the required high temperatures (> 1000 °C); the high loss of the volatile precursors during the melting processes; only a certain range of many multicomponent glass compositions can be melt derived; bioactive molecules such as antibiotics cannot be incorporated into the glass owing to theirs decomposition at high temperature. The traditional melting and slow cooling processes result in materials with very small specific surface area and porosity [10]. Even nowadays a lot of authors use the classic quenching of melts to produce $CaO–SiO_2$ [8, 18-24], $CaO–P_2O_5–SiO_2$ [25, 26] or $CaO–P_2O_5$ [11, 27-32] systems.

The common advantages of sol-gel technique are the low temperature (< 1000 °C); the better quality of products, the good homogeneity, and purity. In the early 1990s the sol-gel procedure was introduced for the synthesis of bioactive glasses. The sol-gel chemistry involved in the process is based on the inorganic polymerization reactions of metal alkoxide (*e.g.* $Si(OR)_4$, $Ca(OR)_4$) or inorganic precursors [*e.g.* $Ca(NO_3)_2$, Na_2SiO_3]. *There* have been some publications given to *exemplars* for using calcium ethylate, $Ca(OEt)_4$ and tetraethoxysilan (TEOS), $Si(OC_2H_5)_4$ in the sol-gel preparation of binary $CaO–SiO_2$ system [33]; calcium nitrate [$Ca(NO_3)_2 \cdot 4\ H_2O$] and TEOS [13, 34-36]; calcium nitrate and tetramethyl orthosilicate, $Si(OCH_3)_4$ [14]; calcium acetate, $Ca(OCH_2CH_3)$ and TEOS [15]; and calcium chloride combined with sodium metasilicate [37]. Vallet-Regí and co-workers have recently published a series of papers on the bioactivity of binary $CaO–SiO_2$ sol–gel glasses [20-23, 38, 39]. All samples were prepared by hydrolysis and polycondensation of TEOS and hydrated calcium nitrate in an acidic aqueous solution.

The aims of this chapter are to present the advantages of sol-gel application recognized up to now and to demonstrate some advantages of sol-gel technique by means of $CaO – SiO_2$ ceramic system.

Experimental

The $CaO – SiO_2$ system were prepared by two routes; via sol-gel technique starting from tetraethoxysilane (TEOS) and calcium nitrate tetrahydrate and via melt-quenching technique using a mixture of $CaCO_3$ and SiO_2. The sol-gel syntheses of calcium silicate glasses were carried out by hydrolysis and polycondensation in an organic solution of stoichiometric amounts of the precursors; TEOS and $Ca(NO_3)_2 \cdot 4H_2O$ [40]. The rate of the hydrolysis of TEOS is very slow in neutral solutions and requires an acid (99-100 m/m% acetic acid) or base (25 m/m% ammonia) catalysis. The gelation, aging as well as drying processes were performed at 80 °C, the heat treatment at 700 °C. A calcium silicate sample of the same composition was also prepared by melting analytical grade reagents $CaCO_3$ and SiO_2 in a platinum crucible in an electrical oven for 3 h at >1000 °C. The particle size was less than 53 and 71 μm, respectively.

The structure characterizations were carried out with x-ray diffraction (XRD with heating cell, using a synchrotron radiation in HASYLAB, DESY); attenuated total reflectance fourier transform infrared spectroscopy (ATR FTIR, Brucker IFS 55 with diamond ATR head); and scanning electron microscopy (SEM, JEOL JSM-5600LV, the samples were sputtered with carbon). The weigh loss during the heat treatment was followed by thermogravimetric analysis (TG, Derivatograph-C System, with heating rate of 6 °C min^{-1}).

Advantages of Sol-Gel Application in Bioceramics` Preparation

Well known advantage of the sol-gel technique is its *low energy requirement*. The sol-gel procedure of $CaO – SiO_2$ ceramic system requires 700 °C to produce bulk ceramics [40], the conventional power technology ≈ 1500 °C. By sol-gel method the decomposition processes finish by 600 °C; the calcium silicate bond system evolves above 500 °C; and by that the mechanical strength increase considerably above 500 °C (Figure 1). On the other hand, the decarboxylation reaction occurs between 600 and 850 °C in the melt-derived samples (Figure 1).

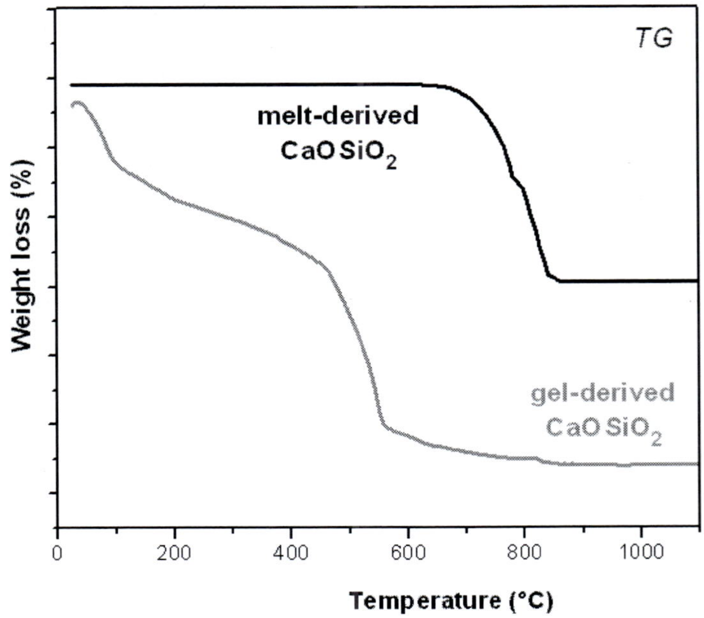

Figure 1. Thermoanalytical measurements of melt- and gel-derived CaO – SiO_2 systems.

By means of sol-gel technique *various compositions* can be obtained (up to 90 mol% SiO_2 in CaO – SiO_2 system). Several compositions cannot be achieved by traditional melting process in silicate systems due to a phase separation occurred during the cooling.

The gel-derived ceramics have a significantly *better bioactivity* compared to melt-derived ceramics [14, 41-43]. According to L.L. Hench no melt-derived glasses with more than 60 mol % silica are always bioactive [44]. In order to obtain a required bioactivity for silica lever higher than 60 mol%, the sol-gel process must be used [44]. The better bioactivity can be explained by the great differences in the textural properties of the gel- and melt-derived materials [41-43].

The natural bone is a nanocomposite material, it consist of hydroxyapatite and collagen fibers. The biological apatites are poorly crystallised, carbonated and non-stoichiometric with calcium deficiency [45]. The natural apatite crystals are smaller than 500 Å in size and contain hydroxyl and carbonate groups [45]. The presence of CO_3^{2-} ions in the structure of apatite result in lattice distortion, creating microstresses and crystalline defects in lattice. The lattice distortion plays a fundamental role in the solubility. [46]. However, the carbonate content of synthetic apatites is always different from the amount of carbonates in natural bone (4 – 8 w/w %) and/or located in different lattice positions [47, 48]. The sol-gel process can help to solve this problem by means to apply low temperature synthesis routes and to *control the amount and positions* of carbonate ions in lattice.

Figures 2 and 3 demonstrate the different textural properties of the materials synthesized by various routes.

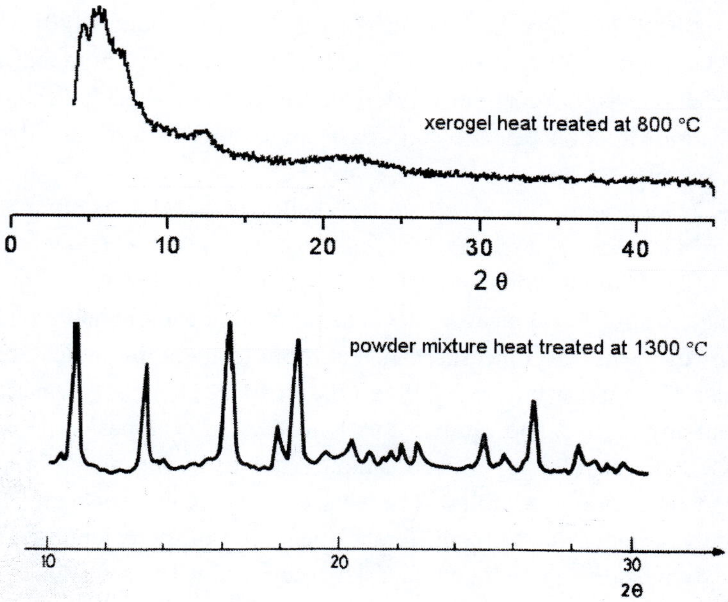

Figure 2. XRD measurements of melt- and gel-derived $CaO - SiO_2$ systems.

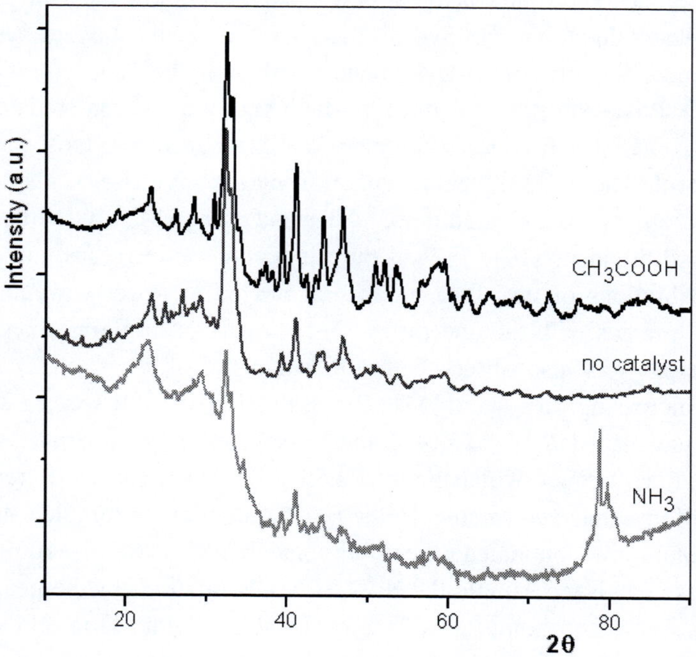

Figure 3. XRD data for $CaO - SiO_2$ systems prepared by sol-gel method using various catalysts and heat treated at 700 °C.

The melt-quenched $CaO - SiO_2$ products prepared in the present work proved to be crystalline materials containing mostly (cyclo)wollastonite phase; the gel derived samples rather amorphous ordered in aggregate structures up to 1000 °C (Figure 2). The heat treatment of ≥1000 °C destroys the structure of gel-derived products [40]. Calcium silicate phases can be identified by XRD from 400 °C in the melt-quenched products and a dicalcium silicate phase from 800-1000 °C in the gel-derived samples as a weekly detectable crystalline phase. Their wide diffraction peaks mean quasi amorphous feature, the size of crystalline particles is less than 10 nm.

The figure 3 represents the *excellent variability* of sol-gel technique. Owing to its variability, this method is eligible for *tailoring the texture* (Figure 3). The XRD diffractograms depict slight volume of $CaCO_3$ as a temporary phase in every sample. According to the "in situ" XRD measurements the appearance temperature range of $CaCO_3$ is 300-500 °C. However, the XRD measurements at room temperature indicate carbonate phase in every sample. The intensity of crystalline phase of $CaCO_3$ is very weak in the samples prepared without any catalyst and catalyzed with acetic acid. The peaks of $CaCO_3$ crystalline phase in the XRD diagram of gel-derived sample catalyzed whit ammonia are stronger and vary from those of previous samples. The peaks in the range between 75° and 80° are disproportionately stronger due to the different orientation of the calcium carbonate crystals. So, varying the catalyst, the amount and the orientation of $CaCO_3$ phase are changing.

The FTIR spectra also exhibit the varied sol-gel technique (Figure 4). Not only the morphology but even the chemical bonds depend strongly on the catalysis applied in the sol-gel process. Alkoxysilanes hydrolyze very slowly without any catalyst, theirs condensation and hydrolysis processes require acid or base catalysis. Acid-catalyzed reactions yield to more linear networks due to the fast hydrolysis. Therefore, acid catalyzed systems have a less completely formed network of Si-O-Si bonds with a higher concentration of unreacted silanols (Si-OH). Base-catalyzed reactions produce highly dense materials due to the longer hydrolysis time. The particles form aggregates and arrange in the most thermodynamically stable arrangement. The SiO_4 stretching vibration modes give rise to a sharp band at 1100 cm^{-1}. By addition of oxide modifiers, the band progressively shifts towards lower wavenumbers and broadens [19]. As well the silica content decreases, the primary peak for the stretching vibrations of the silica tetrahedral moved to lower wavenumbers [34]. This band eventually merges with the one for Si–O, terminal non-bridging oxygen resulting in a peak broadening. It was also observed that the intensity of the O–Si–O stretching modes decreased with increasing Ca content [34]. The evaluation of FTIR spectra was carried out by means of literature data [19, 34, 23, 49] and IR spectra for comparison samples (calcium nitrate, TEOS, silica xerogel, wollastonite). The FTIR spectra show differences between the structures of various catalyzed sample. In the FTIR spectrum for sample catalyzed with acid, the Si-O-Ca bonds are dominated (the vibrational bands at 850 – 1000 cm^{-1}); while in spectrum for base catalyzed sample the Si-O-Si bonds (a strong, wide peak in the range of 950-1150 cm^{-1}). The absorption peaks of sample catalyzed with acetic acid show a very good similarity with those of calcium metasilicate (wollastonite). In contrast to this, the peak of Si-O^-/ Ca^{2+} is very weak in the spectrum for sample catalyzed with ammonia. The chemical bond system of samples prepared without any catalyst presents some difference from the catalyzed bond system. Its IR spectrum indicates the presence of NO_3^- ions (peak at 1400 cm^{-1}) even in the sample heat treated at 700 °C. Otherwise the Si-O-Ca bonds are represented in IR spectrum. Thus, there are a lot of possibilities in the sol-gel method to *tailor the structure* and by that *the properties* of ceramics. The above exemplars show only one possibility, the influence of the catalyst.

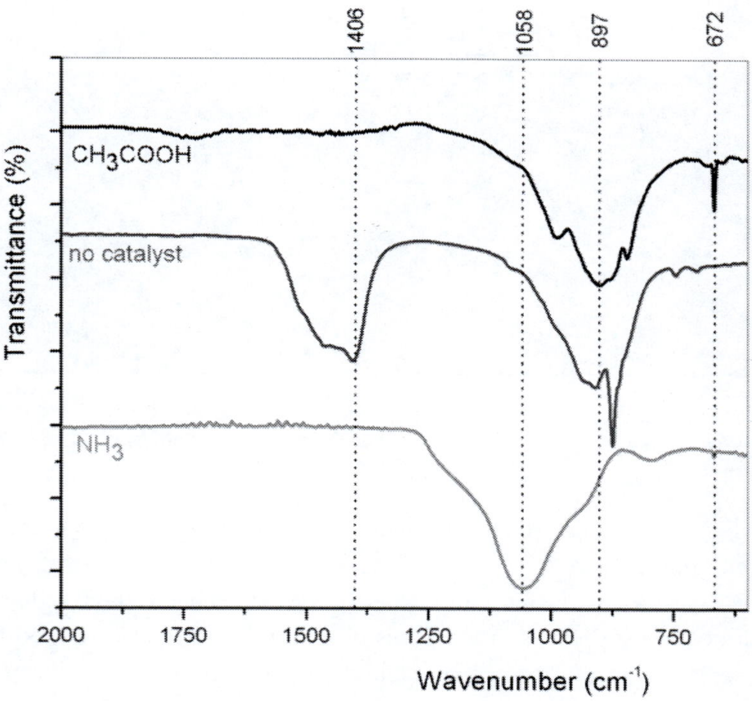

Figure 4. FTIR spectra for CaO – SiO_2 systems prepared by sol-gel method using various catalysts and heat treated at 700 °C.

The next factor, which has influence on the chemical reactivity, i.e. on the bioactivity is the *porosity*. The melt-quenching technique produces ceramics with low porosity. The pore volume of the melt-quenched glasses is generally less than 1 cm^3g^{-1} [11]. The traditional power technology provides the ceramics with a less compact (10-20 % porosity) structure, while the sol-gel method results in the highest porosity (> 20 %). (The porosity is 5-10 % in cortical bone and > 50 % in trabecular bone.) (See the figure 5!) The required porosity can be reliably achieved by using sol-gel process and fitted the pore system of natural bone tissues. The structure can be tailored to provide it with interconnected pores of 10-200 μm, mimicking the architecture of trabecular bone. The high porosity and the high specific surface area of gel-derived glasses faster the formation of the carbonate hydroxyapatite surface layer, formed on the glass surface as a product of the reaction between the glass and the surrounding flowing medium. The hydroxyapatite layer formed at the surface is compact, continuous and composed of many small crystallites, theirs supramolecular structure show similarity to natural cortical bone (Figure 5) [7]. The silica gel and carbonate hydroxyapatite layers provide adsorption sites for the cellular growth factors promoting bone formation [50, 51]. The porous structures allow of the growth of natural tissue inside the pores, to faster and intensify the incorporation of implants [11]. The surface area of gel-glasses has been found to increase with silica content [50]. However, a larger amount of SiO_2 leads to a lower macro- and meso-pore volume in the terner system of SiO_2 – CaO – P_2O_5, and even the pore diameter decreases in both ranges. Despite that, the surface area follows the opposite trend [42, 52].

The other advantage of silica content in bioceramics is that the sol-gel process can provide the surface of silica gel-glasses with silanol groups.

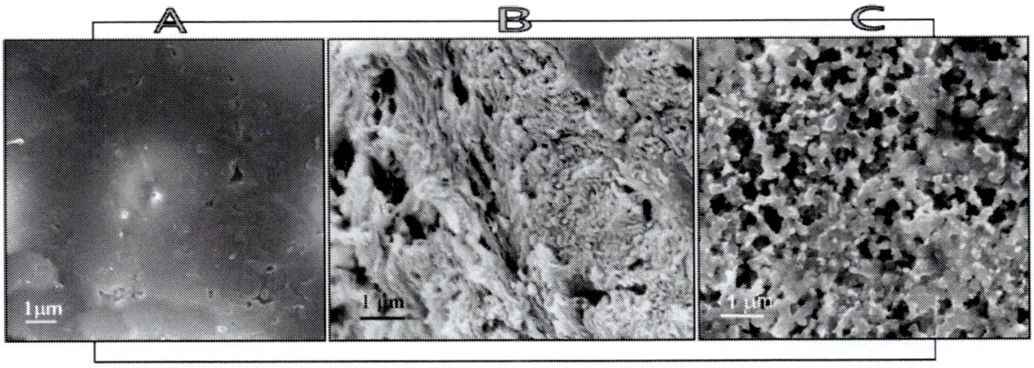

Figure 5. SEM micrograph of melt-derived $SiO_2 - CaO$ ceramic (A); natural bone (B); and gel-derived $SiO_2 - CaO$ ceramic (C).

The silanol groups effect strongly the apatite nucleation [9, 53]. Due to the silanol groups the gel-derived glasses can more rapidly be dissolved and the formation of carbonate hydroxyapatite layer is also faster compared with melt-quenched glasses. The soluble silica nucleates hydroxyapatite crystals in the pores of gel-glass. The network modifiers (*e.g.* Ca^{2+} ions) can be replaced by hydrogen ions resulting silanol group. Thus, the phosphorus and calcium as components of bioactive glasses could be potential nucleation centers for apatite crystallization.

The sol-gel technique can produce materials in bulk as well as *powder* form. The size and shape of powder can be well *controlled* by sol-gel method. The $CaO - SiO_2$ or $SiO_2 - CaO - P_2O_5$ powders can be applied for bone filling. By mineralization, the powder can adapt very well to the profile of each bone defect.

Conclusion

The advantageous of sol-gel application in bioceramics synthesis can be summarized in the following:

- The sol-gel technique is an energy-consuming method. It has low processing temperature (600-700 °C) in contrast to the temperature of melt-quenching process (1500-2000 °C).
- The sol-gel compositions are varied in wide range. Some compositions lied in the liquid–liquid immiscibility dome cannot be produced with melt-quenching technology.
- The sol-gel technique proved the ceramic materials to provide with special components, ions, *e.g.* with important OH^- or CO_3^{2-} ions considering the bio characters. The sol-gel route reliably controls the compositions and morphology; the amount and the ordering of components in the structure. Structural variation can be

produced without compositional changes, only by control of hydrolysis and polycondensation reactions during synthesis.

- Application of sol-gel method leads to the formation of a good homogeneity and purity due to the initial solutions of analytical grade reagents.
- Owing to the variability of sol-gel process, it is eligible for tailoring the textures; *e.g.* the crystallinity and porosity.
- The gel-derived ceramics exhibit much better bioactivity than melt-derived glasses. Composition, particle sizes, surface area, morphology, porosity, defects, and crystallinity have considerable effect on the bioactivity. The higher the porosity and specific surface area the better the bioactivity is. Even the pore size influences the biocompatibility; the pore size can be regulated by sol-gel method and made more similar to that of bone.
- Summarizing the present research work, the ammonia proved to be the most efficient catalyst. The fastest evaporation of vaporizable phases, the lowest temperature range of decomposition processes, the controllable of the calcite phase, the homogeneous structure, and the greatest hardness has been experienced in the use of ammonia catalyst. The homogeneous structure and the more emphatic calcium silicate bond system can be taken into account as advantages of catalysis with acetic acid.

References

[1] Kokubo, T. Surface Chemistry of Bioactive Glass-Ceramics. *J. Non-Cryst. Solids*, (1990) 120, 138-151.

[2] Kokubo, T. An Introduction to Bioceramics. Advanced Series in Ceramics. Eds. Hench, LL; Wilson, J. Singapore: World Scientific Publishing C; 1993.

[3] Kokubo, T; Hayashi, T; Sakka, S; Kitsugi, T; Yamamuro, T. Bonding between bioactive glasses, glass-ceramics or ceramics in a simulated body fluid. *Yogyo-Kyokai-Shi*, (1987) 95, 785-791.

[4] Liu, DM. Bioactive glass-ceramic: Formation, characterization and bioactivity. *Mater. Chem. Phys*., (1994) 36, 294-303.

[5] De Aza, PN; Guitian, F; De Aza, S. Bioactivity of wollastonite ceramics: in vitro evaluation. *Scrip. Metall. Mater.,* (1994) 31, 1001-1005.

[6] Izquierdo-Barba, I; Vallet-Regi, M. In vitro Calcium Phosphate Layer Formation on Sol-Gel Glasses of the CaO-SiO_2 System. *J. Biomed. Mater. Res*., (1999) 47, 243-250.

[7] Alemany, MI; Velasquez, P; de la Casa-Lillo, MA; De Aza, PN. Effect of materials' processing methods on the 'in vitro' bioactivity of wollastonite glass-ceramic materials. *J. Non-Cryst. Solids*, (2005) 351, 1716–1726.

[8] De Aza, PN; Luklinska, ZB; Anseau, M; Guitian, F; De Aza, S. Bioactivity of pseudowollastonite in human saliva. *J. Dentistry*, (1999) 27, 107-113.

[9] Pereira, MM; Hench, LL. Mechanisms of hydroxyapatite formation on porous *gel–* silica substrates. *J. Sol–Gel Sci. Technol.*, (1996) 7, 59-68.

[10] Hench LL; Splinter, RJ; Allen WC; Greenlee TK. Bonding mechanisms at the interface of ceramic prosthetic materials. *J. Biomed. Mater. Res. Symp.*, (1971) 2, 117-141.

[11] Vallet-Regí, M. Ceramics for medical applications. *J. Chem. Soc., Dalton Trans.*, (2001) 97–108.

[12] Hayashi, T; Saito, H. Preparation of CaO-SiO_2 glasses by the gel method. *J. Mater. Sci.*, (1980) 15, 1971-1977.

[13] Bansal, NP. Influence of Several Metal ions on the Gelation Activation Energy of Silicon Tetraethoxide. *J. Am. Ceram. Soc.*, (1990) 73, 2647-2652.

[14] Catauro, M; Laudisio, G. Low Temperature Synthesis, Structure and Bioactivity of 2CaO·3SiO_2 Glass. *J. Sol–Gel Sci. Technol.*, (1997) 10, 231-237.

[15] Catauro, M; Laudisio, G. Sol–gel processing and crystallization of calcium silicate glasses. *J. Mater. Sci. Lett.*, (1998) 17, 311-312.

[16] Li, PJ; Ohtuki, C; Kokubo, T; Nakanishi, K; Soga, N; Nakamura, T; Yamamuro, T. Apatite formation induced by silica gel in a simulated body fluid *J. Am. Ceram. Soc.*, (1992) 75, 2094-2097.

[17] Karlsson, KH; Fröberg, K; Ringbom, T. A structural *approach to bone adhering of bioactive glasses. J. Non-Cryst. Solids*, (1989) 112, 69-72.

[18] Frantz, JD; Mysen, BO. Raman spectra and structure of BaO-SiO_2, SrO-SiO_2, and CaO-SiO_2 Melts to 1600°C. *Chem. Geolog.*, (1995) 121, 155-176.

[19] Branda, F; Arcobello-Varlese, F; Costantini, A; Luciani, G. T_g and FTIR of $(2.5 - x)$CaO·x/3M_2O_3·2SiO_2 (M=Y, La, In, Al, Ga) glasses. *J. Non-Cryst. Solids,* (1999) 246, 27-33.

[20] Vallet-Regí, M; Izquierdo-Barba, I; Salinas, AJ. Influence of P_2O_5 on crystallinity of apatite formed *in vitro* on surface of bioactive glasses. *J. Biomed.Mater. Res.*, (1999) 46, 560-565.

[21] Izquierdo-Barba, I; Salinas, AJ; Vallet-Regí, M. *In vitro* calcium phosphate layer formation on sol-gel glasses of the CaO-SiO_2 system. *J. Biomed.Mater. Res.*, (1999) 47, 243-250.

[22] Izquierdo-Barba, I; Salinas, AJ; Vallet-Regí, M. Effect of continuous solution exchange on in vitro reactivity of a CaO–SiO_2 sol–gel glass. *J. Biomed.Mater. Res.*, (2000) 51, 191-199.

[23] Martínez, A; Izquierdo-Barba, I; Vallet-Regí, M. Bioactivity of a CaO-SiO_2 Binary Glasses System. *Chem. Mater.*, (2000) 12, 3080-3088.

[24] Ebisawa, Y; Kokubo, T; Ohura, K; Yamamuro, T. Bioactivity of CaO·SiO_2-based glasses: in vitro evaluation. *J. Mater. Sci.Mater. Med.*, (1990) 1, 239-244.

[25] Li, PJ; Nakanishi, K; Kokubo, T; Degroot, K. Induction and morphology of hydroxyapatite, precipitated from metastable simulated body fluids on sol-gel prepared silica. *Biomaterials,* (1993) 14, 963-968.

[26] Li, PJ; Ohtuki, C; Kokubo, T; Nakanishi, K; Soja, N; Nakamura, T; Yamamuro, T. Process of formation of bone-like apatite layer on silica gel. *J. Mater. Sci. – Mater. Med.,* (1993) 4, 127-131.

[27] Aoki, H; Kato, K; Ogiso, M; Tabata, T. Sintered hydroxyapatite as a new dental implant material. *J. Dent. Outlook*, (1997) 49, 567-575.

[28] Knaack, D; Aiolova, M; Tofighi, A; Catalano, A; Rey, C; Nies, B; Duke, D. Bioceramics 11. eds. LeGeros, RZ; LeGeros, JP. New York: World Scientific Publishing Co; 1998.

[29] Salih, V; Franks, K; James, M; Hastings, GW; Knowles, JC; Olsen, I. Development of soluble glasses for biomedical use Part II: The biological response of human osteoblast cell lines to phosphate-based soluble glasses. *J. Mater. Sci.: Mater. Med.,* (2000) 11, 615-620.

[30] Franks, K; Abrahams, I; Georgiou, G; Knowles, JC. Investigation of thermal parameters and crytallisation in a ternary CaO-Na_2O-P_2O_5-based glass system. *Biomaterials*, (2001) 22, 497-501.

[31] Ahmed, I; Lewis, M; Olsen, I; Knowles, JC. Phosphate glasses for tissue engineering: Part 2. Processing and characterisation of a ternary-based P_2O_5-CaO-Na_2O glass fibre system. *Biomaterials*, (2004) 25, 501-507.

[32] Bitar, M; Salih, V; Mudera, V; Knowles, JC; Lewis, MP. Soluble phosphate glasses: in vitro studies using human cells of hard and soft tissue origin. *Biomaterials*, (2004) 25, 2283-2292.

[33] Hayashi, T; Saito, H. Preparation of CaO-SiO_2 glasses by the gel method. *J Mater Sci.*, (1980) 15, 1971-1977.

[34] Saravanapavan, P; Hench, LL. Mesoporous calcium silicate glasses. I. Synthesis. *J. Non-Cryst. Solids,* (2003) 318, 1-13.

[35] Iimori, Y; Kameshima, Y; Okada, K; Hayashi, S. Comparative study of apatite formation on $CaSiO_3$ ceramics in simulated body fluids with different carbonate concentrations. *J. Mater. Sci.*, (2005) 16, 73-79.

[36] Chrysafi, R; Perraki, Th; Kakali, G. Sol–gel preparation of $2CaO{\cdot}SiO_2$. *J. Eur. Ceram. Soc.*, (2007) 27, 1707-1710.

[37] Perruchot, A; Massard, P; Lombardi, J. Composition et volume molaire apparent des gels Ca-Si, une approche expérimentale. *C R Geosience*, (2003) 335, 951-958.

[38] Vallet-Regí, M; Ragel, CV; Salinas, AJ. Glasses with Medical Application. *Eur. J. Inorg. Chem.*, (2003) 6, 1029-1042.

[39] Vallet-Regí, M; Salinas, AJ; Martínez, A; Izquierdo-Barba, I; Pérez-Pariente, J. Textural properties of CaO–SiO_2 glasses for use in implants. *Solid State Ionics*, (2004) 172, 441-444.

[40] Meiszterics, A; Sinkó, K. Sol-gel derived calcium silicate ceramic. *Colloid Surface A*, (2008) 319, 143-148.

[41] Vallet-Regí, M; Rámila, A. New Bioactive Glass and Changes in Porosity during the Growth of a Carbonate Hydroxyapatite Layer on Glass Surfaces. *Chem. Mater.*, (2000) 12, 961-965.

[42] Pérez-Pariente, J; Balas, F; Vallet-Regí, M. Surface and chemical study of $SiO_2{\cdot}P_2O_5{\cdot}CaO{\cdot}(MgO)$ bioactive glasses. *Chem. Mater.*, (2000) 12, 750-755.

[43] Vallet-Regí, M; Arcos, D; Pérez-Pariente, J. Surface and Chemical Study of $SiO_2{\cdot}P_2O_5{\cdot}CaO{\cdot}(MgO)$ Bioactive Glasses. *J. Biomed. Mater. Res.*, (2000) 51, 23-.

[44] Hench, LL; Jones, JR; Sepulveda, P. Bioactive materials for tissue engineering scaffolds. Ed: Polak, JM; Hench, LL; Kemp, P. London: Imperial College Press, 2002.

[45] Nainwright, A; Briggs, WD; Currey, JD; Gosline, JM. Mechanical Design in Organisms. Princeton: Princeton University Press, 1976.

[46] Vallet-Regi, M; Elliott, JC. Structure and Chemistry of the Apatites and Other Calcium Orthophosphates. London: Elsevier, 1994.

[47] LeGeros, RZ. Calcium Phosphates in Oral Biology and Medicine. Basle: Karger, 1991.
[48] Elliot, JC; Bond, G; Tombe, JC. Space group and lattice constants of $Ca_{10}(PO_4)_6CO_3$. *J. Appl. Crystallogr.*, (1980) 13, 618-621.
[49] Miyata, N; Fuke, K; Chen, Q; Kawashita, M; Kokubo, T; Nakamura, T. Apatite-forming ability and mechanical properties of PTMO modified CaO–SiO_2 hybrids prepared by sol–gel processing: effect of CaO and PTMO contents. *Biomaterials,* (2002) 23, 3033–3040.
[50] Pereira, MM; Clark, AE; Hench, LL. *Calcium phosphate* formation on sol-gel-derived bioactive glasses in vitro. *J. Biomed. Mater. Res.*, (1994) 28, 693-698.
[51] Vallet-Regí, M; Balas, F; Gil, M; Nogueroles, E; Romero, A; Román, J; Salinas, AJ; Ragel, V. Non-crystalline and Nanoscale Materials. London: World Scientific, 1998.
[52] Pérez-Pariente, J; Balas, F; Román, J; Salinas, AJ; Vallet-Regí, M. Influence of composition and surface characteristics on the *in vitro* bioactivity of SiO_2-CaO-P_2O_5-MgO sol-gel glasses. *J. Biomed. Mater. Res.*, (1999) 47, 170-175.
[53] Karlsson, KH; Fröberg, K; Ringbom, T. A structural approach to bone adhering of bioactive glasses. *J. Non-Cryst. Solids*, (1989) 112, 69-72.

In: Bioceramics: Properties, Preparations and Applications
Editors: W. Kossler, J. Fuchs, pp. 235-252
ISBN: 978-1-60741-056-0

Chapter VI

Two Injectable Calcium Phosphate Cements, Two Approaches: A Review

M. A. Lopez-Heredia[1,a], S. C. G. Leeuwenburgh[1], P. Layrolle[2] and J. A. Jansen[1*]

[1] Department of Periodontology and Biomaterials,
Radboud University Nijmegen Medical Center, 6500 HB,
Nijmegen, the Netherlands

[2] INSERM U791, Laboratory for Osteo-Articular and
Dental Tissue Engineering, Faculty of Dental Surgery, University of Nantes,
1 Place Alexis Ricordeau, 44042 Nantes, France

Abstract

Injectable calcium phosphates cements (ICPC) are an alternative to calcium phosphates preforms, such as granules or blocks, and other bone substitute materials that can not be molded to the defect site they have to fill. In addition they are potential candidates for minimal invasive surgery. Several approaches have been used to accomplish this task. Here we review two approaches that have been studied by two different research groups and that are amply used. The first approach uses the formation of one or more calcium phosphate compounds when mixing a liquid solution, containing or not calcium or phosphate ions, with calcium phosphate compounds. Then, the dissolution-precipitation mechanism, and growth of crystals, governs the setting of the material. The second approach is a composite one, which uses calcium phosphate as a filler material in a polymer matrix; in this situation the stiffness of the cement depends on the polymer properties. The actual state of the art, biphasic concept, mechanical and physical properties, control of porosity, drug delivery capacities, in vivo tests, as well as the future trends and differences for these two approaches are discussed.

* Corresponding author: Prof. John A. Jansen, PhD, DD. Tel: +31(0)243614461; Fax: +31(0)243614657; E-mail: J.Jansen@dent.umcn.nl; a previous address: INSERM U791, Laboratory for Osteo-Articular and Dental Tissue Engineering, Faculty of Dental Surgery, University of Nantes, 1 Place Alexis Ricordeau, 44042 Nantes, France

Keywords: Calcium phosphate cements, hydraulic cement, biphasic concept, macroporous structure, delivery systems.

1. Introduction

There are three key factors for a successful bone graft substitute: i.e. bone forming cells, a suitable scaffold and the presence of biological stimulants [1]. Calcium phosphates (CaP) can possess by themselves the last two mentioned characteristics since their composition is close to that of the mineral phase of bone and they possess an intrinsic capacity to form bone [2]. CaP ceramic, in the right composition, allows the adhesion and differentiation of osteoblasts [3]. Injectable calcium phosphates cements (ICPC) are an alternative to CaP preforms, such as granules or blocks [4], and other bone substitute materials that can not be molded to the defect they have to fill, such as rigid metallic and polymeric preforms [5]. This ability to adapt to the defect is obtained due to the plasticity they exhibit before setting or hardening. This makes them able to conform to the shape of the space they have to fill and act as a transient assembly. The initial contact between the graft material and bone tissue is particularly important in order to obtain a good integration of the graft and a faster establishment of bone formation [6]. These characteristics make ICPC potential candidates for minimal invasive surgery. ICPC require a good control of the resorption of the cement and substitution of them by bone [7]. Nowadays, several commercially ICPC are available. For example, Norian® SRS (Norian), α-BSM® (Etex-Merck), BoneSource® (Orthofix-Howmedica), Calcibon® (Biomet-Merck), Biopex® (Mitsubishi), MBCP Gel® (Biomatlante) or Cementek® (Teknimed).

In a general way, there are four categories of ICPC [8, 9]:

- Calcium phosphate compounds where the mixing liquid is water or solutions containing calcium or phosphate ions. Hardening takes place by the formation of one or more calcium phosphate compounds and the crystal growth of these.
- Calcium phosphates as the solid component with an organic acid as the mixing liquid phase. Hardening occurs by complex formation of the organic acid and the calcium.
- Calcium phosphates as the solid components and a polymer as the "liquid". Hardening occurs by the formation of a calcium phosphate compound, e.g. hydroxyapatite, or formation of a calcium-polymer solution.
- Composites of calcium phosphates and polymers, CaP act as a filler. Hardening takes place by polymerization or crosslinking.

The first and fourth types of cements have been extensively studied by research groups in Nijmegen, the Netherlands and in Nantes, France, respectively. The first research group has focused on the study of a cement that falls in the group of hydraulic cements (H-ICPC). This cement is composed of α-tricalcium phosphate (62.5 wt%), calcium hydrogen phosphate (26.8 wt%), calcium carbonate (8.9 wt%), and precipitated hydroxyapatite (1.8 wt%). The liquid used to create a paste out of these CaP powders is an aqueous disodium hydrogen phosphate solution. The quantity of sodium in the liquid has an influence on the acceleration of the setting reaction [10]. The second research group has focused on the study of a cement, which falls in the category of composite of calcium phosphates and polymers and uses the biphasic concept (B-ICPC). This cement is composed of biphasic calcium phosphate granules (55% of MBCP 80-200 μm granules) in an hydrophilic polymer solution (45% of 2%-Hydroxypropyl Methylcellulose). These two cements are commercially available under the brand names of Calcibon® (Biomet-Merck) and MBCP Gel® (Biomatlante), respectively.

2. Hydraulic Cements (H-ICPC)

Hydraulic cements set and harden after being combined with a liquid phase. Most of the ICPC are Hydraulic cements and they have been studied since the beginning of 1970 [11], but they started to gain more attention in the 1980 [12, 13] and by the end of 1990 they were seen as an emerging technology with impact for many areas in reconstructive surgery [14]. The ICPC is obtained by dissolution-precipitation of CaP compounds when mixed with an aqueous solution around room temperature. In this ICPC, the dissolution-precipitation mechanism and the crystal growth, govern the setting of the material and even if some heat is formed during the setting reaction, this amount of heat is not high enough to damage the surrounding tissue like the exothermic reactions that occur with PMMA cements. In general, depending on the solubility product constant of the calcium phosphates that are mixed and the pH values during mixing, two categories may exist by using this approach, i.e. apatite (AP) and brushite (DCPD) cements. The final-formed crystal phase determines the speed of resorption of the cement [14]. An hydraulic ICPC falls in the first category and has been proven to maintain its dimensional stability, or cohesion, due to the absence of passive dissolution in a liquid [15]. In this ICPC, the microposority is related to the ratio of powder to liquid as used in the mixture. This microporosity can be increased if a CO_2 induction technique is used [16], but the performance of this microporosity can be surpassed by using a macroporous structure by incorporating degradable polymeric microspheres of PLGA (poly (lactic-co-glycolic acid)) [17].

3. Biphasic Concept (B-ICPC)

The biphasic concept has been investigated for almost 20 years [7, 18]. For biomedical applications, hydroxyapatite and/or tricalcium phosphate are the most frequently used materials [19]. The biphasic concept is related to the simultaneous presence of these two CaP phases, i.e. hydroxyapatite (HA) and β-tricalcium phosphate (β-TCP). When present in a certain ratio within the CaP material, this ratio affects, among other factors, the solubility, reactivity, resorption and bonding of the CaP material to the bone tissue [20]. Depending on the properties of the material used for the sintering, i.e Calcium Deficient Apatite (CDA), and the sintering parameters, different HA/β-TCP ratios can be achieved. This biphasic concept has been transmuted into an ICPC by using a polymer carrier [20, 21]. It has been shown that this approach is as good, in terms of biocompatibility, as the use of biphasic calcium phosphates particles [22]. It is important to note that β-TCP cannot be obtained directly from aqueous systems [18] and that the hydroxypropyl methylcellulose (HPMC) used with this approach, when used without modifications, is a non-hardening polymer. The main characteristic provided by the HPMC is the capacity to be resorbed and replaced by newly formed bone in a fast way [21]. HPMC allows the adhesion and growth of bone cells onto the biphasic CaP material [23]. The use of a fibrin glue as the polymer matrix has also been explored, but this approach sometimes shows contradictory results and not a direct growth of bone on the CaP materials [4, 24-27], which is probably related to the hermeticity of fibrin [28]. Two generations of HPMC gels have been explored; the first one consisted of a non-self-hardening HPMC, while the second one is a HPMC grafted by silane and diluted in an aqueous solution at basic pH, which is able to harden *in vivo* [29]. In comparison to the hydraulic cements, biphasic particles with a polymer matrix do not present the same mechanical properties. Their mechanical properties are dependent of the behavior of the polymer matrix. Both of these approaches aim to guide the cells in a three-dimensional (3D) network (Figure 1).

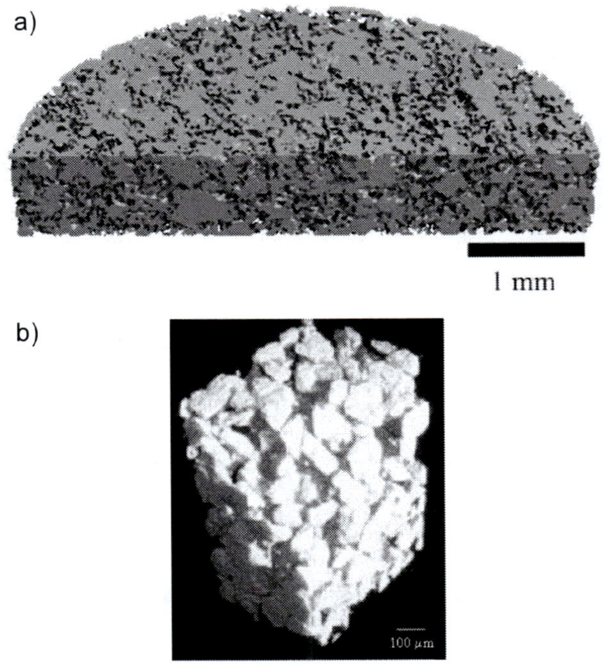

Figure 1. µCT reconstruction of an a) H-ICPC with a 30/70 PLGA/CaP ratio [37] and b) B-ICPC containing 80-200 µm biphasic CaP particles [42].

4. Physical and Mechanical Properties

As mentioned before, for the H-ICPC the initial composition of the solid phase is a mixture of α-tricalcium phosphate, calcium hydrogen phosphate (a.k.a. monetite), calcium carbonate, calcium carbonate and precipitated hydroxyapatite with a 2 wt% Na_2HPO_4 solution used as the liquid mixing phase. 1 to 4wt% Na_2HPO_4 solutions have also been used as the liquid mixing phase [30-33]. After mixing, the resulting cement is mainly composed of α-TCP and monetite (Figure 2a).

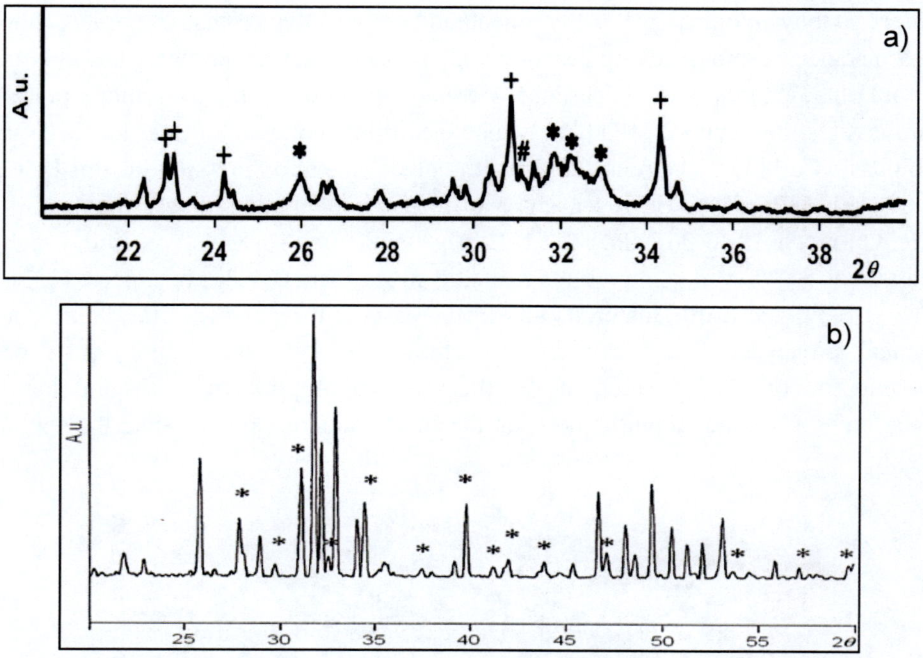

Figure 2. XRD of the Injectable calcium phosphate cements a) H-ICPC; *= Apatite; #= β-Tri calcium phosphate (β-TCP) and += α-TCP [34] and b) B-ICPC; *= β-TCP [41].

These CaP phases start transforming into apatite by hydrolysis after a few days in physiological conditions [34, 35]. The mechanical compression values for this H-ICPC is in average around 50 MPa after immersion for three days in Ringer's solution, which is within the value of human cortical bone [30, 36-38]. For this H-ICPC, injectability and mechanical properties can be changed by modifying the percentage and type of Na_2HPO_4, by using a pore generator or by changing the liquid to powder ratio [30, 37] without affecting the final obtained CaP phase. For a particle-filled H-ICPC, compression values can be reduced to an 80%, or more, of the value for a cement without particles [30, 37]. The mechanical values of the porous H-ICPC will be dependent on the size and distribution of the pores within the cement [30], as well as in their compositions [39]. An agglomeration of particles within the cement can result in zones with lower mechanical properties, which affects the overall mechanical properties of the cement [40].

In case of the B-ICPC, the main components are hydroxyapatite (HA) and β-tricalcium phosphate (β-TCP) [41] (Figure 2b). These particles are fabricated by sintering a Calcium Deficient Apatite (CDA) at high temperatures. The level of calcium deficiency is related, after sintering, to the percentage of HA and β-TCP obtained. If there is more β-TCP, the particles are more reactive, hence more resorbable. These properties are maintained when the particles are deposited in the polymer matrix [42]. It is the role of the polymer matrix to provide the cohesion properties to the CaP particles. The polymer matrix prevents phase segregation between particles and the aqueous phase by increasing the viscosity of the paste and ensures its injectability. Since the used HPMC is a non-hardening polymer, the mechanical values are very low. This can be changed by adding silane grafts in the HPMC [29, 43, 44]. Cross-linking reactions between silane groups grafted on HPMC polymer chains take place at physiological pH. After injectability, the polymer matrix hardens into a gel through acido-basic cross-linking reactions. Composites of CaP particles and this polymer matrix are obtained with various particles sizes and quantities. The maximum reported value for hardness test is around 2 MPa [29], which is still low compared to the 196 MPa value of solid biphasic CaP [45]. The reported strength values under compression for this B-ICPC are lower than 1 MPa [46]. However, after different implantation times, the B-ICPC/bone mixture can reach 18 to 26 MPa [46, 47]. In general, for hydrogels containing high water concentrations (> 95wt%), compressive strengths lower than 0.01 Pa are expected [23].

The H-ICPC are brittle materials and in the case of the polymer filled ICPC they lack mechanical properties. As a consequence, they will not possess an elastic behavior comparable to bone [36], which makes them less appropriate to withstand load. Bone regeneration will depend, among others, on the structural stress patterns and the applied load [48, 49].

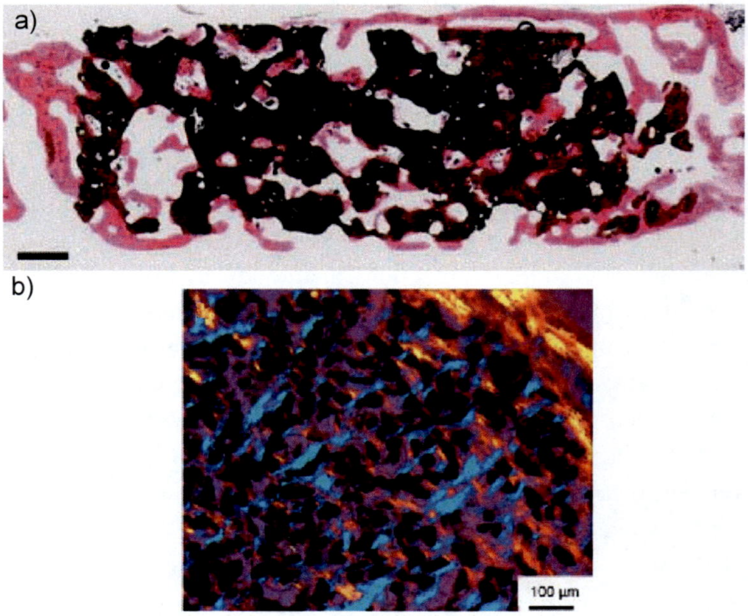

Figure 3. Histology after implantation of Injectable Calcium Phosphate Cements a) H-ICPC; Undecalcified section of porous CaP cement loaded with rhBMP-2 in a rabbit skull defect (bar=1 mm), the defect was closed via the growth of bone through the cement porosity [84] and b) B-ICPC; Polarized light micrograph of a B-ICPC-filled bone defect in rabbit femurs after 8 weeks with new bone formation, Haversian structures and osteocytes between the BCP granules (black) [46].

5. Cell Interaction and Macroporous Structures

Both ICPC are designed to act as a support that provides the right vector for biological processes after implantation in the body. ICPC present a large specific surface area, which affects their reactivity [39]. The main interesting features of ICPC are their ability to fill the defect in which they are injected, their ability to form a direct bond with the host bone, and thus a strong interface, and the capacity to be replaced in time by bone. This ICPC-bone interface is created by the conversion of the dissolved Ca and P ions into a carbonated apatite and then integration with bone tissue. Osteoclast activity is influenced by the solubility of the ceramic [50].

Bone remodeling is a complex process that involves the participation of proteins and cells [51]. The combination of an adequate architecture, implant contact and composition results in a sequence of events, which ends with the formation of bone [52-54]. Interconnected micro- and macroporosity of the ICPC allows the invasion of biological fluid through the micro- and macrochannels of the cement. This first fluid contact creates a protein coverage of the material, which is used by cells to colonize the surface. The inclusion of porosity affects the degradation rate and is used to increase the bone ingrowth response since a porous structure increases the surface of contact for proteins and exchange of ions in the implant. The bone formation is activated by the participation of dissolved calcium and phosphorus ions. If the ICPC does not present a porosity with pore sizes large enough to enable bone ingrowth, they resorb in a layer by layer process [39]. However, the degradation of the material should not be too fast in order to avoid the collapse of the structure and the prevention of nutrients supply, protein adsorption, cell adhesion and differentiation and hence osteoinduction [55]; neither it has to be too slow, otherwise the resorption is limited [32].

Porosity allows, within implantation time, ingrowth of bone into the structure making the bone-cement interface stronger [40]. It has been observed that the bone formation in the CaP cement implants starts at the surface of implants and proceeds to the interior [2]. The recommended pore size for cell invasion and nutrient distribution has been suggested to be 100 to 150 μm [56, 57], and between 200 and 400 μm for bone formation in osseous sites [58, 59], but lower sizes have been recently proven to be also good for bone ingrowth [60, 61]. If the pore size is not adequate, it takes longer for the material to resorb and to allow bone ingrowth.

H-ICPC have an intrinsic microporosity due to their fabrication process [62]. In order to create a macroporosity in the hydraulic cement structure the introduction of degradable particles has been investigated [17, 63, 64]. This approach aims to use degradable polymer microspheres made of PLGA, or other biodegradable polymers [62, 63, 65, 66], which within time disappear and create a spherical pore. In the case of the PLGA particles, these are obtained by a double emulsion process ([water-in-oil]-in water). The size of the particles can be modified by using specific parameters in this procedure or by sieving at the end of this procedure [31, 37, 64, 67, 68]. A spherical particle shape has been reported to be positive for the resorption of the material and the subsequent bone ingrowth [69, 70]. The maximal amount of particle/CaP ratio that can be used without compromising the mechanical integrity of the composite has been reported to be 30/70 [37]. Nevertheless, it is important to remember that with an increase in the porosity the mechanical properties will be diminished, as mentioned in the previous section. The formed phase after the dissolution-precipitation process has crystals with Ca/P ratios similar to those of bone apatite. These crystals have a small needle-like shape and, when precipitated into the micropores, they can provide bone cell adhesion and hence allow bone ingrowth [71]. Small crystals facilitate the resorption process, which also involves dissolution and precipitation of the crystals. These crystals are not dependent of the implantation site, subject and the type of the CaP [52, 72]. The right balance between the transformation speed of the ICPC and tissue ingrowth is a key factor for their structural maintenance and a support for the start of the tissue formation. For the B-ICPC, the macro and microporosity is determined by the sintering process that the biphasic particles have followed. In the B-ICPC, the polymer matrix dissolves and is invaded by cells, which react with the particles and start the remodeling process [42]. The hydrogel material dissolves in harmony with the new tissue regeneration, which allows maintenance of the 3D network and brings the biphasic particles in contact with the physiological environment. After implantation, the polymer matrix maintains intergranular spaces for the invasion of cells while CaP particles serve as scaffolds for bone ingrowth.

The first cells that interact with the material are multinucleated cells, such as macrophages and foreign body giant cells. These cells phagocitize the small particles of the ICPC [7, 8, 73]. Later on, mesenchymal stem cells, osteoblast and osteoclasts interact with the material. These cells can penetrate into the macropores, if the size is optimal for their passage [7, 17, 74]. The chemistry of the pore surface plays also a role, as it has been reported that CaP in combination with a good pore-architecture can attract mesenchymal stem cells and induce their phenotype into an osteogenetic type [53]. In this way, after some months bone remodeling occurs through cellular activity by the action of osteoclast resorption and bone ingrowth. This process proceeds continuously. Porosity and architecture of the material are known to play an important role in bone induction in muscle sites [51].

The PLGA particles, as used in the H-ICPC, can also be used as a delivery system for growth factors, such as rhBMP-2 or TGF-β1 [2, 37, 62, 67, 75-79] as alternative to load the ceramic material by itself [78]. Whatever the type of cement, with a polymer carrier or precipitation of CaP, the particle size and porosity (micro and macro) play an important role in the reactivity of the ICPC [7, 17, 72]. The reaction of cells with the material in an *in vitro* environment differs from their *in vivo* behavior since only a few parameters can be controlled in the former compared to the latter. It is accepted that CaP materials *in vitro* can release calcium and phosphorus ions, which will have an effect on the pH of the medium. If the pH is outside the 6.8 - 7.2 range, cells are hammered, which results in limited viability, proliferation and differentiation [34, 74]. In *in vivo* conditions, potential toxic products are rapidly washed away, since body fluids are under constant renewal so that insignificant or no harm is done. Preclinical and/or clinical applications have proven the biocompatibility and bioactivity of these two ICPC.

6. Implantation and Loaded-ICPC

In vivo, the H-ICPC can reach a degradation of 80% after 10 weeks [80]. Subcutaneous implantation in rats of porous and non-porous H-ICPC, has shown that the presence of porosity allows the invasion of fibrous tissue, blood vessels and bone [17, 64]. In a subcutaneous goat model, no bone formation was observed, but this response was probably related to the mechanical instability of the material and its degradation rate [55]. When using PLGA as a pore generator, it has been seen that a PLGA/CaP ratio of 30/70 exhibits better characteristics with respect to the consistency and abundance of bone formation and with a ratio of 20/80 there is enough the interconnectivity, degradation rate and structural consistency [30, 64]. By using a femoral goat model the capacity of H-ICPC to fixate and allow the ingrowth of simple oral implants with standard gaps has been evaluated [15]. After

12 weeks CaP cement was covered with new bone and no fibrous tissue or inflammatory response was observed. The difficulty observed here was the slow resorption rate of the ICPC.

When tested in a femoral rabbit defect, B-ICPC has shown osteoconduction, apposition of new bone and also presented greater resorption compared to the biphasic particles alone, allowing a more homogenous and earlier bone substitution than biphasic particles alone [22]. B-ICPC creates a network with the hydrogel, which keeps the space between particles. Subsequently, the gel is rapidly resorbed allowing the contact of body fluids and particles, which may favor the osteoblastic activity, bone formation and ceramic resorption. H-ICPC and B-ICPC have already been tested in human clinical and preclinical trials and they have shown potential to be resorbed and replaced by newly formed bone tissue, which makes them promising materials in orthopedic and dental applications [81-83].

Bone healing is a complex process in which a lot of growth factors are involved [77]. For a small bone defect, an ICPC can be used, but for larger defects it is necessary to increase the bone forming capacity of the ICPC. This can be done by the inclusion of growth factors such as TGF-β1 and rhBMP-2 [84]. TGF-β1 and rhBMP-2 belong to the transforming growth factor-β (TGF-β) family, which is involved in the morphogenesis of tissue and can induce *de novo* bone formation [70]. Factors inducing bone formation can be important in large size defects or when the healing conditions of the surrounding tissue are not favorable. The two mentioned factors have been studied in a great extent when associated to an H-ICPC (Table 1 and 2).

Table 1. Studies that have used of rhBMP-2 growth factor in the H-ICPC

Method of loading	Release analysis	Animal Model
•Adsorption + lyophilisation. Dose : 10 μg and 2μg /implant [67]	• In vivo by using ^{131}I labeling	• Wistar Rats, Cranial defect implantation
•Adsorption + lyophilisation. Dose : 10 μg/implant [75]	•Not available	•New Zealand White Rabbits, subcutaneous implantation
•Entrapment, adsorption + lyophilisation in PLGA particles. Dose : ≈ 0.7 μg/implant [77]	•In vivo by using ^{131}I labeling	• Sprague Dawley Rats, subcutaneous implantation
•Adsorption + lyophilisation. Dose : 10 μg/implant [78]	•In vitro by using ^{125}I labeling.	• New Zealand white rabbits, Cranial defects implantation

By associating a growth factor with an ICPC, it is attempted to alter the local milieu of cells to evoke a specific reaction (bone formation) via a cascade of cellular events [1, 70]. TGF-β1 and rhBMP-2 show osteogenic properties and/or accelerate the formation of new bone. Even in extra-skeletal ectopic implantation sites, their osteoinductive properties have been confirmed. The response of these factors will depend on the amount of factor loaded, the interaction between the carrier and factor, the chemistry and dissolution of the scaffold, its porosity, the site and size of defect and the animal model used [2, 55, 85]. Further, biphasic CaP by themselves also shows osteoinductive properties [86]. However, it has to be noticed that today the optimal concentration and release kinetics of these factors to induce bone formation is not known.

Table 2. Studies that have used of TGF-β1 growth factor in the H-ICPC

Method of loading	Release analysis	Animal Model
•Adsorbtion + lyophilisation. Dose : 0.75 μg/implant [2]	•By using an Enzyme-Linked Immmunosorbent Assay (ELISA)	• Wistar Rats, parietal calvaria implantation
•Adsorbtion + lyophilisation. Dose : 250 ng/implant [62]	• Not available	•New Zealand White Rabbits, femoral defect implantation
•Adsorbtion + lyophilisation. Dose : 200 ng/implant. [76]	• Not available	• Wistar Rats, cranial implantation
•Adsorbtion + lyophilisation. Dose : 20 and 400 ng/implant [79]	• Not available	• Saanen Goats, pulp capping implantation in incisors

When using the ICPC for drug/growth factor release, the objective is to distribute signals homogeneously into the scaffold in a 3D network [87]. The release of growth factors, drugs or bone proteins will be depending on the mode of inclusion, e.g. absorbtion on the cement surface, encapsulation in degradable microparticles or mixture through the cement paste. Further, growth factors show a high affinity for CaP ceramics [2, 77]. In case of the use of PLGA microspheres to include the growth factors, the molecular weight of the PLGA used will play a role in the release of growth factors, drugs or proteins [88]. The release will be dependent on the degradation rate of the polymer [77, 89-93]. This parameter does not play a role when factors are adsorbed onto the surface of PLGA particles [77]. However, high-dosed implants will perform better than low-dosed ones and show a same percentage of retention than the latters [67].

When H-ICPC was implanted in cranial defects in rabbits with or without rhBMP-2, bone formation was observed at the implant periphery, being this formation more important at longer implantation delays and when rhBMP-2 was present [78]. The inclusion of rhBMP-2 also allowed a better pore filling by bone compared to non-loaded CaP cement, i.e. 53% *vs.* 43.1 %. When loaded in the CaP cement (10 μg/ implant) and implanted in a rabbit cranial defect after 28 days an accumulative release of 9.7 ± 0.9 % was reached [78].

Subcutaneous implantation in New Zealand white rabbits [75] showed that when the H-ICPC was loaded with rhBMP-2 (10 μg/implant), blood vessels and loose connective tissue were present in all macropores after two weeks of implantation. After 10 weeks of implantation, bone formation had occurred; bone pore filling for the rhBMP-2-loaded scaffolds was about 18%.

TGF-β1 has also been loaded into H-ICPC by adsorption (0.75 μg) and implanted in the parietal calvaria of rats. The release observed was of 1.1 ± 0.5 % after 1 week. The CaP carrier showed a high retention since after 1 week no further release was seen without really improving the osteogenic properties of the CaP cement [2]. Other studies with this model have shown that TGF-β1-loaded implants performed better than non-loaded H-ICPC [76]. When used in pulp capping it was shown that an amount of 400 ng was able to enhance tertiary denting formation [79]. However, the method needs to be improved for this application. When using gelatin particles as a carrier and implanted in femoral defects in rabbits, TFG-β1-loaded implants enhanced the bone remodeling process [62].

The use of particles as drug delivery systems in the B-ICPC is a not well-explored area [94]. However, this approach or using the hydrogel as the delivery system, can be useful to introduce growth factors or cells in a three dimensional culture and increase the ostogenicity of this ICPC [23, 51, 95].

7. Future Trends

Since osteogenesis is related to the species and their reactions with materials [14, 25, 51] different animal models will give different results. Extensive research work has been carried out by both research groups. However, there are still some points that need to be studied. For example, independent of the approach that is used for the preparation of an ICPC, the actual mechanical behavior of these materials not allow their use for load bearing applications since the required values (shear strength and tension) are lower than required, which plays an important role *in vivo* [39, 96]. The option of giving some elastic or rigidity properties to the CaP cements (depending on the approach) without inducing toxic responses and to provide the ICPC with mechanical characteristics similar to the surrounding bone tissue is very challenging. However, this lack of mechanical strength can be compensated by an excellent bone ingrowth of the material. Other issue that needs further studying is improving the release of growth factors and their effectiveness or stability [97]. There is also a need to understand the interaction/release mechanism of the factors, or drugs, with their carrier and the CaP cement. The order of release -when using multiple growth factors-, the rate of release, the optimal dose and a way to verify the retention of their bioactivity must be studied more precisely. The use of cell-loaded particles within ICPC or cell embedding in the hydrogel matrix has also to be studied in order to assure the viability of this approach by the transportation of oxygen and nutrients to the cells and to protect them from aggressive conditions, such as low pH values, during the first hours after implantation. Finally, in a general aspect, improving of their contrast is also a requirement, specially if ICPC are intended to be used in minimal invasive surgery in order to have a safe clinical application.

Conclusion

ICPC are good candidates for minimal invasive surgery. Although the ICPC presented here use different approaches to create a 3D network, their potential applications are similar. These ICPC have suitable chemical properties and all animal models used with these two ICPC show their capacities reconstruct a small critical size defects. ICPC studied by both research groups do not produce harmful degradation products nor they elicit inflammatory responses or immunogenicity or cytotoxicity. This review presented in a summarized form the work done by these groups. Other groups around the world are working also on these or other ICPC categories, exploring different or similar aspects. Additional work is still needed to understand better the processes involved in bone regeneration. When predictable and reproducible results after application of the ICPC in a bone defect can be obtained, both H-ICPC and B-ICPC are excellent candidates for a successful bone graft substitute.

References

[1] Hartman EH, Vehof JW, Spauwen PH, Jansen JA. Ectopic bone formation in rats: the importance of the carrier. *Biomaterials*. 2005;26(14):1829-35.

[2] Huse RO, Quinten Ruhe P, Wolke JG, Jansen JA. The use of porous calcium phosphate scaffolds with transforming growth factor beta 1 as an onlay bone graft substitute. *Clin. Oral Implants Res*. 2004;15(6):741-9.

[3] Anselme K. Osteoblast adhesion on biomaterials. *Biomaterials*. 2000;21(7):667-81.

[4] Le Nihouannen D, Saffarzadeh A, Gauthier O, Moreau F, Pilet P, Spaethe R, et al. Bone tissue formation in sheep muscles induced by a biphasic calcium phosphate ceramic and fibrin glue composite. *J. Mater. Sci. Mater. Med*. 2008;19(2):667-75.

[5] Denissen HW, Kalk W, Veldhuis AA, van den Hooff A. Eleven-year study of hydroxyapatite implants. *J. Prosthet. Dent*. 1989;61(6):706-12.

[6] Gosain AK, McCarthy JG, Staffenberg D, Glat PM, Simmons DJ. The histomorphologic changes in vascularized bone transfer and their interrelationship with the recipient sites: a 1-year study. *Plast Reconstr Surg*. 1996;97(5):1001-13.

[7] Daculsi G, Laboux O, Malard O, Weiss P. Current state of the art of biphasic calcium phosphate bioceramics. *J. Mater. Sci. Mater Med.* 2003;14(3):195-200.

[8] Chow LC. Calcium phosphate cements. *Monogr. Oral Sci.* 2001;18:148-63.

[9] Ooms E. Thesis. *Injectable calcium phosphate cement for bone repair and implant fixation.* Katholieke Universiteit Nijmegen; 2003.

[10] Khairoun I, Boltong MG, Driessens FC, Planell JA. Some factors controlling the injectability of calcium phosphate bone cements. *J. Mater. Sci. Mater. Med.* 1998;9(8):425-8.

[11] Higashi S, Yamada I, Satomura A, Anzai M, Nishijima K. Studies on water-settable cement. Preparatory experiments on water-settable phosphate cement and properties of water-settable primary calcium phosphate. *J. Nihon Univ Sch. Dent*. 1972;14(2):58-63.

[12] Brown WE, Chow LC. Patent No. 4518430. American Dental Association Health Foundation, assignee. *Dental resptorative cement pastes*. U.S.A. 1985.

[13] LeGeros RZ, Chohayeb A, Shulman A. Apatitic calcium phosphates: Possible restorative materials. *J. Dent Res*. 1982;61:343.

[14] Schmitz JP, Hollinger JO, Milam SB. Reconstruction of bone using calcium phosphate bone cements: a critical review. *J. Oral Maxillofac Surg*. 1999;57(9):1122-6.

[15] Comuzzi L, Ooms E, Jansen JA. Injectable calcium phosphate cement as a filler for bone defects around oral implants: an experimental study in goats. *Clin. Oral Implants Res*. 2002;13(3):304-11.

[16] del Real RP, Wolke JGC, Vallet-Regí M, Jansen JA. A new method to produce macropores in calcium phosphate cements. *Biomaterials.* 2002;23(17):3673-80.

[17] Ruhe PQ, Hedberg-Dirk EL, Padron NT, Spauwen PH, Jansen JA, Mikos AG. Porous poly(DL-lactic-co-glycolic acid)/calcium phosphate cement composite for reconstruction of bone defects. *Tissue Eng.* 2006;12(4):789-800.

[18] LeGeros RZ. Calcium phosphates in oral biology and medicine. *Monogr. Oral Sci.* 1991;15:1-201.

[19] Bodde EW, Wolke JG, Kowalski RS, Jansen JA. Bone regeneration of porous beta-tricalcium phosphate (Conduit TCP) and of biphasic calcium phosphate ceramic (Biosel) in trabecular defects in sheep. *J. Biomed. Mater. Res. A.* 2007;82(3):711-22.
[20] Daculsi G. Biphasic calcium phosphate concept applied to artificial bone, implant coating and injectable bone substitute. *Biomaterials.* 1998;19(16):1473-8.
[21] Daculsi G, Weiss P, Bouler JM, Gauthier O, Millot F, Aguado E. Biphasic calcium phosphate/hydrosoluble polymer composites: a new concept for bone and dental substitution biomaterials. *Bone.* 1999;25(2 Suppl):59S-61S.
[22] Gauthier O, Goyenvalle E, Bouler JM, Guicheux J, Pilet P, Weiss P, et al. Macroporous biphasic calcium phosphate ceramics versus injectable bone substitute: a comparative study 3 and 8 weeks after implantation in rabbit bone. *J. Mater. Sci. Mater. Med.* 2001;12(5):385-90.
[23] Vinatier C, Guicheux J, Daculsi G, Layrolle P, Weiss P. Cartilage and bone tissue engineering using hydrogels. *Biomed. Mater Eng.* 2006;16(4 Suppl):S107-13.
[24] Jegoux F, Goyenvalle E, Bagot D'arc M, Aguado E, Daculsi G. In vivo biological performance of composites combining micro-macroporous biphasic calcium phosphate granules and fibrin sealant. *Arch Orthop Trauma Surg.* 2005;125(3):153-9.
[25] Le Guehennec L, Layrolle P, Daculsi G. A review of bioceramics and fibrin sealant. *Eur. Cell Mater.* 2004;8:1-10.
[26] Le Nihouannen D, Saffarzadeh A, Aguado E, Goyenvalle E, Gauthier O, Moreau F, et al. Osteogenic properties of calcium phosphate ceramics and fibrin glue based composites. *J. Mater. Sci. Mater. Med.* 2007;18(2):225-35.
[27] Le Guehennec L, Goyenvalle E, Aguado E, Pilet P, Bagot D'Arc M, Bilban M, et al. MBCP biphasic calcium phosphate granules and tissucol fibrin sealant in rabbit femoral defects: the effect of fibrin on bone ingrowth. *J. Mater Sci. Mater. Med.* 2005;16(1):29-35.
[28] Nakamura K, Koshino T, Saito T. Osteogenic response of the rabbit femur to a hydroxyapatite thermal decomposition product-fibrin glue mixture. *Biomaterials.* 1998;19(20):1901-7.
[29] Bourges X, Gauthier O, Grimandi G, Daculsi G, Legeay G, Weiss P. Développement d'un hydrogel autodurcissant in vivo, en perspective d'un usage biomédicalA new self-hardening gel in prospect of biomedical use. *ITBM-RBM.* 2003;24(4):185-91.
[30] Habraken WJ, Wolke JG, Mikos AG, Jansen JA. Injectable PLGA microsphere/calcium phosphate cements: physical properties and degradation characteristics. *J. Biomater Sci. Polym Ed.* 2006;17(9):1057-74.
[31] Link DP, van den Dolder J, van den Beucken JJ, Cuijpers VM, Wolke JG, Mikos AG, et al. Evaluation of the biocompatibility of calcium phosphate cement/PLGA microparticle composites. *J. Biomed. Mater. Res. A.* 2008, in press.
[32] Link DP, van den Dolder J, van den Beucken JJ, Habraken W, Soede A, Boerman OC, et al. Evaluation of an orthotopically implanted calcium phosphate cement containing gelatin microparticles. *J. Biomed. Mater. Res. A.* 2008, in press.
[33] Ooms EM, Wolke JG, van der Waerden JP, Jansen JA. Trabecular bone response to injectable calcium phosphate (Ca-P) cement. *J. Biomed. Mater Res.* 2002;61(1):9-18.

[34] Link DP, van den Dolder J, Wolke JG, Jansen JA. The cytocompatibility and early osteogenic characteristics of an injectable calcium phosphate cement. *Tissue Eng.* 2007;13(3):493-500.

[35] Ooms EM, Wolke JG, van de Heuvel MT, Jeschke B, Jansen JA. Histological evaluation of the bone response to calcium phosphate cement implanted in cortical bone. *Biomaterials.* 2003;24(6):989-1000.

[36] Gibson LJ, Ashby MF. *Cellular solids - Structure and properties.* 2nd ed. Cambridge: Cambridge University Press; 1997.

[37] Ruhe PQ, Hedberg EL, Padron NT, Spauwen PH, Jansen JA, Mikos AG. rhBMP-2 release from injectable poly(DL-lactic-co-glycolic acid)/calcium-phosphate cement composites. *J. Bone Joint Surg. Am.* 2003;85-A Suppl 3:75-81.

[38] Jarcho M. Calcium phosphate ceramics as hard tissue prosthetics. *Clin. Orthop Relat Res.* 1981;(157):259-78.

[39] Bohner, Bohner M. Physical and chemical aspects of calcium phosphates used in spinal surgery. *European Spine Journal.* 2001;10(0):S114-S21.

[40] Link DP, van den Dolder J, Jurgens WJ, Wolke JG, Jansen JA. Mechanical evaluation of implanted calcium phosphate cement incorporated with PLGA microparticles. *Biomaterials.* 2006;27(28):4941-7.

[41] Dupraz A, Nguyen TP, Richard M, Daculsi G, Passuti N. Influence of a cellulosic ether carrier on the structure of biphasic calcium phosphate ceramic particles in an injectable composite material. *Biomaterials.* 1999;20(7):663-73.

[42] Gauthier O, Khairoun I, Bosco J, Obadia L, Bourges X, Rau C, et al. Noninvasive bone replacement with a new injectable calcium phosphate biomaterial. *J. Biomed. Mater Res.* A. 2003;66(1):47-54.

[43] Bourges X, Weiss P, Coudreuse A, Daculsi G, Legeay G. General properties of silated hydroxyethylcellulose for potential biomedical applications. *Biopolymers.* 2002;63(4):232-8.

[44] Bourges X, Weiss P, Daculsi G, Legeay G. Synthesis and general properties of silated-hydroxypropyl methylcellulose in prospect of biomedical use. *Adv Colloid Interface Sci.* 2002;99(3):215-28.

[45] Nicolazo C, Gautier H, Brandao MJ, Daculsi G, Merle C. Compactibility study of calcium phosphate biomaterials. *Biomaterials.* 2003;24(2):255-62.

[46] Fellah BH, Weiss P, Gauthier O, Rouillon T, Pilet P, Daculsi G, et al. Bone repair using a new injectable self-crosslinkable bone substitute. *J. Orthop. Res.* 2006;24(4):628-35.

[47] Gauthier O, Muller R, von Stechow D, Lamy B, Weiss P, Bouler JM, et al. In vivo bone regeneration with injectable calcium phosphate biomaterial: a three-dimensional micro-computed tomographic, biomechanical and SEM study. *Biomaterials.* 2005;26(27):5444-53.

[48] Burger EH, Klein-Nulen J. Responses of bone cells to biomechanical forces in vitro. *Advances in dental research.* 1999;13:93-8.

[49] Chao EY, Inoue N. Biophysical stimulation of bone fracture repair, regeneration and remodelling. *Eur. Cell Mater.* 2003;6:72-84; discussion -5.

[50] Yamada S, Heymann D, Bouler JM, Daculsi G. Osteoclastic resorption of calcium phosphate ceramics with different hydroxyapatite/[beta]-tricalcium phosphate ratios. *Biomaterials*. 1997;18(15):1037-41.

[51] Le Nihouannen D, Daculsi G, Saffarzadeh A, Gauthier O, Delplace S, Pilet P, et al. Ectopic bone formation by microporous calcium phosphate ceramic particles in sheep muscles. *Bone*. 2005;36(6):1086-93.

[52] Le Guehennec L, Goyenvalle E, Aguado E, Houchmand-Cuny M, Enkel B, Pilet P, et al. Small-animal models for testing macroporous ceramic bone substitutes. *J. Biomed. Mater. Res. B Appl Biomater*. 2005;72(1):69-78.

[53] Yuan H, Kurashina K, de Bruijn JD, Li Y, de Groot K, Zhang X. A preliminary study on osteoinduction of two kinds of calcium phosphate ceramics. *Biomaterials*. 1999;20(19):1799-806.

[54] Yuan H, Yang Z, Li Y, Zhang X, De Bruijn JD, De Groot K. Osteoinduction by calcium phosphate biomaterials. *Journal of Materials Science: Materials in Medicine*. 1998;9(12):723-6.

[55] Bodde EW, Cammaert CT, Wolke JG, Spauwen PH, Jansen JA. Investigation as to the osteoinductivity of macroporous calcium phosphate cement in goats. *J. Biomed. Mater. Res. B Appl. Biomater*. 2007;83(1):161-8.

[56] Habibovic P, Yuan H, van der Valk CM, Meijer G, van Blitterswijk CA, de Groot K. 3D microenvironment as essential element for osteoinduction by biomaterials. *Biomaterials*. 2005;26(17):3565-75.

[57] Park JB, Lakes RS. *Biomaterials: an introduction 2nd ed*. 2nd ed. New York: Plenum Press; 1992.

[58] Karageorgiou V, Kaplan D. Porosity of 3D biomaterial scaffolds and osteogenesis. *Biomaterials*. 2005;26(27):5474-91.

[59] Tsuruga E, Takita H, Itoh H, Wakisaka Y, Kuboki Y. Pore size of porous hydroxyapatite as the cell-substratum controls BMP-induced osteogenesis. *J. Biochem*. 1997;121(2):317-24.

[60] Bobyn JD, Pilliar RM, Cameron HU, Weatherly GC. The optimum pore size for the fixation of porous-surfaced metal implants by the ingrowth of bone. *Clin. Orthop. Relat. Res*. 1980;(150):263-70.

[61] Itala AI, Ylanen HO, Ekholm C, Karlsson KH, Aro HT. Pore diameter of more than 100 microm is not requisite for bone ingrowth in rabbits. *J. Biomed. Mater. Res*. 2001;58(6):679-83.

[62] Link DP, van den Dolder J, van den Beucken JJ, Wolke JG, Mikos AG, Jansen JA. Bone response and mechanical strength of rabbit femoral defects filled with injectable CaP cements containing TGF-beta 1 loaded gelatin microparticles. *Biomaterials*. 2008;29(6):675-82.

[63] Habraken WJ, Zhang Z, Wolke JG, Grijpma DW, Mikos AG, Feijen J, et al. Introduction of enzymatically degradable poly(trimethylene carbonate) microspheres into an injectable calcium phosphate cement. *Biomaterials*. 2008;29(16):2464-76.

[64] Ruhe PQ, Hedberg EL, Padron NT, Spauwen PH, Jansen JA, Mikos AG. Biocompatibility and degradation of poly(DL-lactic-co-glycolic acid)/calcium phosphate cement composites. *J. Biomed. Mater. Res A*. 2005;74(4):533-44.

[65] Habraken WJEM, Wolke JGC, Jansen JA. Ceramic composites as matrices and scaffolds for drug delivery in tissue engineering. *Advanced Drug Delivery Reviews*. 2007;59(4-5):234-48.

[66] Young S, Wong M, Tabata Y, Mikos AG. Gelatin as a delivery vehicle for the controlled release of bioactive molecules. *Journal of Controlled Release*. 2005;109(1-3):256-74.

[67] Bodde EW, Boerman OC, Russel FG, Mikos AG, Spauwen PH, Jansen JA. The kinetic and biological activity of different loaded rhBMP-2 calcium phosphate cement implants in rats. *J. Biomed. Mater. Res A*. 2008, in press.

[68] Le Ray AM, Chiffoleau S, Iooss P, Grimandi G, Gouyette A, Daculsi G, et al. Vancomycin encapsulation in biodegradable poly([var epsilon]-caprolactone) microparticles for bone implantation. Influence of the formulation process on size, drug loading, in vitro release and cytocompatibility. *Biomaterials*. 2003;24(3):443-9.

[69] Bohner M, Baumgart F. Theoretical model to determine the effects of geometrical factors on the resorption of calcium phosphate bone substitutes. *Biomaterials*. 2004;25(17):3569-82.

[70] Ripamonti U. Soluble, insoluble and geometric signals sculpt the architecture of mineralized tissues. *J. Cell Mol. Med*. 2004;8(2):169-80.

[71] LeGeros RZ. Calcium phosphate materials in restorative dentistry: a review. *Advances in dental research*. 1988;2(1):164-80.

[72] Daculsi G, LeGeros RZ, Heughebaert M, Barbieux I. Formation of carbonate-apatite crystals after implantation of calcium phosphate ceramics. *Calcif Tissue Int*. 1990;46(1):20-7.

[73] Fellah BH, Josselin N, Chappard D, Weiss P, Layrolle P. Inflammatory reaction in rats muscle after implantation of biphasic calcium phosphate micro particles. *J. Mater Sci Mater. Med*. 2007;18(2):287-94.

[74] Benahmed M, Bouler JM, Heymann D, Gan O, Daculsi G. Biodegradation of synthetic biphasic calcium phosphate by human monocytes in vitro: a morphological study. *Biomaterials*. 1996;17(22):2173-8.

[75] Kroese-Deutman HC, Ruhe PQ, Spauwen PH, Jansen JA. Bone inductive properties of rhBMP-2 loaded porous calcium phosphate cement implants inserted at an ectopic site in rabbits. *Biomaterials*. 2005;26(10):1131-8.

[76] Plachokova A, Link D, van den Dolder J, van den Beucken J, Jansen J. Bone regenerative properties of injectable PGLA-CaP composite with TGF-beta1 in a rat augmentation model. *J. Tissue Eng Regen Med*. 2007;1(6):457-64.

[77] Ruhe PQ, Boerman OC, Russel FG, Spauwen PH, Mikos AG, Jansen JA. Controlled release of rhBMP-2 loaded poly(dl-lactic-co-glycolic acid)/calcium phosphate cement composites in vivo. *J. Control Release*. 2005;106(1-2):162-71.

[78] Ruhe PQ, Kroese-Deutman HC, Wolke JG, Spauwen PH, Jansen JA. Bone inductive properties of rhBMP-2 loaded porous calcium phosphate cement implants in cranial defects in rabbits. *Biomaterials*. 2004;25(11):2123-32.

[79] Zhang W, Walboomers XF, Jansen JA. The formation of tertiary dentin after pulp capping with a calcium phosphate cement, loaded with PLGA microparticles containing TGF-beta1. *J. Biomed. Mater Res A*. 2008;85(2):439-44.

[80] del Real RP, Ooms E, Wolke JG, Vallet-Regi M, Jansen JA. In vivo bone response to porous calcium phosphate cement. *J. Biomed Mater Res A*. 2003;65(1):30-6.

[81] Grafe IA, Baier M, Noldge G, Weiss C, Da Fonseca K, Hillmeier J, et al. Calcium-phosphate and polymethylmethacrylate cement in long-term outcome after kyphoplasty of painful osteoporotic vertebral fractures. *Spine*. 2008;33(11):1284-90.

[82] Maestretti G, Cremer C, Otten P, Jakob RP. Prospective study of standalone balloon kyphoplasty with calcium phosphate cement augmentation in traumatic fractures. *Eur Spine J.* 2007;16(5):601-10.

[83] Weiss P, Layrolle P, Clergeau LP, Enckel B, Pilet P, Amouriq Y, et al. The safety and efficacy of an injectable bone substitute in dental sockets demonstrated in a human clinical trial. *Biomaterials*. 2007;28(22):3295-305.

[84] Jansen JA, Vehof JW, Ruhe PQ, Kroeze-Deutman H, Kuboki Y, Takita H, et al. Growth factor-loaded scaffolds for bone engineering. *J. Control Release*. 2005;101(1-3):127-36.

[85] Ripamonti U. Osteoinduction in porous hydroxyapatite implanted in heterotopic sites of different animal models. *Biomaterials*. 1996;17(1):31-5.

[86] Fellah BH, Gauthier O, Weiss P, Chappard D, Layrolle P. Osteogenicity of biphasic calcium phosphate ceramics and bone autograft in a goat model. *Biomaterials*. 2008;29(9):1177-88.

[87] Hou Q, De Bank PA, Shakesheff KM. Injectable scaffolds for tissue regeneration. *J. Mater. Chem.* 2004;14(14):1915-23.

[88] Shive MS, Anderson JM. Biodegradation and biocompatibility of PLA and PLGA microspheres. *Adv. Drug Deliv. Rev*. 1997;28(1):5-24.

[89] Hedberg EL, Kroese-Deutman HC, Shih CK, Crowther RS, Carney DH, Mikos AG, et al. In vivo degradation of porous poly(propylene fumarate)/poly(DL-lactic-co-glycolic acid) composite scaffolds. *Biomaterials*. 2005;26(22):4616-23.

[90] Hedberg EL, Shih CK, Lemoine JJ, Timmer MD, Liebschner MA, Jansen JA, et al. In vitro degradation of porous poly(propylene fumarate)/poly(DL-lactic-co-glycolic acid) composite scaffolds. *Biomaterials*. 2005;26(16):3215-25.

[91] Lu L, Stamatas GN, Mikos AG. Controlled release of transforming growth factor beta1 from biodegradable polymer microparticles. *J. Biomed. Mater. Res*. 2000;50(3):440-51.

[92] Lu L, Yaszemski MJ, Mikos AG. TGF-beta1 release from biodegradable polymer microparticles: its effects on marrow stromal osteoblast function. *J. Bone Joint Surg Am*. 2001;83-A Suppl 1(Pt 2):S82-91.

[93] von Recum HA, Cleek RL, Eskin SG, Mikos AG. Degradation of polydispersed poly(L-lactic acid) to modulate lactic acid release. *Biomaterials*. 1995;16(6):441-7.

[94] Iooss P, Le Ray AM, Grimandi G, Daculsi G, Merle C. A new injectable bone substitute combining poly([var epsilon]-caprolactone) microparticles with biphasic calcium phosphate granules. *Biomaterials*. 2001;22(20):2785-94.

[95] Le Nihouannen D, Guehennec LL, Rouillon T, Pilet P, Bilban M, Layrolle P, et al. Micro-architecture of calcium phosphate granules and fibrin glue composites for bone tissue engineering. *Biomaterials*. 2006;27(13):2716-22.

[96] Yaszemski MJ, Payne RG, Hayes WC, Langer R, Mikos AG. Evolution of bone transplantation: molecular, cellular and tissue strategies to engineer human bone. *Biomaterials*. 1996;17(2):175-85.

[97] Fu K, Klibanov AM, Langer R. Protein stability in controlled-release systems. *Nat Biotech.* 2000;18(1):24-5.

In: Bioceramics: Properties, Preparations and Applications
Editors: W. Kossler, J. Fuchs, pp. 253-267
ISBN: 978-1-60741-056-0

Chapter VII

Corrosion Behavior and Biofriction and Wear Property of the AlTiN Coating Deposited on the Surface of Ti6Al4V Alloy in Simulated Physiological Environment

Zhu Weidong[1], Zhu Tao[1], Wang Xudong[2], Su Xiangdong[3] and Jiang Xiaoying[4]

[1] College of materials science and metallurgy engineering, Guizhou University, Guiyang 550003, China

[2] Department of physiology, Guiyang medical college, Guiyang 550004, China

[3] College of Science, Beijing University of aeronautics and astronautics, Beijing 100083, China

[4] College of Science, Guizhou University, Guiyang 550025, China

Abstract

An AlTiN ceramic coating was deposited on the surface of biomedical Ti6Al4V alloy by high ionic pulse (H.I.P) technology; The electrochemical corrosion test indicated that the Ti6Al4V-AlTiN coating material basically kept to a passivation state in the range of current density -0.4~0.25A/m^2, but the current density increased suddenly at 0.5V potential while Ti6Al4V alloy sample tested, and its oxidation film broken; The chemical immerssion test also displayed that the coated material effectively blocked the release of Al and V ions; And the property of biofriction and wear of AlTiN coating in simulated serum lubrication at 37^{0}C was investigated and compared with that of non-coating Ti6Al4V alloy. It shows that under the same conditions, the wear loss of the sample deposited AlTiN was 1.2% of the substrate, and the friction coefficient was only 0.007. A significant approach to the mechanism of the property is discussed with the aid of SEM, EDS and XRD.

Keywords: AlTiN coating; Ti6Al4V alloy; Release of Al and V ions; Biofriction and wear; H.I.P technology.

Preface

Titanium and its alloys have a lot of excellent properties such as high strength, fatigue capability, corrosion resistance and good biocompatibility, so they have been applied widely in the medical field. But the Ti6Al4V most in use has a disadvantage of poor wear resistance. When it is transplanted into a body, a black and brown-sticky substance would formed around the joint due to wear. Aroused pain may lead to re-operate and re-transplanted, thus worsening the patient suffering. It is reported [1] that the average life-span of artificial hip-joint made from American titanium alloy is less than 10 years. Ludama [2] reported that under conditon of lubricating, it is easy to strip and cause the surface roughness because of poor hardness and wear resistance of TiO_2 procuct on the Ti6Al4V surface. Therefore, it is a goal to prepare a ceramic coating on a metallic substrate which can be as a plant with metallic strength and toughness, and also with ceramic hagh hardness, low wear loss and good biocompatibility. In recent years, an AlTiN ceramic coating gradually spreaded in surface engineering, coincides with the ceramic features very much because of its high hardness, excellent property of friction and wear, good chemical inertness and strong adhesive force [3, 4]. After Ti6Al4V was deposited with AlTiN, the Ti6Al4V-AlTiN coating material so formed displayed a better corrosion behavior than Ti6Al4V substrate's [5]. Moreover, it can be very convenient for the concave, convex and back to deposit due to H.I.P's good diffraction. For the AlTiN coating surface modification of titanium alloy, which can be used as the skelecton's, especially the complicated places as joint's substitute material, it is easy to accomplish in technics. Until now there have been very few reports on the AlTiN preparation of Ti6Al4V alloy. In the present paper, from the testing results of electrochemical corrosion, ion release and friction and wear in simulated body fluid (37^0C), for the AlTiN coating deposited on the surface of biomedical titanium alloy Ti6Al4V, a possibility that the ceramic coating can be used as a biomaterial with a potential application prospect has been investigated.

1. Materials and Methods

1.1. The Preparation of Ti6Al4V-AlTiN Ceramic Coating Samples

The biomedical titanium alloy was linear-cut into the sizes 10mm×10mm×3mm (the samples for electrochemical corrosion and chemical immersion) and 30mm×7mm×6mm (the samples for friction and wear) respectively. The AlTiN deposition of the Ti6Al4V substrate surface worked well was performed in CC800®/9 XL coating system made in German CemeCon company by H.I.P technology based on compound cathode, bipole and unbalanced magnetron sputtering. Deposition time 2h; Al content of the ceramic coating 60% (high aluminum); Thickness of the ceramic layer 4μm (measured by calotte grinder); Adhesive force between ceramic coating and substrate: grade 2 (standard of CemeCon company: adhesive force is divided into 1~11, grade 1 highest).

1.2. Electrochemical Corrosion Test in Simulated Physiological Environment

The experimental medium was simulated physiological serum, and its composition was [6]: NaCl 6.800g/l + $CaCl_2$ 0.200g/l + KCl 0.200g/l + $MgSO_4$ 0.100g/l + $NaHCO_3$ 2.200g/l + Na_2HPO_4 0.126g/l + NaH_2PO_4 0.026g/l + $C_6H_{12}O_6$ 1.000g/l, PH6.88.

A standard of three-electrode system was used for electrochemical corrosion testing, as shown in figure 1.1. The power supply was a DJS-292 potentiostat; The reference electrode was the saturated calomel one; The auxiliary electrode was a platinum one; And the working electrode was Ti6Al4V alloy sample or Ti6Al4V-AlTiN coating one which was rinsed with distilled water and acetone. The working face area was $1cm^2$, and the non-working faces were sealed with silica gel. And the surface morphology was observed with the aid of OLYMPUS SZX-STAD2 optical microscope.

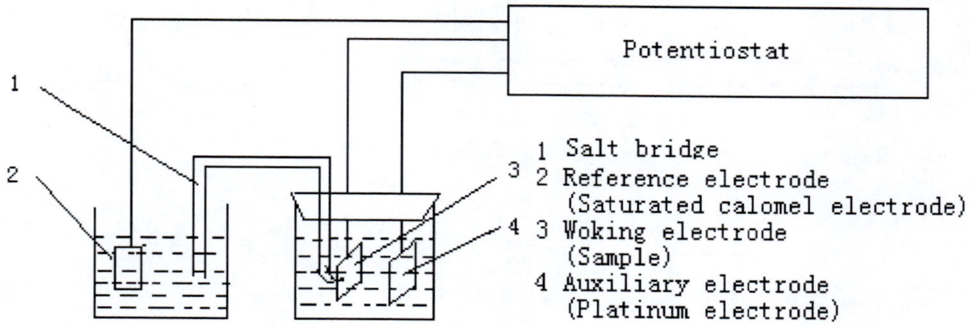

Figure 1.1. Schematic plan of three-electrode system.

1.3. Release Test of Al, V Ions in Simulated Physiological Environment

Taking a Ti6Al4V alloy sample and a Ti6Al4V-AlTiN coating sample respectively into a thermostat-controlled water bath, each sample was immersed in the simulated physiological serum of 25ml at 37^0C for 7 days. The sample size was 10mm×10mm×3mm. The contents of Al and V eleaments in the solution were detected with IRIS intrepid II ICP after immersion. And the surface of Ti6Al4V-AlTiN coating sample was analysized with EMPA-1600.

Taking a Ti6Al4V alloy sample and a Ti6Al4V-AlTiN coating sample respectively into a water bath, in which a sample was immersed in a simulated physiological balanced saline Hank's solusion of 25ml for 100 days. The sample size was the same as above, temperature kept at 37^0C $+1^0$C. With ICP the contents of Al and V eleaments in the solution were detected after immersion.

The composition of Hank's solusion was [7]: NaCl 8g/l + Na_2HCO_3 0.35g/l + Na_2HPO_4 0.0475g/l + KCl 0.4g/l + KH_2PO_4 0.06g/l + $MgCl_26H_2O$ 0.10g/l + $MgSO_4$ $7H_2O$ 0.10g/l + $CaCl_2$ 0.18g/l + Glucose 1g/l , PH7.45.

1.4. Test of Biofriction and Wear

The test of the friction and wear for the material was performed with an MM-200 friction tester. The samples tested were Ti6Al4V's and Ti6Al4V-AlTiN's. The size was a stripe sample of 30mm×7mm×6mm (wearing face: 30mm×7mm). The opposite sample was an annular one. The material was GCr15 (experienced treatments of quenching and tempering), hardness HRC62. And its testing sketchs are as shown in figures 1.2 and 1.3 (the temperature-controlled heating device illustration omitted).

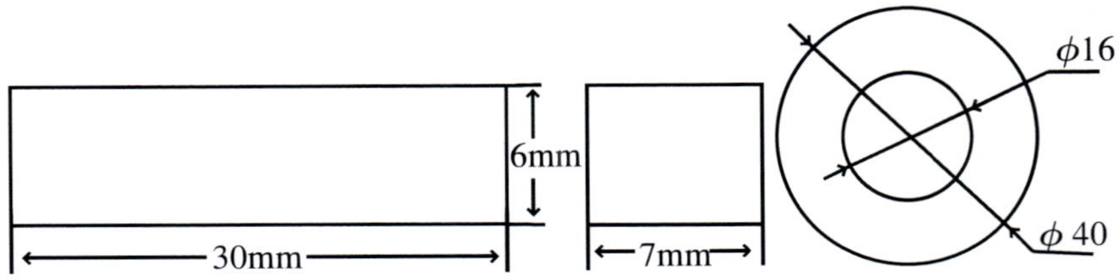

Figure 1.2. Schematic diagram of sample and anti-wear ring.

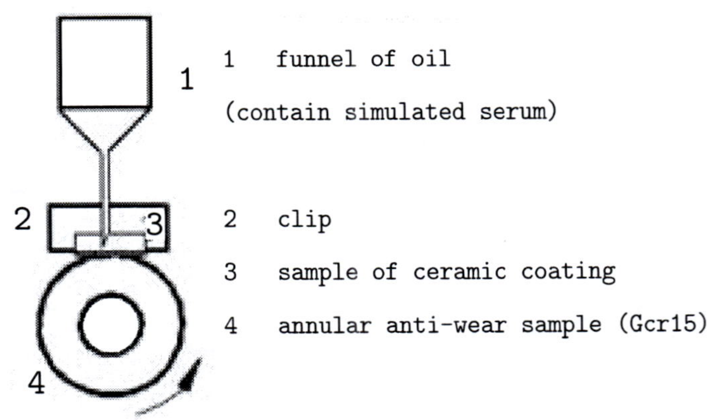

Figure 1.3. Schematic diagram of friction and wear.

Because the joint synovium is excised totally or greater partially after an artificial joint operation, the body lubricant should be a tissue fluid which resembles serum extremely [8]. The lubricant used in this experiment was a simulated physiological serum compounded with the analytically pure chemical agents, PH6.86, and the composition sees [6] in 1.2.

2. Results and Analysis

2.1. The Test of Potentiodynamic Polarization in Simulated Physiological Environment

Figure 2.1 shows the curves of potentiodynamic polarization of the Ti6Al4V alloy and Ti6Al4V-AlTiN coating samples in simulated physiological serum. It can be seen from the figure that under the experimental condition, the current density changed not greatly when the potentioal of Ti6Al4V-AlTiN coating material from -1.5V went to 1.5V, basically in an inert state from -0.4A/m^2 to 0.25A/m^2; But the current density suddenly increased from 0.25A/m^2 when the potential of Ti6Al4V was at 0.5V, its oxidation film was broken, and the Eb was 0.5V.

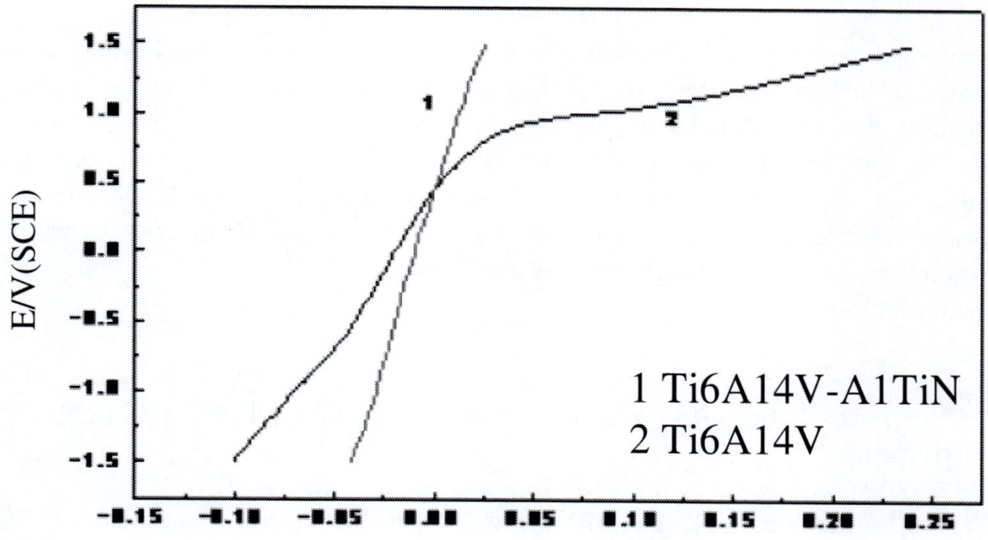

Figure 2.1. Polarization curve of coated and uncoated Ti6Al4V alloy.

The result from figure 2.1 shows that Ti6Al4V-AlTiN has a better corrosion resistance. The polarized Ti6Al4V alloy surface appeared golden yellow under sunlight, and color stripes partially. Through anodizing, different color titanium can be prepared [9]. Obtaining a compact anodized film of Ti alloy can improve the surface properties of the alloy as well as the corrosion resistance of the substrate. In the same electrolyte, the color of a anodized film mainly depends on voltage. Different oxidation film thicknesses can be got in different voltages, thus color different [10]. Under this experimental condition, the oxidtion film producted on the surface of Ti6Al4V alloy might be very thin, neither compact nor even. So, the corrosion resistance was increased to a certain extent, but not ideal.

Figure 2.2 shows the optical microphotos of Ti6Al4V and Ti6Al4V-AlTiN coating samples after electrochemical corrosion. It can be seen from the figure 2.2(a) that though uneven oxidation film existed on the rugged surface of Ti6Al4V alloy, it was not enough to have a good protedtion effect.

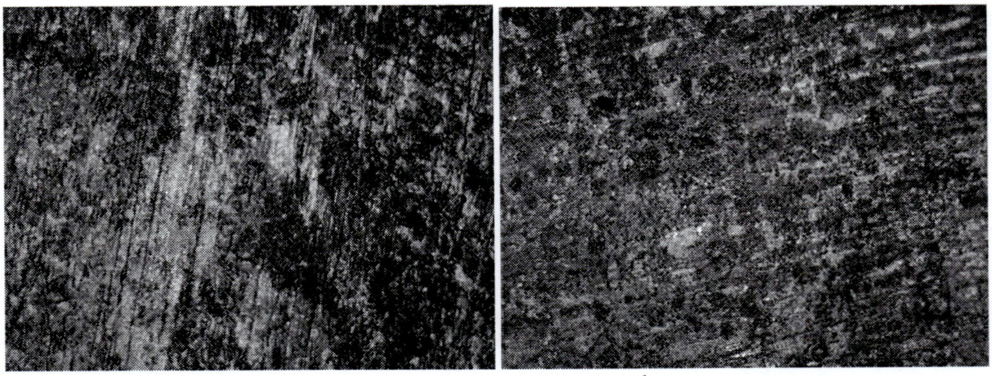

a b

Figure 2.2. Optical microscope results of Ti6Al4V alloy and Ti6Al4V-AlTiN samples after electrochemical corrosion (1000×) a: Ti6Al4V alloy; b: Ti6Al4V-AlTiN sample.

Furthermore, the partial corrosion after the oxidation film was brokendown speeded up corrosive disruption. Therefore, the releases of the harmful ions of Al and V have been accelerated, thus the material's structural strength would be weakened. It can be seen from figure 2.2b that the surface of Ti6Al4V-AlTiN coating material is even, no major peeling off, and displays a better corrosion resistance. This is why a coated sample in electrochemical corrosion had been being in an inert state under the experimental condition. And this is inseparable with that the compact and even structure of an AlTiN coating has a good bonding strength with substrate.

2.2. The Test of Ionic Release of Al and V in Simulated Physiological Environment

Table 2.1 shows the contents of Al and V of repectively uncoated and coated Ti6Al4V alloy samples immersed in the simulated physiological serum of 25ml for 7 days. It can be seen from it that the ionic release amounts of Al and V of Ti6Al4V-AlTiN coating sample in the serum are lower than those of Ti6Al4V alloy. That illustrates that the AlTiN coating is acting as a very good protection.

Table 2.1. Contents of Al, V in simulated physiological serum after immersed for 7 days

Materials	Ti6Al4V alloy	Ti6Al4V-AlTiN
Al(mg/l)	0.2	<0.1
V(mg/l)	0.03	<0.03

Note: Detectability of IRIS Intrepid □ S-92 plasma emission spectrometer: Al(0.1 mg/l), V(0.03 mg/l).

In Ti6Al4V alloy, Al and V respctively accelerates the formations of α phase and β one. And β phase occupies over 10%, presenting a structure of α+β phases. The b.c.c β phase in Ti6Al4V alloy existes in different phase areas. Due to the differences of interphase thermodynamic stabilities, it is easy to form a corrosion micro-cell, thus bringing about partially anodic action to release the metallic ions. But an AlTiN ceramic coating possesses a hard, compact and even structure, which acts as a very good protection. Because the research into biology of AlTiN coating material is still at an exploratory stage, detailed theoretical explanation needs further exploration.

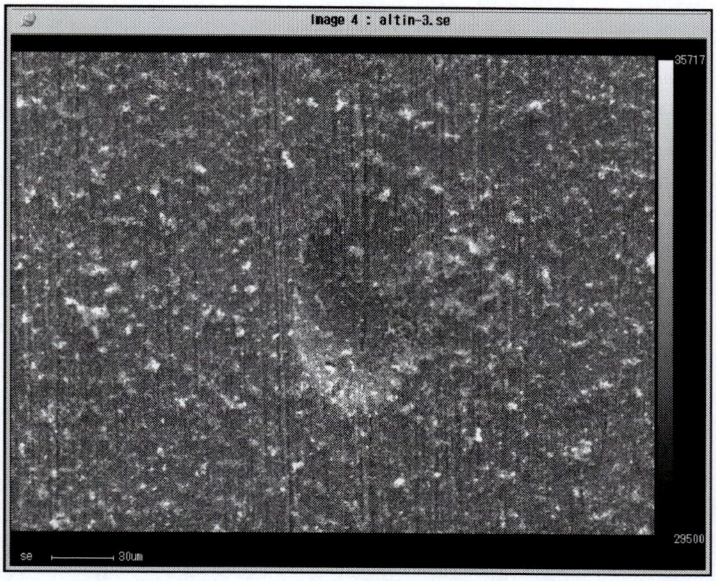

Figure 2.3. EPMA result (se) of Ti6Al4V-AlTiN sample after immersed for 7 days.

Taking the Ti6Al4V-AlTiN coating sample after immersed in the serum (PH6.88), constant temperature at 37 ± 1^0C for 7 days, to observe with EPMA (secondary electron image, as shown in figure 2.3), the surface constitutent content tested sees table 2.2. It can be seen from figure 2.3 that there is much deposition arosen on the surfce of Ti6Al4V-AlTiN coating material.

Table 2.2. Elemental composition of Ti6Al4V-AlTiN surface after immersed for 7 days

Element	Wt%	At%
N	2.79	6.17
O	9.66	18.68
Al	36.31	41.62
P	0.93	0.93
Ca	0.98	0.76
Ti	49.33	31.85

Wt%: Weight percent, At%: Atomicity percent.

The composition of the deposition can be known from table 2-2. There are the elements of Ca and P in it. Both the two elements are the major constituted composition of hydroxyapatite (HA) $Ca_{10}(PO_4)_6(OH)_3$. Moreover, HA is the major constitutent composition of skeleton and teeth also.

The formation of Ca/P layer may be due to the negative charge OH^- binding with on the surface of titanium alloy in the solution. Thus the PH value of the solution near by the alloy surface layer may be increased. The increase of PH will bring about calcium ions and phosphorus-bearing groups near the surface to oversaturate, and thus to promote the ions and groups to nucleate on the surface of AlTiN coating which bears rich negative charges of OH^-. At the beginning of the surface C/P layer growth, P deposited quickly, the ratio of Ca/P increased gradually with time. It is usually easier for HPO_4^{2-} and PO_4^{3-} to exist in an alkline environment. Besides, the solubility product of HA is far lower than that of other phosphates. And in the same concentration of calcified solution, the oversaturation of HA is over than that of other phosphates. So, the deposition of the elements of Ca and P on the surface of Ti6Al4V-AlTiN coating material is an important condition to form HA. Moreover, the formtion of Ca/P layer on the surfce makes the ions of Al and V migrate more difficultly, it is contributory to restrain the ionic release of Al and V. Similarity, there will be Ca/P layer appearing when the Ti6Al4V alloy is immersed in the solution of calcium and phosphorus-rich-bearing. About this, there have been some literatures reported [11, 12].

Nevertheless, through XRD testing, no HA was found to form on the surface of Ti6Al4V-AlTiN. The deposition of Ca/P layer for the most of biomaterials would arise on the surface in the Ca and P-rich-bearing simulated body fluid. Although there was a trace Ca/P layer deposition on the surface, it was not enough to form HA in a shorter time, that is without bioactivity.

Table 2.3 shows the elemental contents of Al and V of the Ti6Al4V alloy, before and after was coated respectively, immersed in the Hank's solution (PH7.54) for 100 days. It can be seen from it that the elemental release amounts of Al and V, especially Al, obviously lower than those of Ti6Al4V alloy samples. This further illustrates that the AlTiN coating has an effective check to the harmful elements. And this is born out again that after immersed for long, Al and V in AlTiN coating did not release a lot, this may closely relate to the microstructure, and the structure needs further research.

Table 2.3. Release amounts of Al and V ions in Hank's solution (PH7.45) after immersed for 100 days

Materials	Ti6Al4V alloy	Ti6Al4V-AlTiN
Al(mg/l)	0.122	0.061
V(ug/l)	8.0	6.7

2.3. Analysis of AlTiN Ceramic Coating Surface and Discussion of Wear Result

The test was performed on a wear tester of MM-200, under the condition of simulated physiology, and its testing principle is as shown in figure 1.3. The testing parmeters were: rotational speed 200r/min, pressure 196N, wear time 2h, and temperature 37^0C. The simulated serum lubricated gravitionally on the strip sample by dripping through the funnel drip hole, about 130 drips per min. The kinetic friction coefficient at a stable state was recorded, and the wear loss was weighed with an analytical balance. The weared surfaces were analized with SEM, EDS and XRD. The tested surfaces hardnesses, wear losses and coefficients of the materials are shown in table 2.4. It can be seen from the table that the hardness of an AlTiN coating was very high, the wear loss was only 1.2% of Ti6Al4V substrate's, and the friction coefficient was only 0.0070.

Table 2.4. Microhardness, wear loss and friction coefficient of samples

Materials	Hardness (HV)	Wear loss (g)	Friction coefficiant
Ti6Al4V	319	0.0167	—
Ti6Al4V-AlTiN	3000	0.0002	0.0070

Hardness is one of the major factors to influence wear resistance. Generally, the higher the hardness, the better the wearability [13]. As the hardness of the material and the bonding strength (grade 2) between the coating and substrate increased, the anti-stripping property of the material would get hightened. The high hardness indicated that the material has a strong bearing capacity, the surface deforms little, and correspondingly the contact area for friction decreases. The kinetic friction coefficient indicated that under the condition of gravity lubricating of the simulated physiological serum, the coated sample had been running at a stable-wear-state, without friction coefficient and wear loss changing suddenly. That indicated that without changing the lubricating form in the test, the coating of the sample did not rupture and peel off. Ti6Al4V-AlTiN has a good bearing and anti-stripping capacities. But the uncoated Ti6Al4V substrate lost too much in the process of friction and wear, so that a friction coefficient at stable state was not recored down.

Figure 2.4 shows the SEM morphology and EDS spectrum of the right surface (30mm×7mm) of the ceramic coating befor wearing. It can be seen from the SEM photo that the coating is composed of a lot tiny particles united closely.

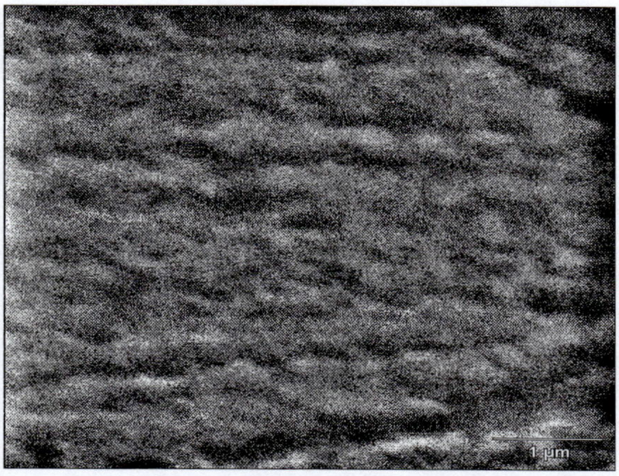

Figure 2.4. (Continued).

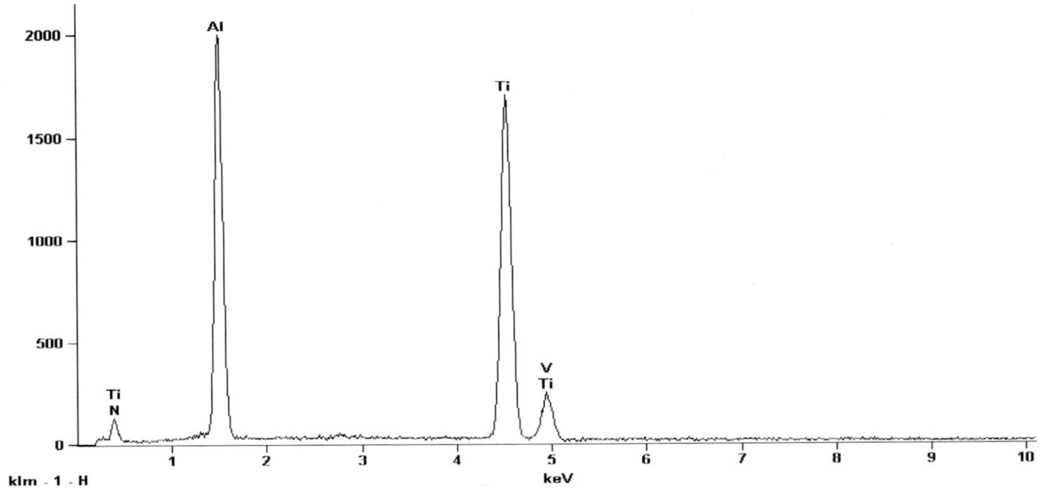

Figure 2.4. SEM morphology and EDS of bioceramic coating before wearing (30mm×7mm).

These nano and micro structures are very helpful for blood and nutrition to transport. AlTiN, called a super nitride, is a tiny particle's, compact cubic lattic's and metallic base's hard coating [14]. But a cubic nitride is fairly effective to heighten wear risistance. It is seen from the EDS spectrum that the major composition of the ceramic coating coincides with that of AlTiN, a little V element (from the substrate, mainly existing in the form of VN) can make a contribution to wearability also.

Figure 2.5 is a SEM morphology of the bonding place between ceramic layer and substrate. It can be seen from the figure that the coating bonds compactly, no obvious boundary was found. Figure 2.6 is a surface morphology of a coated sample after wearing. It can be obversed from the figure that there are some slight weared traces in the direction of wearing (vertical direction).

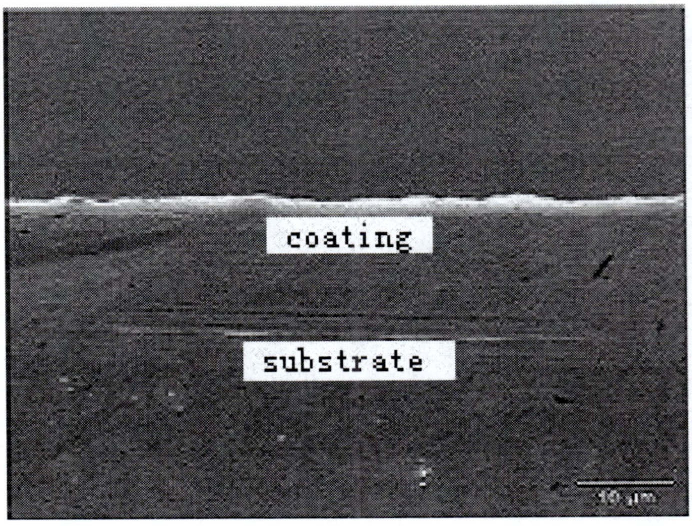

Figure 2.5. SEM morphology of connected area of bioceramic coating and substrate (6mm×7mm).

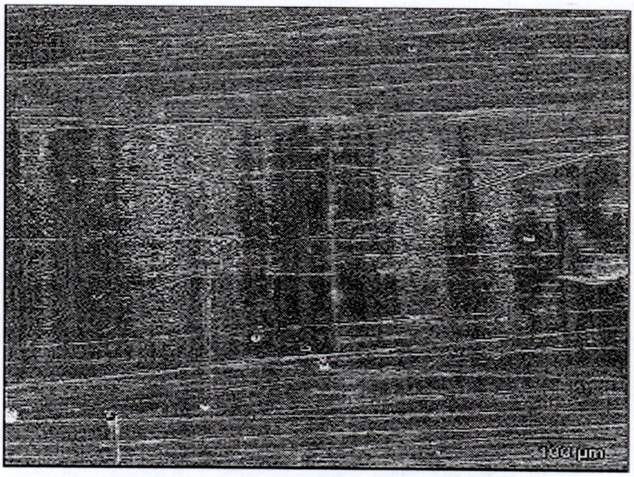

Figure 2.6. SEM morphology of Ti6Al4V-AlTiN after weared.

Generally speaking, surface fatigue wear will be unavoidable even under the condition of a good lubrication [15]. But this surface fatigue is just at a stage of running-in, belongs to a non-developing wear. Because the extremely dense plasma produced by H.I.P directly guided to the deposited surface, and high-ionizedly bombarded the growing film, that made the hardness of AlTiN coating extremely high, the bonding strength with substrate very strong, oxidation resistance and adhesion resistance excellent, and the coating presented a very good wearability.

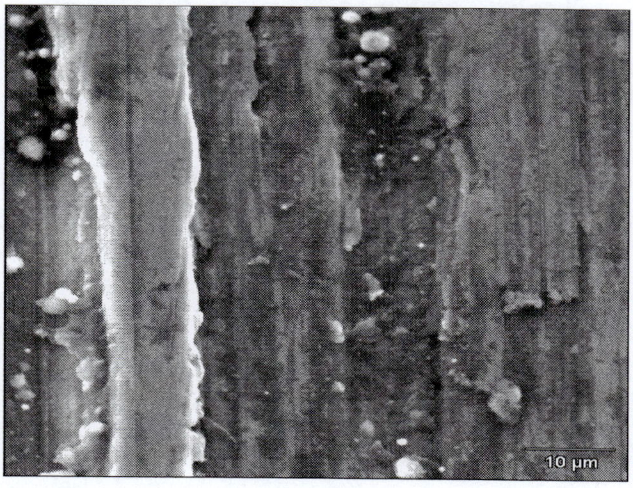

Figure 2.7. SEM morphology of Ti6Al4V alloy after wearing.

Figure 2.7 is an SEM morpholoy of Ti6Al4V sample, undeposited treatment, under the same condition. It is seen from the figure that there are many deep ploughings and different sizes of debris adhered on the surface, it displyed an obvious character of adhesive wear. It is easy for Ti6Al4V surface to produce a layer of oxidation film. The film, with brittleness, fatiguely cracked in the process of wearing, then the crack would propagate with the particles peeling off to form the debris [16]. And then the action of rolling and grinding on the wearing surface would create a serious phenomenon of abrasive wear. It was seen from EDS analyses of the debris (point 1, figure 2.8), white area (point 2) and black area (point 3) that the elements of Fe and Cr came out on the weared surface, thus indicated a severe materials transfer occurred between the sample Ti6Al4V and the opposite wearing piece GCr15. Both the debris and the plough had the phenomena of oxidation, there was oxidation wear existing traced. The elements of C and Ca were the remains of simulated physiological fluid (Mo was the external pollution when the sample line cut).

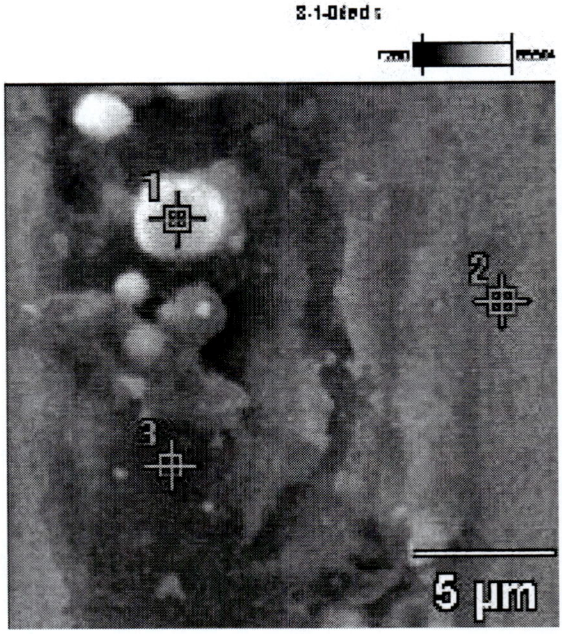

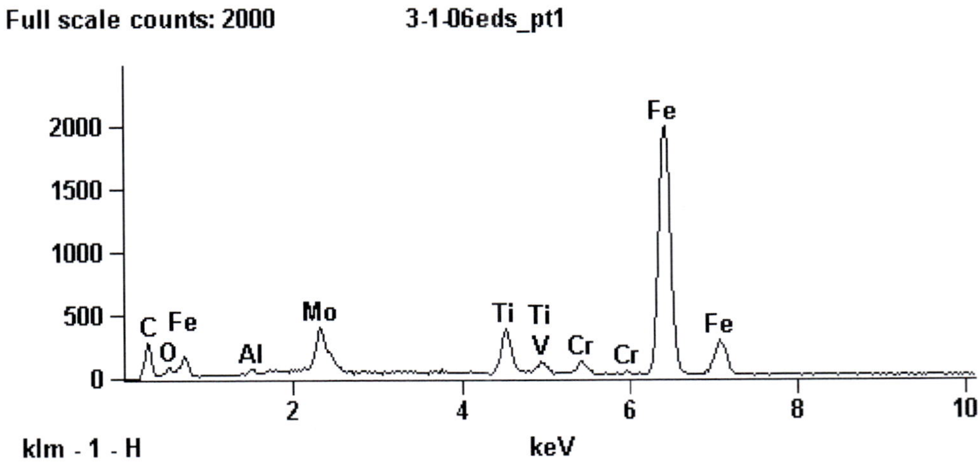

Figure 2.8. (Continued on next page).

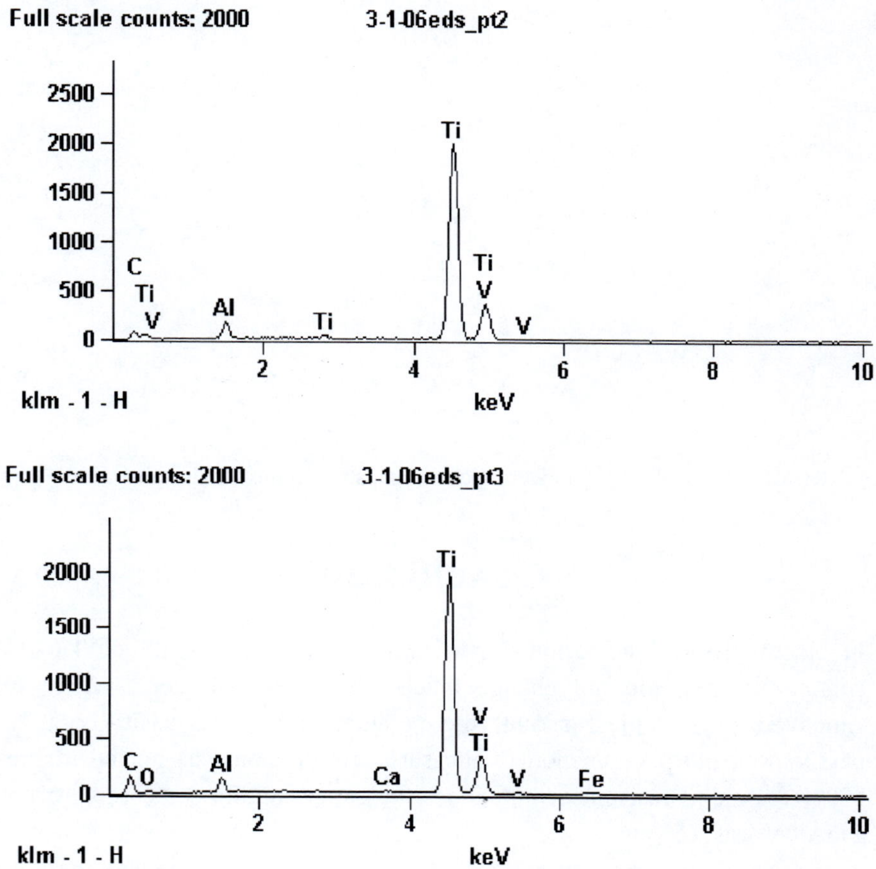

Figure 2.8. EDS of micro-area of wear trace of Ti6Al4V alloy.

Figure 2.9 is an XRD result of the ceramic coating. The phases of $AlTi_3$ and Ti_2AlN on the surface of the ceramic coating belong to a hexagonal system. And the hexagonal structure is the most effective to reduce friction coefficient, and has a minor tendence to adhere also [17]. Moreover, a firm and close bonding among the phases as well as with the substructure is beneficial to bear a high fatigue stress in human joints. It is also advantageous to improve fatigue wearability, a reflection of the weared face is even, fine and smooth (in comparision with the substrate Ti6Al4V). It is necessary to explain that the AlTiN, as an independent phase, has not been included in PDF (The Powder Diffraction File) yet, and has not been searched out in the spectrum of diffraction, especially in the range of small angles in which the unknown peaks came out. For the high Al coating of over 50% content, many companies including CemeCon have changed the standard to AlTiN, and differentiated it from TiAlN [18]. Due to the effectiveness to increase wearability and the confinement of the harmful elements in AlTiN to release, these testing results have indicated that the AlTiN modification on the Ti6Al4V surface can be developed as a bio-wearbility material with a potential application prospect.

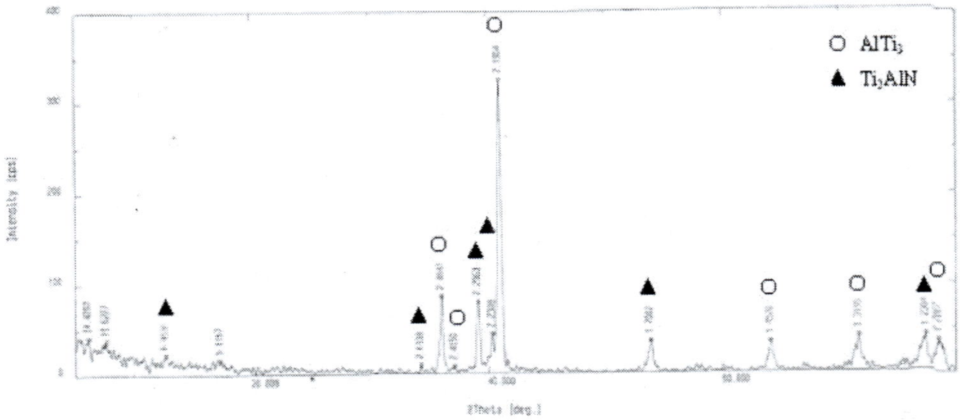

Figure 2.9. XRD of connected area of bioceramics and substrate (6mm×7mm).

Conclusion

(1) In electrochemical corrosion experiment, the current density of Ti6Al4V-AlTiN coating material did not change much with protential increasing in PH6.88 of simulated physiological serum, the potential 1.5V was basically at a state of passivation, the phenomenon of the surface corrosion was not clear, presenting a better corrosion resistance; but under the same condition the rupture potential of Ti6Al4V was 0.5V.

(2) In the test of ionic release, the coated material effectively reduced the release of Al and V ions. After Ti6Al4V alloy was immersed in PH6.88 of the simulated physiological serum for 7 days, the ionic release amount of Al and V was 0.2mg/l and 0.03mg/l respectively. Under the same condition, the release amount of Al and V ions of the coated sample was all lower than the testing limit. After the Ti6Al4V alloy was immersed in the PH7.45 of Hank's solution for 100 days, the release amount of Al ion was 0.122 mg/l, that of V one 8.0μg/l. Under the same condition, the release amount of Al ion was 0.061mg/l, that of V one 6.7μg/l. So, comparing the two testing results, it can be elucidated that the coated alloy would increase the safety of long transplanting in human body.

(3) After an AlTiN ceramic coating deposited on the surface of Ti6Al4V by H.I.P technology, the surface hardness increased greately. The coating bonded with substrate strongly, having an excellent bio-wearbility and anti-stripping. And the weared face would just occur slight weared traces, belong to non-developing fatigue wear.

(4) The Ti6Al4V substrate occured severe adhesive wear and abrasive wear under the testing condition, and was accompanied by oxidation wear, belonging to a compound action of the three.

(5) The AlTiN ceramic coating on the Ti6Al4V substrate had not been cracked, stripped and worn out, it indicated that the coated material is a good way to reduce friction coefficient and to increase the wear resistance of Ti6Al4V.

References

[1] R. Hurchings. A tem investigation of the structure of nitrogen-implanted Ti-6Al-4V[J]. *Materials Letters*. 1983, 1(5-6): 137-140.

[2] K. C. Ludema. A review of scuffing and running-in of lubricated surfaces, with asperities and oxides in perspective[J]. *Wear,* 1984, 100: 315-331.

[3] Han Rongdi, Hu Guangyi, Han Bin. Experimental investigation on coating technology and cutting performance of coated tool[J]. *Manufacturing Technology and Machine Tool,* 2004, (10): 17-19.

[4] Ye Weichang. A new type of AlTiN coating[J]. *Machine Design and Manufacturing Engineering,* 1998, 27(5): 12.

[5] Tian Bo, Zhu Weidong, Su Xiangdong, et al. Corrosion resistance of Ti6Al4V-AlTiN in artificial biological environment[J]. *Journal of Clinical Rehabilitative Tissue Engineering Research,* 2007, 11(18): 3468-3471.

[6] Wang Ju'ru, Zhang Chaowu, Wod. J. V. Investigation of composite ceramic coatings on CoCrMo alloy substrates[J]. *Journal of Chinese ceramic society*, 1996, (2): 14-18

[7] ZD. Cui, HC. Man, XJ. Yang. The corrosion and nickel release behavior of laser surface-melted NiTi shape memory alloy in Hanks solution[J]. *Surface and Coatings Technology*, 2005, 192: 347-353.

[8] Yang Min, Zheng Changqiong, Ran Junguo, et al. Studies on properties of biofriction and wear for friction paris of UHMWPE and Ti matrix-TiN-TiC gradient film materials[J]. *Journal of Biomedical Engineering*, 2000, 17(1): 1-4.

[9] Delplancke JL, Degrez M, Fontana A, et al. Self-color anodizing of titanium[J]. *Surf Technol,* 1982, 16(2): 153-162.

[10] Du Zhihui, Cui Zhenduo, Zhu shengli, et al. Corrosion behavior in Hank's solution of the anodic oxide film on Ti alloy[J]. *Transactions of materials and heat treatment,* 2004, 25(6): 101-103.

[11] F.Barrere, C.A van Blitterswijk, K. de Groot, P. Layrolle. Nucleation of biomimetic Ca-P Coatings on Ti6Al4V from a SBF×5 solution: influence of magnesium[J]. *Biomaterials*, 2002, 23: 2211-2220.

[12] Boon Sing Ng, Ingegerd Annergren, Andrew M. Sotar, et al. Characterisation of a duplex TiO_2/CaP coating on Ti6Al4V for hard tissue replacement[J]. *Biomaterials,* 2005, 1087-1095.

[13] Liu Jiajun. *The wear principle and resistance of materials*[M]. Beijing: Tsinghua University Press, 1993.

[14] Shen Zhuangxing translated. Development status of the cutting tool coating of Al-Ti-N[J]. Cutting Tool View, 2004, (1): 8-10.

[15] Wen Shizhu, Huang Ping. Elements of tribology[M]. Beijing: Tsinghua University Press, 2002.

[16] Zhang Li, Yin Guangfu, Zheng Changqiong, et al. The appraisal of biotribological properties of DLC gradient film on titanium alloy substrate[J]. *Journal of Functional Materials,* 2003, 34(3): 278-280.

[17] Karl-Heina, habig. VerschleiB und Harte von Werkstoffen[M]. Translated by Yan Li. Beijing: Mechanical Industry Press, 1987.

[18] Vetter J., Kayser O., Krug T. AlTiN – A universal coating for different applications[C]. *International Surface Engineering Congress - Proceedings of the 1st Congress*, 2003, 635-639.

In: Bioceramics: Properties, Preparations and Applications
Editors: W. Kossler, J. Fuchs, pp. 269-279
ISBN: 978-1-60741-056-0

Short Communication

Bone Regeneration with β-Tricalcium Phosphate: New Aspects

Fabian Peters* and Wolf-Dietrich Hübner
Curasan AG, Lindigstraße 4,
D-63801 Kleinostheim, Germany

Abstract

Nearly 40 years of intensive research on bone regeneration, biomaterials, material characteristics and predictable medical results led to a number of different synthetic bone substitution and bone regeneration materials. Due to their risks of immunoresponse, inflammation and disease transfer caused by remaining proteins, xenografts (from other animals, e.g. cows) or allografts (chemically treated bone from human cadavers) should be avoided. Even if autologous bone is still used in most of the clinical cases, an increasing number of bone defects is filled with resorbable synthetic biomaterials from β-tricalcium phosphate (β-TCP). In the past years over 600.000 cases were treated with the β-TCP biomaterial Cerasorb® (curasan AG, Kleinostheim, Germany) in the whole skeletal system. Different sizes, shapes and porosities were manufactured specifically adapted to the clinical case so that today the knowledge about the use of β-TCP is elevated.

1. Introduction

Biodegradable materials from β-tricalcium phosphate (β-TCP, $Ca_3(PO_4)_2$) are widely used as bone augmentation materials. However, the success of bone regeneration by using different β-TCP products has not always been comparable. Since the first experiments with implantable β-tricalcium phosphates the knowledge about the material characteristics has

* Correspondence to: Dr. Fabian Peters, Curasan AG, Lindigstraße 4, D-63801 Kleinostheim, Germany. Tel.: 06027 / 40 900-0. Fax: 06027 / 40 900-19. Email: fabian.peters@curasan.de

been more and more completed. Today, β-TCP products are available which fulfil strict requirements as regards to the quality and reproducibility and comprise all the knowledge from the past 30 years' clinical and scientific research. Especially in the dental field bone defects can be treated with β-TCP successfully and substitute the use of autologous bone [1].

In the following, the different material characteristics and principles are described to reach the target of complete bone regeneration.

2. Biomaterial Characteristics

2.1. Porosity

Pores and cavities are important for the inflow of blood, body fluids, proteins and cells in the augmentation material, for cell growth and nutrition and in the following for the dissolution of the material. Also blood vessels and young, newly formed bone should grow along and through the biomaterial. A minimum pore size of 60 µm was found for supporting bone ingrowth [2]. Other authors found a bone ingrowth supported by interconnections of 20 µm with a pore size of 50-100 µm [3]. Also the spaces in between the granules can act as "pores" and support their biological functions. Long winding pores cannot be completely filled with bone because nutrition of cells is not possible at the far end of the pores. Therefore de Groot formulated a rule that the maximum length for open pores should not exceed ten times the width [4]. For the treatment of different bone defects different resorption/degradation speeds are preferable. Mandibular defects for preparing implantations demand a fast resorption/degradation speed and therefore a higher inner surface and porosity. For the treatment of periodontal defects a lower porosity of a beta-TCP biomaterial supports a lower resorption/degradation speed for a complete bone healing.

2.2. Phase Purity

Tricalcium phosphate can be divided into two main phases with only mineralogical differences with respect to the atomic positions of the atoms in the crystal lattice. The material with the chemical formula $Ca_3(PO_4)_2$ will be transformed from the beta (β) phase to the alpha (α) phase by heating it higher than 1125°C. The mineralogical difference of the material leads to basic changes of the material characteristics. The alpha phase is thermodynamically more instable and therefore more soluble than the beta phase [5]. After implantation of α-TCP biomaterials the material changes to a dissolution-recrystallisation process. The material recrystallizes to the thermodynamically most stable calcium phosphate phase: the heavily soluble and non resorbable hydroxyapatite (HA, $Ca_{10}(PO_4)_6(OH)_2$).

Other calcium phosphate phase impurities are increasing the risk of non successful bone regeneration. Calcium phosphate phases slower resorbable than β-TCP like hydroxyapatite can remain left after resorption of the β-TCP. If it is finely dispersed in the β-TCP biomaterial the fine particles can provoke inflammatory reactions. More soluble calcium phosphate phases like Calcium pyrophosphate or α-TCP can lead to particular disintegration of the material. The placeholder function of the material is not fulfilled anymore, fibrous tissue can grow into the defect and hinder the bone growth. Also giant cell reactions might be activated caused by fine particles. Moreover, every impurity in a substance has different densities and coefficients of expansions and therefore weakens the β-TCP scaffold. Micro cracks in the material and mechanical instabilities will follow and increase the risk of particular disintegration as well.

Caused by these facts the American Society for Testing and Materials (ASTM) demands a phase purity of ≥ 95% [6]. In sense of reproducible results the phase purity should be ≥ 99%.

2.3. Chemical Purity

Impurities of heavy metals are strictly regulated by normative and regulatory provisions [6]. As well as the *pro analysi* grade of the raw materials is recommended, also possible influences of auxiliary materials, machines and tools which come in touch with the product have to be analyzed and validated. With an abrasive biomaterial like calcium phosphate the possibility of contamination with chemical traces can be minimized by using machinery and tools from mineral (agate mortars), coated (diamond-like) or from plastics as far as possible. For fast and reproducible risk free predictable bone regeneration it is essential to minimize the chemical impurities to a minimum.

Small traces of silicon in biomaterials have been shown as positive in terms of promoting bone formation. Higher amounts of silicon have shown to be toxic [7]. Foreign body giant cells have been observed on Si-rich areas of bioglasses with high silica content whereas bone bonding was only observed on Ca- and P-rich surfaces [8]. Silica has also been shown to induce sclerodermia *in vitro*: in serum free supernatant high doses of cytokines like interleukines, quantikines as well as TNF alpha were found in silica exponated cultures of leukocytes, monocytes and endothelial cells. Therefore, it could be shown that silica can induce diseases like sclerodermia [9].

2.4. Particle Size and Mechanical Stability

In 1985 de Groot detected that some implants made of macro- and microporous β-TCP disintegrated very rapidly into particles that could be found in the neighbouring lymph nodes [4]. The particular disintegration of these materials resulted in mechanical stress during implantation caused by a very low mechanical stability of the material. Examinations about the relationship between particle size and foreign body reactions showed that smaller particles ranging in particle sizes of a few μm were phagocytosed by macrophages [10, 11]. These giant cell reactions can lead to inflammatory reactions of the surrounding tissue. The phagocytosed particles will be transported to the lymphatic system. To prevent such reactions and therefore to minimize the risk of inflammatory reactions the average size of the primary particles should be about 7-10 μm. A β-TCP material built up by particles with a smaller size has to have a high mechanically stable interconnection to prevent disintegration into small particles in the way de Groot described. While forming new bone the material has to degrade but not to disintegrate into small particles that can provoke inflammatory reactions.

2.5. Resorption and Degradation

Biomaterials *degrade* by hydrolysis, i.e. dissolution in blood and body fluids. β-tricalcium phosphate will be metabolized completely. Tracer studies with ^{45}Calcium marked β-TCP biomaterials have shown that the calcium from the biomaterial will also be involved in the local mineralization process as well as in the metabolism [12]. Osteoclasts are the only cells that *resorb* bone and/or resorbable biomaterials [13]. The interactions between osteoblasts and osteoclasts are still not known. The degradation and resorption speed from β-TCP biomaterials is adapted to the bone regeneration and can be directed by fine tuning of the inner surface with pores [14, 15] (*Figure 1*).

The solubility of two β-TCP Cerasorb® modifications was tested. In a batch system the granulates were incubated in TRIS/HCl buffer solution. In defined time steps 1000 µl solution was removed and the sum of ions (calcium and phosphate) was measured by Atomic Adsorption Spectroscopy (AAS). The removed solution was replaced by fresh buffer solution. It could be shown that 1g Cerasorb® granulate (porosity about 35%) is completely dissoluted in 6 months in this system, Cerasorb® M has, caused by its higher porosity of 65%, a dissolution rate of 1g in 4 months (*Figure 2*).

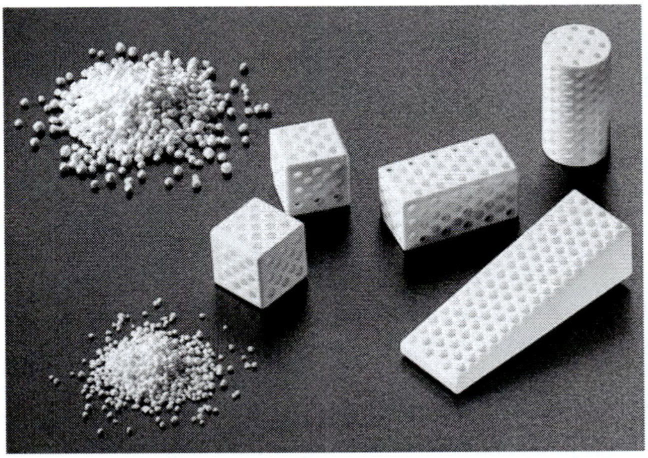

Figure 1. The Cerasorb® product range: granulas and morsels in different sizes as well as block forms in nearly every shape from pure phase β-TCP are available.

2.6. Bioactivity

A Biomaterial has to be bioactive in sense of supporting bone growth. Also osteoconductivity (forming a "guide rail" for bone forming in and along the biomaterial) is recommended. β-TCP has shown both characteristics.

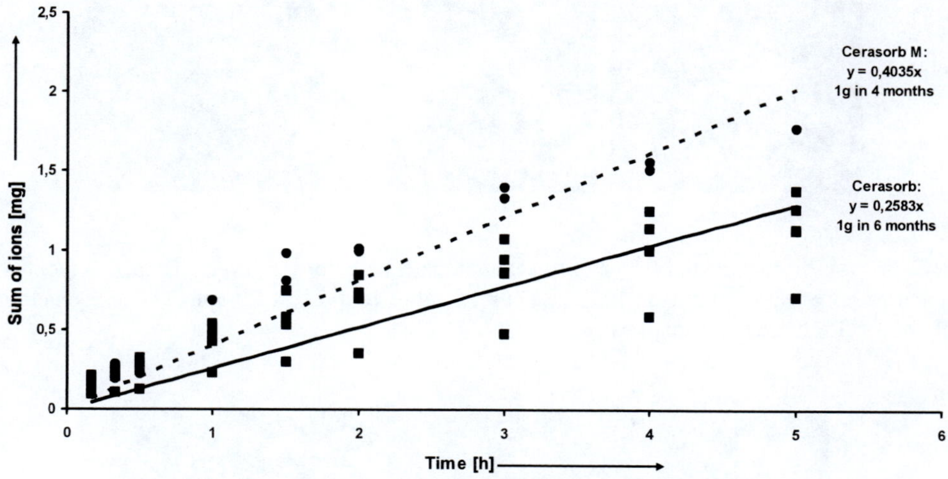

Figure 2. Solubility diagram of Cerasorb® granulate (solid line) and Cerasorb® M granulate (dotted line).

The induction of bone formation means that stem cells will be stimulated to differentiate into osteoblasts. This stimulation will be performed by growth factors such as BMPs. Therefore, ceramics are not osteoinductive by itself. Ectopic bone formation after implantation of substances in muscle tissue was observed since 1969 [16]. Depending from the animal species, the implantation site, the ceramic (mainly the surface characteristics) and the porosity, ectopic bone formation can be observed by intramuscular implantation of nearly all substances. From this observation it was concluded that the adsorption of stimulating proteins in and on a microporous biomaterial out from blood and body fluids leads to a higher concentration of stimulating proteins in the surrounding tissue of the material. So stem cells can differentiate to osteoblasts and form bone [17, 18]. Also with this effect only the proteins are osteoinductive. Therefore the definition of the term "osteoinduction" must not be used in combination with ceramics alone.

3. Cases

3.1. Dental Surgery with Cerasorb® Granulate

In a 35 year old male patient a fibromixoma mandibulae was excised and the defect filled with Cerasorb® granulate 1000-2000 μm. The original defect size was about 8 x 3 cm. The clinical follow-up was uneventful. CT scans after 15 months showed complete bone regeneration (*Figures 3-4*).

Generally, different stages of resorption of Cerasorb® granulate at the same time are visible in biopsy specimen. It can be shown that the resorption/degradation of the material starts from the outer parts of the Cerasorb granules. Outgoing from small areas the material will be made accessible inside for degradation. After 6 months only small amounts of material remains are visible [19] *(Figure 5)*.

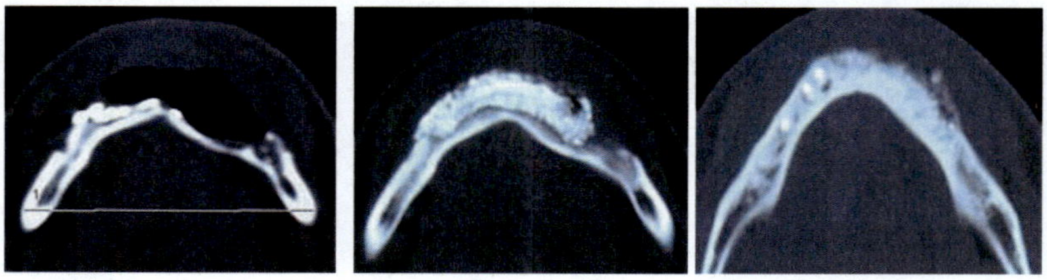

A B C

Figure 3. CT scan from a case of fibromixoma mandibulae. A: before treatment, B: after 4 months implanted with Cerasorb® granulate 1000-2000 µm, C: after 15 months. Complete bone regeneration can be shown [Prof. Szabo, Budapest].

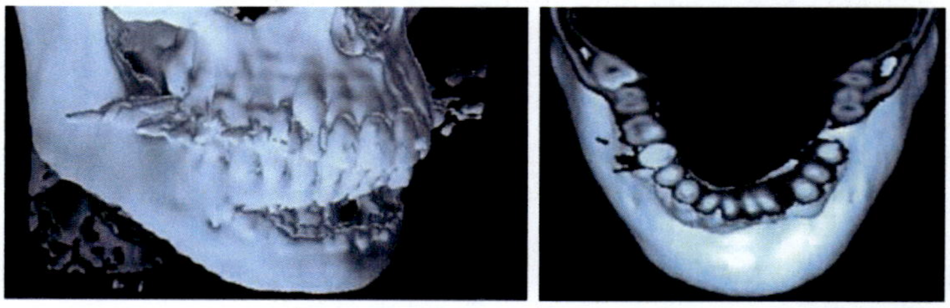

A B

Figure 4. High resolution 3D CT scan of the fibromixoma mandibulae case (figure 3): A: situation before augmentation with Cerasorb®, B: 15 months after Cerasorb® implantation: full recovery.

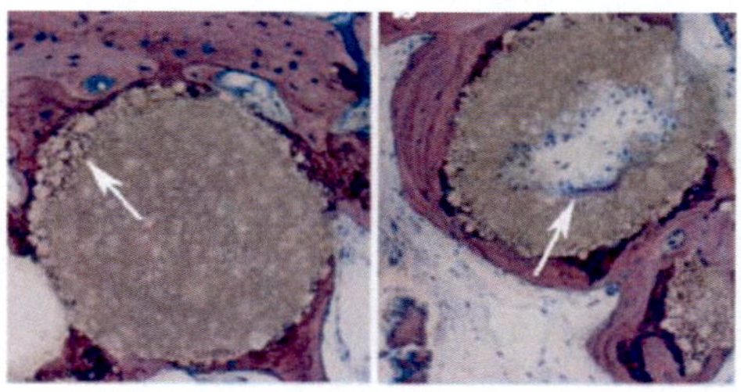

A B

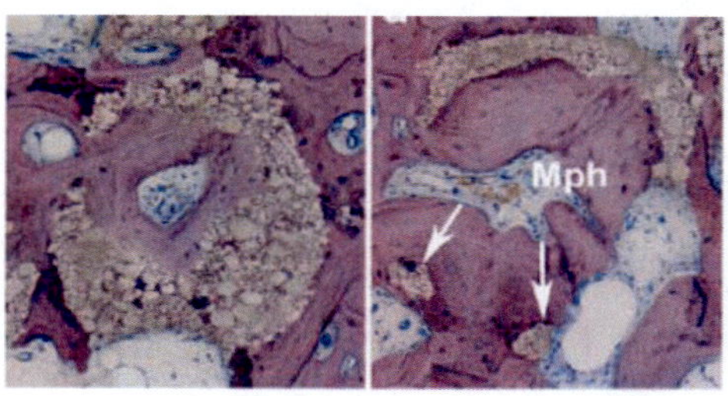

C D

Figure 5. Histological examination of a sinus graft drillcore 4,5 months after implantation. Different stages of resorption can be seen: A: beginning bone matrix substitution and ceramolysis at the outer part of Cerasorb® granulate, B: Resorption/degradation from inside to outside, bone forming in the center of the pure phase β-tricalcium phosphate, C: Resorption/degradation from outside to inside, central building of osteons, D: Complete new bone in former granulate area. Only a thin hull of Cerasorb® is visible [Prof. Plenk, Vienna].

Due to its radio opacity these partly resorbed materials might show a similar x-ray photo like post implantation (*Figure 6*) but consist of stable tissue of new bone, connective tissue and β-TCP remains. Knowing this fact, experienced users place dental implants, finding the described histological situation during surgery.

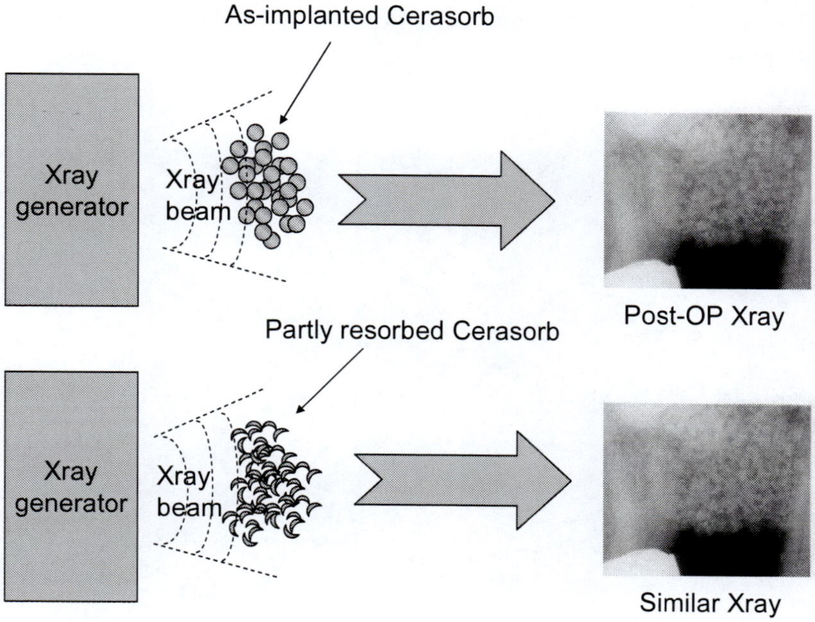

Figure 6. Possible findings in X-ray photographs as shown in figure 5 (partly resorbed β-Tricalcium phosphate Cerasorb®).

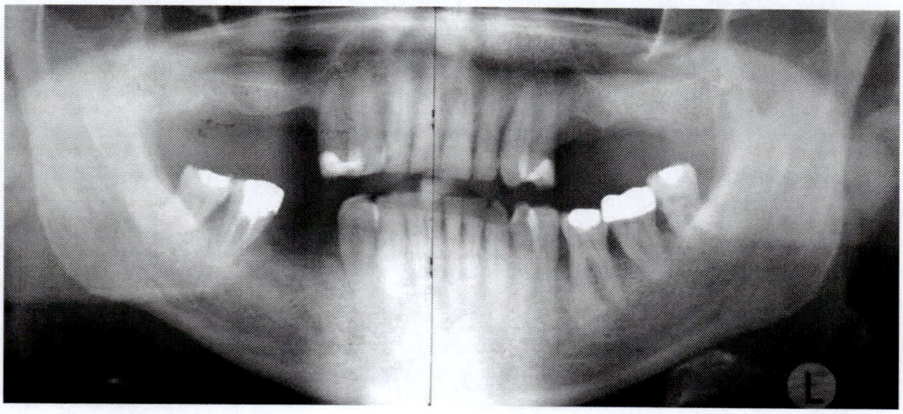

Figure 7. Preoperative Orthopantomogram before treatment with Cerasorb® M granulate [Dr. Palm, Konstanz].

3.2. Dental Surgery with Cerasorb® M Granulate

In a 68 years old male patient bilateral sinus lifting and simultaneous placement of three implants in the right and another three in the left maxilla, as well as two implants in the right mandible was done. For sinus lifting with Cerasorb® M in a granule size of 1000-2000 μm was used alone at a volume of 2 cc in the right and 1,5 cc in the left maxilla. Follow-up radiographs were recorded immediately after the procedure (*Figure 8*), and at 4 months (*Figure 9*). At 6 months the implants were exposed and loaded. The radiographs showed progressive obliteration of the defects by bone and simultaneous resorption of the grafting material [20].

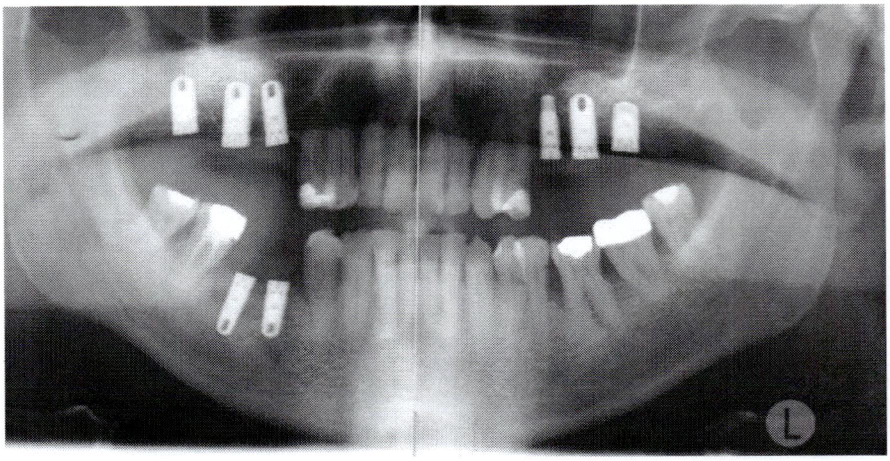

Figure 8.. Condition after bilateral sinus lifting with Cerasorb® M and simultaneous placement of three implants in the right and another three in the left maxilla, as well as two implants in the right mandible.

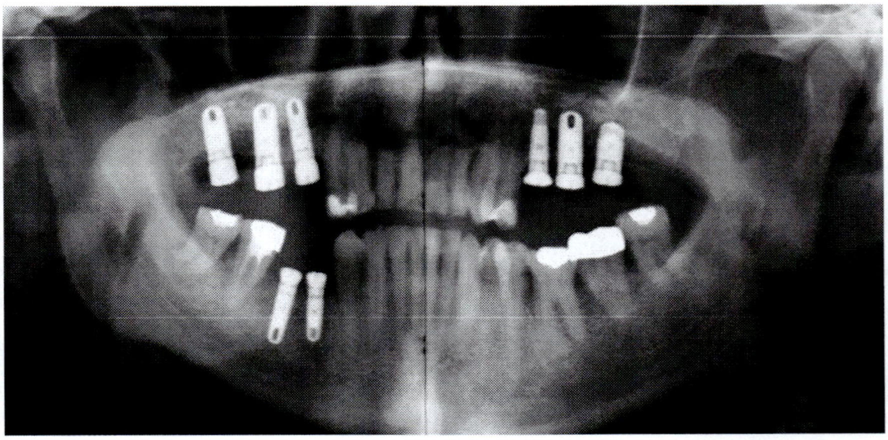

Figure 9. Follow-up radiograph at 4 months. Note clearly visible resorption of bone regenerating material which has been largely substituted by newly formed bone.

3.3. Orthopedic Surgery with Cerasorb® Block Forms

In a one year old girl with dysplasia of the right hip Salter's osteotomy and insertion of a Cerasorb® wedge was performed. To avoid dislocation, the wedge was fixed with two k-wires, which could be removed after three months. After 15 months the Cerasorb® block was largely resorbed and substituted by bone. The clinical follow-up was inconspicuously and showed the usefulness of the Cerasorb® wedge in this indication (*Figure 10*).

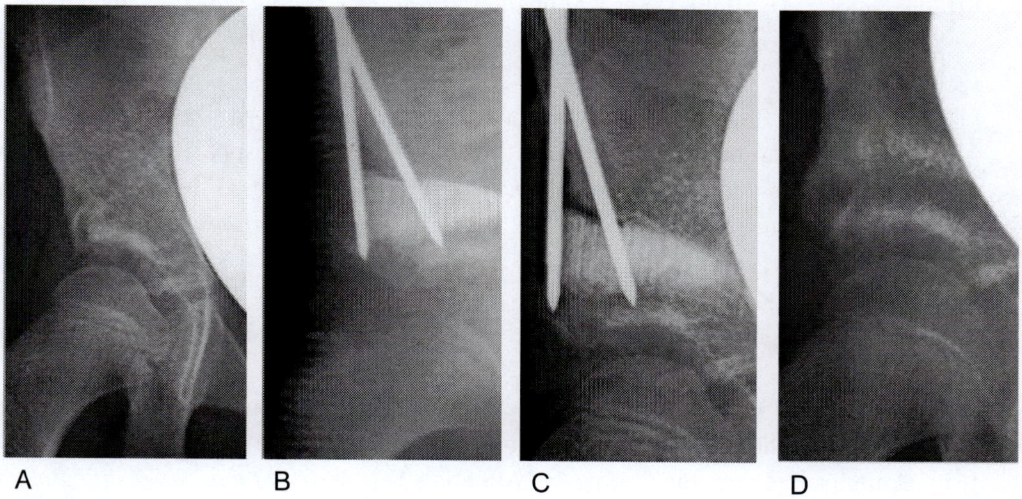

Figure 10. Salters osteotomy after hip dysplasia with a Cerasorb® wedge. A: pre OP, B: after 1 month post OP, C: after 3 months post OP, D: after 15 months post OP [Prof. Behrendt, Lübeck].

Conclusion

The detecting and the combination of the requirements for a successful bone augmenting material have directed the development of β-TCP biomaterials over the past 30 years. In the early 1970s the research of synthetic biomaterials took place at the Battelle Institute in Frankfurt/Germany [21]. In the middle of the 1990s the collected knowledge led to a β-TCP biomaterial program called Cerasorb®. Granular materials as well as block forms are available for a complete regeneration in the entire skeletal system. All modifications consist of β-TCP with a validated phase purity of ≥ 99% [22]. For different indications different granular materials are available: round granules with a porosity of 30 ± 5% (pore size 0.1-50 μm) with higher mechanical stability, the rounded broken Cerasorb® M with a porosity of 60 ± 5 % (pore size 0.1-500 μm) for a fast resorption and the polygonal broken Cerasorb® Perio with a porosity of 20 ± 5%, a slower resorption rate and a higher mechanical stability for the treatment of periodontal defects.

In near future research and studies of patient individual resorbable implants from pure phase β-TCP are planned. CT data shall be sent to the CAD CAM device for shaping implants fitting individual defects. [23].

References

[1] Szabo, G; Huys, L; Coulthard, P; Maiorana, C; Garagiola, U; Barabas, J; Nemeth, Z; Hrabak, K; Suba, Z. A Prospective Multicenter Randomized Clinical Trial of Autogenous Bone Versus β-Tricalcium Phosphate Alone for Bilateral Sinus Elevation: Histologic and Histomorphometric Evaluation. *Int J Oral Maxillofac Implants* 2005, *20*: 371-381.

[2] Klawitter, JJ; Hulbert, SF. Application of Porous Ceramics for the Attachment of Load Bearing Internal Orthopedic Applications. *J. Biomed Mater. Res. Symposium* 1971, *2*, 161-229.

[3] P. S. Eggli, PS; Mueller, W; Schenk, RR. The role of pore size on bone ingrowth and implant substitution in hydroxyapatite and tricalcium phosphate ceramics; A histologic and morphometric study in rabbits. In: A. Pizzoferrato, P. G. Marchetti, A. Ravigiolo, A. J. C. Lee (eds.): *Biomaterials and clinical applications*, Elsevier Science Publ. Amsterdam 1987, 53-56.

[4] De Groot, K. Effect of Porosity and Physicochemical Properties on the Stability, Resorption and Strength of Calcium Phosphate Ceramics. *Ann. N. Y. Acad. Sci.* 1988, 227.

[5] Elliott JC. Structure and Chemistry of the Apatites and Other Calcium Orthophosphates, *Studies in Inorganic Chemistry* 18, Elsevier 1994.

[6] American Society for Testing and Materials F 1088-04, *Standard Specification for Beta Tricalcium Phoshate for Surgical Implantation.*

[7] Nagase, M; Abe, Y; Chigira, M; Udagawa, E. Toxicity of silica-containing calcium phosphate glasses demonstrated in mice, *Biomaterials* 1992, *13 (3)*, 172-175.

[8] Vogel, M; Voigt, C; Knabe, C; Radlanski, RJ; Gross, UM; Müller-Mai, CM. Development of multinuclear giant cells during the degradation of Bioglass® particles in rabbits. *J. Biomed. Mater. Res.* 2004, *70A*, 370-379.

[9] Anderegg, U; Haustein, UF. Experimentelle Untersuchungen zur quarzinduzierten Sklerodermie. *Deutsches Ärzteblatt,* 1998, *95 (8)*, A-1099.

[10] Lu, J; Descamps, M; Dejou, J; Koubi, G; Harduin, P; Lemaitre, L; Proust, JP. The biodegradation mechanism of calcium phosphate biomaterials in bone. *J. Biomed. Mater. Res. (Appl. Biomater.)* 2002, *63*, 408.

[11] Shimizu, S. Subcutaneous tissue responses in rats to injection of fine particles of synthetic hydroxyapatite ceramic. *Biomed. Res.* 1988, *9 (2),* 95-111.

[12] LeHuec, JC; Clement, D; Brouillaud, B; Barthe, N; Dupuy, B; Foliguet, B; Basse-Cathalinat, B. Evolution of the local calcium content around irradiated β-tricalcium phosphate ceramic implants: in vivo study in the rabbit. *Biomaterials* 1998, *19*, 733-738.

[13] Schilling, AF; Linhart, W; Filke, S; Gebauer, M; Schinke, T; Rueger, JM; Amling, M. Resorbability of bone substitute biomaterials by human osteoclasts. *Biomaterials* 2004, *25 (18)*, 3963-38972.

[14] Wiltfang, J; Merten, HA; Schlegel, KA; Schultze-Mosgau, S; Kloss, FR; Rupprecht, S; Kessler, P. Degradation Characteristics of α and β Tri-Calcium-Phosphate (TCP) in Minipigs. *J. Biomed. Mater. Res. (Appl. Biomater)* 2002, 63, 115.

[15] Peters, F; Reif, D. Functional Materials for Bone Regeneration from Beta-Tricalcium Phosphate. *Mat.-wiss. u. Werkstofftech.* 2004, *35 (4)*, 203-207.

[16] Winter, GD; Simpson, BJ. Heterotopic Bone formed in a Synthetic Sponge in the Skin of Young Pigs. *Nature* 1969, *223 (201)*, 88.

[17] Ripamonti, U. Ostroinduction in porous hydroxyapatite implanted in heterotopic sites of different animal models. *Biomaterials* 1996, *17*, 31-35.

[18] Yuan, H; Yang, Z; de Bruijn, JD; de Groot, K; Zhang, X. Material-dependent bone induction by calcium phosphate ceramics: a 2.5-year study in dog. *Biomaterials* 2001, *22*, 2617-2623.

[19] Plenk, H; Lederer, J. Histomorphologie der Knochenregeneration nach Sinusbodenaugmentation mit zwei Formen eines TCP-Granulates – ein Fallbericht. *Z Oral Implant* 2005, *1*, 32.

[20] Palm, F. Cerasorb®M – a new synthetic pure-phase β-TCP ceramic material in oral and maxillofacial surgery – An open study of 121 patients. IMOI 2006, 3: 24-27.

[21] Köster, K; Karbe, E; Kramer, H; Heide, H; König, R. Experimenteller Knochenersatz durch resorbierbare Calciumphosphat-Keramik. *Lang. Arch. Chir.* 1976, 341, 77-86.

[22] Tadic, D; Epple, M.A Thorough physicochemical characterisation of 14 calcium phosphate-based bone substitution materials in comparison to natural bone. *Biomaterials* 2004, *25*, 987-994.

[23] Peters, F; Groisman, D; Davids, R; Hänel, T; Dürr, H; Klein, M. Comparative Study of patient individual implants from β-tricalcium phosphate made by different techniques based on CT data. *Mat.-wiss. u. Werkstofftech.* 2006, *37(6)*, 457-461.

Index

B

C

D

E

F

G

H

I

J

K

L

M

N

Q

R

S

T

U

V

W

X

Y

Z